Foot and Ankle Athletic Injuries

Guest Editor

BOB BARAVARIAN, DPM, FACFAS

CLINICS IN PODIATRIC MEDICINE AND SURGERY

www.podiatric.theclinics.com

Consulting Editor
THOMAS ZGONIS, DPM, FACFAS

January 2011 • Volume 28 • Number 1

SAUNDERS an imprint of ELSEVIER, Inc.

W.B. SAUNDERS COMPANY
A Division of Elsevier Inc.

1600 John F. Kennedy Boulevard • Suite 1800 • Philadelphia, Pennsylvania 19103-2899

http://www.theclinics.com

CLINICS IN PODIATRIC MEDICINE AND SURGERY Volume 28, Number 1
January 2011 ISSN 0891-8422, ISBN-13: 978-1-4557-0494-1

Editor: Patrick Manley

Clinics in Podiatric Medicine and Surgery (ISSN 0891-8422) is published quarterly by Elsevier Inc., 360 Park Avenue South, New York, NY 10010-1710. Months of issue are January, April, July, and October. Business and Editorial Offices: 1600 John F. Kennedy Blvd., Ste. 1800, Philadelphia, PA 19103-2899. Customer Service Office: 3251 Riverport Lane, Maryland Heights, MO 63043. Periodicals postage paid at NewYork, NY and additional mailing offices. Subscription prices are $270.00 per year for US individuals, $385.00 per year for US institutions, $137.00 per year for US students and residents, $324.00 per year for Canadian individuals, $477.00 for Canadian institutions, $384.00 for international individuals, $477.00 per year for international institutions and $193.00 per year for Canadian and foreign students/residents. To receive student/resident rate, orders must be accompanied by name of affiliated institution, date of term, and the *signature* of program/residency coordinator on institution letterhead. Orders will be billed at individual rate until proof of status is received. Foreign air speed delivery is included in all *Clinics* subscription prices. All prices are subject to change without notice. POSTMASTER: Send address changes to *Clinics in Podiatric Medicine and Surgery*, Elsevier Health Sciences Division, Subscription Customer Service, 3251 Riverport Lane, Maryland Heights, MO 63043. **Customer Service: 1-800-654-2452 (US). From outside of the US, call 314-447-8871. Fax: 314-447-8029. E-mail: JournalsCustomerService-usa@elsevier.com (for print support); JournalsOnlineSupport-usa@elsevier.com (for online support).**

Reprints. For copies of 100 or more of articles in this publication, please contact the Commercial Reprints Department, Elsevier Inc., 360 Park Avenue South, New York, NY 10010-1710. Tel.: 212-633-3812; Fax: 212-462-1935; E-mail: reprints@elsevier.com.

Clinics in Podiatric Medicine and Surgery is covered in *MEDLINE/PubMed (Index Medicus)* and *EMBASE/Excerpta Medica.*

Printed and bound by CPI Group (UK) Ltd, Croydon, CR0 4YY
Transferred to Digital Print 2011

CLINICS IN PODIATRIC MEDICINE AND SURGERY

CONSULTING EDITOR
THOMAS ZGONIS, DPM, FACFAS

Contributors

CONSULTING EDITOR

THOMAS ZGONIS, DPM, FACFAS
Director, Podiatric Surgical Residency and Reconstructive Fellowship Programs;
Chief, Division of Podiatric Medicine and Surgery; Associate Professor,
Department of Orthopedic Surgery, The University of Texas Health Science
Center at San Antonio, San Antonio, Texas

GUEST EDITOR

BOB BARAVARIAN, DPM, FACFAS
Co-Director, University Foot and Ankle Institute, Santa Monica; Chief of Podiatric Foot and
Ankle Surgery, and Assistant Clinical Professor, Santa Monica/UCLA Medical Center and
Orthopedic Hospital, Santa Monica, California

AUTHORS

BOB BARAVARIAN, DPM, FACFAS
Co-Director, University Foot and Ankle Institute, Santa Monica; Chief of Podiatric Foot and
Ankle Surgery, and Assistant Clinical Professor, Santa Monica/UCLA Medical Center and
Orthopedic Hospital, Santa Monica, California

PATRICK R. BURNS, DPM, FACFAS
Clinical Assistant Professor, Division of Foot and Ankle, Department of Orthopaedic
Surgery, University of Pittsburgh School of Medicine; Director, Podiatric Surgical
Residency Program, University of Pittsburgh Medical Center, Pittsburgh, Pennsylvania

ZACHARIA FACAROS, DPM
Fellow, Reconstructive Foot and Ankle Surgery; Clinical Instructor, Division of Podiatric
Medicine and Surgery, Department of Orthopaedic Surgery, University of Texas Health
Science Center at San Antonio, San Antonio, Texas

JUSTIN FRANSON, DPM, FACFAS
University Foot and Ankle Institute, Valencia; Attending Surgeon, West Los Angeles
Veterans Affairs Medical Center, Los Angeles, California

SUZANNE T. HAWSON, PT, MPT, OCS
Physical Therapist, Physical Therapy Department, University Foot and Ankle Institute,
Valencia, California

MATTHEW J. HENTGES, BA
College of Podiatric Medicine and Surgery, Des Moines University, Des Moines;
Des Moines, Iowa

JOSHUA C. HUNT, BA
Medical Student, College of Podiatric Medicine, Western University of Health Sciences,
Pomona, California

DANIEL K. LEE, DPM, PhDc, FACFAS
Assistant Clinical Professor of Orthopaedic Surgery, Department of Orthopaedic Surgery, School of Medicine, University of California, San Diego, California

MICHAEL S. LEE, DPM, FACFAS
Capital Orthopaedics and Sports Medicine, PC; Associate Clinical Professor, Des Moines University, Des Moines, Iowa

NICHOLAS LOWERY, DPM
PGY-4, Podiatric Surgical Residency Program, University of Pittsburgh Medical Center, Pittsburgh, Pennsylvania

GERIT D. MULDER, DPM, MS, PhDc, FAPWCA, FRCST
Professor of Surgery and Orthopaedics; Director of Wound Treatment and Research Center, Division of Trauma, Department of Surgery, School of Medicine, University of California, San Diego, California

DORON NAZARIAN, DPM
Fellow, University Foot and Ankle Institute, Los Angeles, California

CRYSTAL L. RAMANUJAM, DPM
Fellow, Postgraduate Research; Clinical Instructor, Division of Podiatric Medicine and Surgery, Department of Orthopaedic Surgery, University of Texas Health Science Center at San Antonio, San Antonio, Texas

BORA RHIM, DPM
Assistant Professor, Department of Podiatric Medicine, Surgery, and Biomechanics, College of Podiatric Medicine, Western University of Health Sciences, Pomona, California

KEVIN B. ROSENBLOOM, CPed
Kevin Orthotics, Foot In Motion, Santa Monica, California

ALEXANDRA K. SCHWARTZ, MD
Associate Clinical Professor of Orthopaedics; Chief of Orthopaedic Trauma, and Director of Orthopaedic Residency Program, Department of Orthopaedic Surgery, School of Medicine, University of California, San Diego, California

DAVID J. SOOMEKH, DPM, FACFAS
Diplomate, American Board of Podiatric Surgery; Faculty, University Foot and Ankle Institute, Santa Monica; Attending Staff, Department of Surgery, University of California Los Angeles Medical Center; Attending Staff, Department of Surgery, Cedars-Sinai Medical Center, Los Angeles, California

JONATHAN THOMPSON, DPM
Clinician, University Foot and Ankle Institute, Private Practice, Manhattan Beach; Department of Surgery, Veterans Affairs Greater Los Angeles Healthcare System, Los Angeles, California

BRUCE WERBER, DPM, FACFAS
InMotion Foot and Ankle Specialists, Scottsdale; Adjunct Assistant Professor, Arizona School of Podiatric Medicine, Midwestern University, Glendale, Arizona

THOMAS ZGONIS, DPM, FACFAS
Director, Podiatric Surgical Residency and Reconstructive Fellowship Programs; Chief, Division of Podiatric Medicine and Surgery; Associate Professor, Department of Orthopedic Surgery, The University of Texas Health Science Center at San Antonio, San Antonio, Texas

Contents

The majority of injuries during sport are to the lower extremity (more than 50%), most of which occur in children and young adults younger than 25 years and involve fractures, ligament injuries, or tendon injuries. This article discusses the etiology of some of the most common foot and ankle sports-related injuries. The authors focus on clinical findings, associated injuries, pathophysiology, and current trends. Many of these factors are discussed in detail elsewhere in this issue.

The advancement of new technologies in the treatment of foot and ankle injuries seems exponential over the last several years. As surgeons expand their knowledge of the pathology and improve their treatment techniques, they come upon new and different ways to treat the same pathologic conditions. Foot and ankle injuries are commonplace in competitive sports. This article provides an overview of the diagnosis and treatment, including surgical techniques, of common foot and ankle injuries.

Hallux, sesamoid, and first metatarsal injuries are common foot injuries and have implications in the biomechanical functionality of the first ray and foot. They are essential for propulsion in normal gait. As part of the first ray, it is an important contributor to normal locomotion. Any structure disruption or injury can create angular changes or arthritis, which can have biomechanical implications, including pain, disability, compensation, swelling, and reduced range of motion.

Forefoot pain is one of the most common presenting problems in a foot and ankle practice. One of the most common presenting problems, yet most commonly missed problems, is a plantar plate tear. Often the problem is considered to be potential neuroma, fat pad atrophy, or a generalized diagnosis of metatarsalgia or metatarsal head overload. Unfortunately, not enough attention is placed on the plantar and medial/lateral ligamentous structures of the metatarsal-phalangeal joints. This lack of attention results in poor diagnosis, lack of care, treatment for the wrong condition, and ultimate frustration for the patients and doctor.

New surgical approaches, including percutaneous and mini-open techniques, are being introduced to potentially diminish perioperative complications. Advent of early protective range of motion and rehabilitation has
shown a potential for earlier return to sporting activities for Achilles ruptures.

this article is to (1) raise awareness for using physical therapy for treatment of foot and ankle injuries in athletes, (2) discuss considerations specific to athletes during the rehabilitation process, and (3) increase the reader's knowledge about the in-depth role of physical therapy in the management of foot and ankle injuries in athletes.

Current Concepts and Techniques in Foot and Ankle Surgery

Comminuted, intra-articular calcaneal fractures can cause severe lower extremity impairment and have devastating effects on a patient's well being. Diabetes is a multisystem process that may cause neuropathy and loss of protective sensation further complicating the prognosis. Not all calcaneal fractures are created equal and when considering the patient's overall presentation and extent of injury, the combined approach of internal and external fixation for fracture reduction may be beneficial for restoration of anatomic alignment and function.

Early and aggressive treatment of diabetic foot wounds is imperative for the reduction of amputation risk. Whereas sound local wound care is important for successful management; chronic wounds often reach a stagnant point in healing because of diabetic vasculopathy, immunopathy, or neuropathy. The type, size, shape, and location of wound may not always allow primary closure or grafting. In patients with adequate perfusion and in the absence of infection, local advancement flaps are suitable for durable closure. A review and case report demonstrating the use of these flaps with external fixation as an adjunctive therapy for surgical off-loading is presented.

RELATED INTEREST

Foot and Ankle Clinics Volume 15, Issue 4, Pages 543–688 (December 2010)
Orthobiologic Concepts in Foot and Ankle
Edited by Stuart D. Miller, MD

THE CLINICS ARE NOW AVAILABLE ONLINE!

Access your subscription at:
www.theclinics.com

Foreword

Athletic Foot and Ankle Injuries

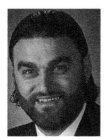

Thomas Zgonis, DPM, FACFAS
Consulting Editor

This issue of *Clinics in Podiatric Medicine and Surgery* is devoted to the overall management of sports-related foot and ankle injuries. Choosing the most effective treatment modalities for restoring normal function following major ligamentous and tendon injuries, fractures, and osteochondral defects requires not only an understanding of the injury but also the sport involved. Dr Baravarian, who has extensive experience in this area, has put together an all-star team, providing us with the most current and rational approaches to treat these challenging athletic injuries.

The articles in this issue focus on ankle and subtalar joint instability, peroneal and achilles tendon pathology, heel pain, osteochondral injuries, midfoot trauma, stress fractures, forefoot pathology, and dance injuries. The invited authors have submitted their work with concise evidence-based recommendations while sharing their personal experience and insight into new technology and advances in this field.

A comprehensive approach to the conservative and surgical treatment of sports-related foot and ankle injuries is essential for the athlete to improve function and return to their respective sport while preventing further injury. I thank you for your continuous efforts and your outstanding submissions.

Thomas Zgonis, DPM, FACFAS
Division of Podiatric Medicine and Surgery
Department of Orthopaedic Surgery
The University of Texas Health Science Center at San Antonio
7703 Floyd Curl Drive–MSC 7776
San Antonio, TX 78229, USA

E-mail address:
zgonis@uthscsa.edu

Clin Podiatr Med Surg 28 (2011) xiii
doi:10.1016/j.cpm.2010.12.002   **podiatric.theclinics.com**
0891-8422/11/$ – see front matter © 2011 Elsevier Inc. All rights reserved.

Preface

Athletic Injuries of the Foot and Ankle

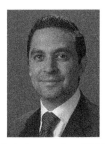

Bob Baravarian, DPM
Guest Editor

Ten years and so much has changed.

I am privileged and proud to be asked to be a guest editor for this *Clinics in Podiatric Medicine and Surgery* on athletic injuries of the foot and ankle. What is amazing is that I was a guest editor for a *Clinics in Podiatric Medicine and Surgery* 10 years ago and how much has changed in that short period of time.

I am proud to be the director of University Foot and Ankle Institute with 11 locations in Southern California. We have a team of 7 podiatric foot and ankle surgeons, 1 fellow, 3 physical therapists, and extensive foot and ankle services as part of our establishment. I am also proud to still be involved with UCLA as the chief of podiatric foot and ankle surgery at Santa Monica/UCLA Medical Center and Orthopedic hospital as well as an assistant clinical professor.

We have published over 100 articles in the past 10 years and multiple book chapters and taught dozens of seminars. We have helped educate hundreds of doctors and residents from all over the world and tried to improve our profession to the best of our abilities.

Ten years seems like a long time, but it has passed faster than I could ever imagine. What has been a constant and a rock in my life has been the love of my family. I want to thank Yas, my wife, Haley, my daughter, and Michael, my son, for their love, laughter, and constant praise in the past 10 years. I also want to thank my partner and co-director of University Foot and Ankle Institute, Gary B. Briskin, for taking a chance and opening the new practice with me. Who would have thought 2 guys could grow so much in just 7 years. Finally, I want to thank the doctors at the University of Pittsburgh residency program who helped train me. You are truly in my thoughts daily and I often thank you in my head for all the lessons and guidance. You have made me the surgeon I am and I thank you from the bottom of my heart.

Clin Podiatr Med Surg 28 (2011) xv–xvi
doi:10.1016/j.cpm.2010.12.001   **podiatric.theclinics.com**

Finally, let me add that what I have done in the past year is what all of us need to do. We all need to train young residents, whether with 1 surgery, 1 patient, or 1 article. We all need to improve ourselves through courses and education. It is not enough to be a good doctor; you need to think about being a good doctor and a good member of your profession. Give back and it will come back to you multiple folds over. I hope the topics presented today help guide you in your patient care and also help you delve deeper into critical thinking on the topics presented.

Bob Baravarian, DPM
University Foot and Ankle Institute
2121 Wilshire Boulevard
Suite 101
Santa Monica, CA 90403, USA

Santa Monica/UCLA Medical Center and Orthopedic Hospital
1250 Sixteenth Street
Santa Monica, CA 90404, USA
E-mail address:
BBaravarian@mednet.ucla.edu

Etiology, Pathophysiology, and Most Common Injuries of the Lower Extremity in the Athlete

Patrick R. Burns, DPM[a,b,]*, Nicholas Lowery, DPM[b]

KEYWORDS

• Sports injury • Foot injury • Ankle injury • Lower extremities

The number of participants in sport activities continues to increase. Approximately 6 million adolescents now participate in school-sponsored activities alone, with many more participating in after-school and community leagues. In the past 10 years, participation in these activities is on the rise; there is as much as a 10% increase for boys and 40% for girls.[1] At the other end of the spectrum, older individuals are also increasing their participation in sport. Many, on the advice of their primary care physicians, are doing so for health benefits such as reducing medications and limiting arthritic complaints.

It is well known that participation in these activities instills positive habits and has many benefits. Learning to be active begins a habit of health maintenance and fosters the concept of teamwork. Participation in sports allows one to acquire these traits early in life along with other physical and mental benefits. Physical activity aids growth and development, helps control weight, and can decrease chances for certain illnesses. What is less clear is the effect on risk-taking behavior as well as the impact of both short- and long-term injuries. Some studies show increased alcohol abuse as well as increased emphasis on self-image and possible eating disorders associated with sport participation.[2] Most of these studies have focused on athletics at the collegiate level. What is known is that the majority of injuries during sport are to the lower extremity (more than 50%), most of which occur in children and young adults younger

[a] Division of Foot and Ankle, Department of Orthopaedic Surgery, University of Pittsburgh School of Medicine, 2100 Jane Street, Roesch-Taylor Medical Building N7100, Pittsburgh, PA 15203, USA
[b] Podiatric Surgical Residency Program, University of Pittsburgh Medical Center, Pittsburgh, PA, USA
* Corresponding author. Division of Foot and Ankle, Department of Orthopaedic Surgery, University of Pittsburgh School of Medicine, 2100 Jane Street, Roesch-Taylor Medical Building N7100, Pittsburgh, PA 15203.
E-mail address: burnsp@upmc.edu

Clin Podiatr Med Surg 28 (2011) 1–18
doi:10.1016/j.cpm.2010.11.003   **podiatric.theclinics.com**
0891-8422/11/$ – see front matter © 2011 Elsevier Inc. All rights reserved.

than 25 years.[3] These injuries make up as much as 20% of the emergency room visits in that age range.

Sports injuries are broadly divided into overuse or traumatic as well as either acute or chronic. Traumatic injuries are more typical in collision or contact sports such as football and soccer, due to their nature. Overuse injuries are seen mostly in training situations and sports that require endurance or repetitive activities such as gymnastics and track. The most common injuries to the lower extremity associated with sport involve fractures, ligament injuries, or tendon injuries.

The current trend of increasing participation in sporting activities among adolescents can lead to fatigue, which plays a large role in overuse injuries. If the body cannot recover, the risk for injury increases. As muscle fatigues, increased stress shifts to the ligaments and bony architecture. This shift plays a large role in overuse injuries. Fatigue may come in 2 ways, the first of which is pure overuse. Participation in various sporting activities on a daily basis with training, practice, scrimmage, and games does not leave adequate time to recover. This situation is especially apparent in adolescents as they and their parents try to maintain a rigorous schedule. The second form of fatigue is seen in the participant with a single sporting interest. In years past activity and participation changed with the seasons, allowing for the use of different muscle groups and different stresses to the body as seasons change. Someone participating in baseball one season and basketball the next would use different skills, with different movements and muscles to fit the requirements of the sport. In some ways this is thought to have helped minimize overuse to any one area. The increase in the number of stress fractures reported recently is in some cases thought to be a reflection of a single activity repeated all year. Specialization in one sport is more common, as there are opportunities for the same sport all year with indoor leagues, outdoor leagues, travel leagues, camps, and tournaments. The same activity using the same muscles, same ligaments, and same motions may be one reason for overuse and subsequent fatigue injury.

It is estimated that high school athletes account for more than 2 million sport-related injuries each year requiring over 500,000 office visits, while children of ages 14 and under produce more than 3 million injuries.[3] Most adolescents want to play and be on the field. Their cartilage is softer and muscles not fully developed, and their ligaments may be stronger than the bone to which they are attached. When these factors are combined with adolescents being unaware of the clues their body is giving them during overuse, delays are made in diagnosis and treatment. Parents, coaches, and trainers need to look for signs of injury early, such as favoring one side, slowing down, difficulty sleeping, and aches and pains including headaches.

Certain injuries are more common with particular sports and seem to be more common in competition than in practice.[4–6] This situation is obviously a result of the training involved as well as the type of impact. Football and soccer tend to have the highest rate of lower extremity injuries, with sprain being the most common at 50%.[3] The ankle is the most often involved, at 42% of all injuries, followed by the knee at 25%. When it comes to fracture, again the ankle is the most likely to be involved, at 42% of all sport-related fractures.[3] Girls tend to have more significant injuries requiring surgical intervention. Approximately 13% of injuries to the lower extremity in girls lead to a "season-ending" decision, which is 1.5 times that of boys at 8%.[3]

In recent years, many simple sports-related injuries were treated with the "RICE" protocol. More recently, this has been modified to include protection ("P") and referral ("R"), now deemed the "PRICER" protocol. For organized sports, many schools and organizations have athletics trainers available to guide practice and physical activity, who are also useful in early diagnosis and treatments. However, if the athlete is not responding to typical conservative therapies then referral should be made to a specialist.

Prevention of injury has been an important development regarding warm-up and bracing in particular. Because ankle injuries are so common, much investigation has been done on the effects of ankle bracing. It appears that ankle taping and bracing provides a benefit in prevention for athletes with chronic sprains, but it is not cost effective to brace or tape every participant. Other conservative treatments such as proprioceptive training may be more cost effective and still may provide significant risk reduction in preventing sprains. Some concerns exist, however, about bracing interfering with activity. In a meta-analysis on the effects of ankle support on function, lace-up bracing showed a negative effect of only approximately 1% impairment of a sprinter's speed (meta 6). Warm-up exercise is also debatable, but it is still thought that most warm-up activities should include 3 parts: increasing heart rate, static stretches, and dynamic stretches. Proper equipment is also paramount. New technologies in helmet design and protective padding are currently being tested with hopes of protecting athletes as they start at younger ages, play and practice faster and more aggressively, and continue sports year-round.

This article discusses the etiology of some of the most common foot and ankle sports-related injuries. The authors focus on clinical findings, associated injuries, pathophysiology, and current trends. Many of these factors are discussed in detail elsewhere in this issue.

LIGAMENT INJURIES

Ligaments are a dense connective tissue composed of collagen fibers connecting bone to bone. Due to their collagen fibers, they are elastic under tension but the cross-linking enables ligaments to remain strong enough to maintain structure and prevent dislocation. Within this tissue, feedback from stretch receptors and other proprioceptors allow for the body to monitor itself to maintain position. This second and possibly more important function of ligaments is commonly overlooked.

The most common sports-related injuries are ligament sprains. As much as 45% of all injuries reported in a 12-year high school analysis involved ligament injuries.[1] Of those the majority were ankle sprains, comprising 15% of all sports injuries.[3,4] The most common sport for ligament sprain was basketball. Although most injuries were minor, the average return to sport was 8 days. Common ligament injuries to the foot and ankle include lateral ankle sprains, Lisfranc complex sprains, and first metatarsal phalangeal (MTP) joint or "turf toe" (**Fig. 1**).

Lateral ankle instability and sprain is one of the most common emergency room and office complaints. Approximately 25,000 of these injuries occur each day in the United States. Many are caused by shoe gear or falling from a curb or into a pothole, but sport activity is another frequent cause. Fortunately the majority are more of a nuisance, requiring therapy and time. Only 15% of ankle sprains include a significant fracture, chondral lesion, or more significant issue requiring further imaging and surgical intervention (**Fig. 2**). The lateral ankle ligament complex comprises the anterior talofibular ligament, calcaneofibular ligament, and posterior talofibular ligament. The syndesmotic ligament between the tibia and fibula completes the complex and when injured is termed a "high" ankle sprain; this may be involved in as many as 10%.[7]

Instability of the lateral ankle is a common problem and can lead to a history of sprain. Instability itself has many causes. It is crucial to look for this instability when examining patients, and in particular when treating athletes and those participating in sports. Ankle sprains are common and continued sprain will eventually lead to

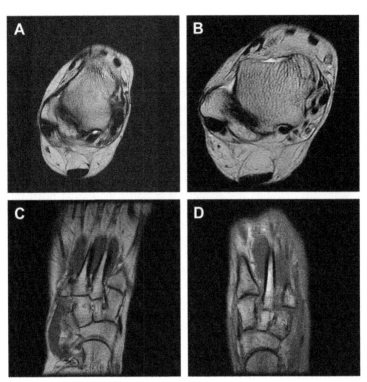

Fig. 1. Magnetic resonance imaging (MRI) examples of normal (*A*) and torn (*B*) anterior talofibular ligament, and normal (*C*) and torn (*D*) Lisfranc ligament after sprain injuries.

a more significant injury. Identifying those at risk is essential for proper treatment and attempted prevention.

Clinically one must look for mechanical causes of instability such as tibial varum, calcaneal varus, cavus foot type, forefoot valgus, plantarflexed first metatarsal, or

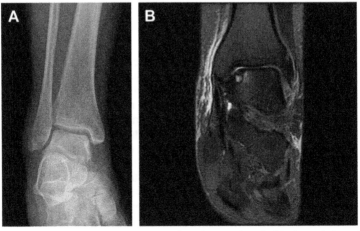

Fig. 2. Radiographic (*A*) and MRI (*B*) examples of osteochondral lesion of the talus after sprain.

any deformity that would contribute to ankle inversion. These deformities increase momentum through the lateral ankle and foot, and predispose to lateral injury. If present, addressing them may be required for chronic injuries.

Weak evertors and ligaments must be identified. The lateral muscle and ligament complex must possess enough physical strength to resist lateral stresses. Physical therapy is mandatory to ensure adequate lateral muscle strength. An often overlooked second function of therapy is to "strengthen" the proprioceptive abilities of the lateral complex. Without proper feedback from this complex, even with adequate "physical" strength of the lateral muscles, an athlete can continue to invert and sprain. This important difference of functional and mechanical instability must be understood and addressed.

For most, the first week or two after sprain is the acute phase with swelling, bruising, and difficulty bearing weight and participating in sport. During this acute phase, athletes are treated with appropriate offloading and rest. At times ankle sprains can have quite significant clinical swelling and bruising, making the patient and family skeptical of the diagnosis. One must perform an adequate examination, ensure no associated injuries exist, and perform standard radiographs if the clinical suspicion is high. Although ankle radiographs are some of the most commonly ordered series, the vast majority of sprains have no radiographic findings. It is still the standard of care at this point and may help rest the minds of those in the treatment room. Bruising along the lateral foot and at the base of the lesser digits is common, explained by the typical pattern of blood pooling after ligament tearing around the lateral ankle (**Fig. 3**).

During the acute injury phase one must carry out a basic examination to rule out associated injuries. This examination should be quick, reproducible, and start in areas that are pain free. One needs to rule out high fibula fractures, fractures of the lateral process of the talus, and anterior process of the calcaneus, fifth metatarsal, and Lisfranc injuries. The examination moves on to the peroneal tendons for subluxation and discomfort as well as the ankle for effusion, clicking, tenderness, and laxity. Laxity may be difficult to assess on initial visit because of guarding as well as difficulty in

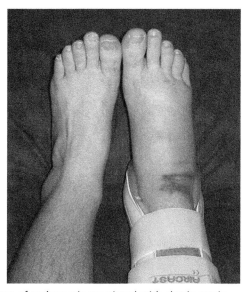

Fig. 3. Clinical pictures of ecchymosis associated with classic sprain.

performing the test in general. The examiner must stabilize the tibia and perform an anterior drawer, looking for puckering in the area of the anterior talofibular ligament. The examination must be performed without twisting the skin during the maneuver, thus avoiding a false test. A simple tip is to practice this maneuver on all patients coming to the office, so as to gain an appreciation of normal and abnormal (**Fig. 4**).

Standard treatment then permits weight bearing and activity as tolerated over the next few weeks, with physical therapy mandatory. This process can be difficult with frequent sprains because therapy is a time commitment and may seem unimportant, but every injury every time must be rehabilitated in attempts to reduce recurrence.

For the patient not responding at 2 months, magnetic resonance imaging (MRI) may be necessary. An MRI scan done during the initial stage will show subcutaneous edema and torn ligaments, which are treated conservatively. There is no role for MRI in the initial visit unless the clinical examination or radiographs reveal concerns (**Fig. 5**). With elite athletes and overbearing parents, this can be difficult to rationalize.

Without associated injuries, and continued symptoms after sprain, thoughts shift to the ankle joint itself as well as to the lateral ligament complex. For those athletes not responding, some require primary ligament repair. Repair for initial injury is not typically necessary. For athletes with continued symptoms from chronic instability leading to chronic tear and thickening of the lateral ligaments, repair may be required. It is becoming more standard at this point to perform arthroscopy of the ankle joint at the same setting (**Fig. 6**). It seems as though a majority of these patients have some intra-articular pathology, including chondral lesions not seen on MRI, meniscoid lesions, adhesions, and impingements from ligament such as the Bassett lesion from the inferior portion of the anterior inferior tibiofibular ligament.[8] These associated findings have been reported in as many as 95% of chronic sprain cases.[9]

Few athletes require more aggressive secondary repairs, but it is important to recognize associated deformities. Secondary repairs in athletes are avoided until necessary, due to the longer recovery and more inconsistent return to prior level. In a patient with chronic instability, calcaneal osteotomies may be necessary to address structural varus. The peroneal tendons, which also frequently have tendinosis issues after multiple sprains, should be evaluated (see later discussion).

For some sports including football and soccer, other sprains are becoming increasingly common. Lisfranc injuries are on the increase, partly due to participation in sport but also due to awareness and improvements in imaging. Direct blow injuries to the midfoot and Lisfranc region are a growing issue, in particular with regard to football and soccer. Injuries to this area without fracture have been described by Nunley and Vertullo.[10] This injury can become quite complicated to treat and even more

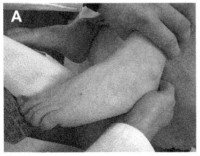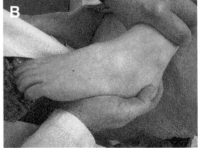

Fig. 4. (*A, B*) Clinical pictures of anterior drawer examination. Note loss of skin lines and puckering of lateral ankle corresponding to anterior talofibular ligament insufficiency.

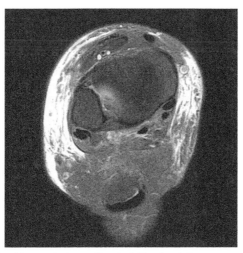

Fig. 5. MR image of ankle sprain immediately following injury. Note subcutaneous edema without more extensive pathology.

complicated to discuss with an athlete. Without large fracture fragments or changes that are easily seen on radiographs or other imaging, it can be difficult to convey the true nature of these injuries. For a high school senior who will miss his last football season, it takes confidence and knowledge of the anatomy, biomechanics, and current literature to convey one's point. These situations are delicate, and the clinician must do what is best for the patient long term, not what is desired in the short term.

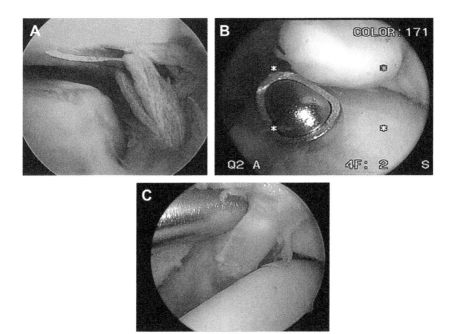

Fig. 6. Arthroscopic images in patients with sprain history. Note acute synovitis (*A*), loose body (*B*), and Bassett (*C*).

The Lisfranc sprain clinically has possible instability, clicking, and discomfort with stress. Plantar ecchymosis is many times present but not necessary. Any "odd" injury from twisting, a fall, or being stepped on creates high suspicion for a Lisfranc injury; this must be ruled out and documented. A simple "sprained foot" from the emergency room should be examined carefully. Radiographs for ligamentous Lisfranc injuries are typically seen as subtle shifts in the normal alignment. Weight-bearing films are essential. One must not settle for non–weight-bearing emergency room views (**Fig. 7**).

Not many Lisfranc injuries respond to conservative treatment. For true incomplete tears, non–weight bearing for 6 to 8 weeks can be recommended. Slow progression and rehabilitation is essential to give adequate time to heal. This complex requires absolute stability. Without it, the bony architecture cannot stabilize itself, leading to chronic instability and pain. Unfortunately, the amount of abnormal motion may be minimal, but is magnified by the load and force generated and accounting for symptoms.

More often this becomes a surgical problem. Stress radiographs can help determine the extent of injury, but they are not used often. MRI has become standard for these sprains. MRI is much more sensitive for bone edema, which signifies injury from ligaments avulsing from bone, thus giving more information about how many ligaments and joints are involved. These joints must be stabilized for long periods of time, allowing the ligaments and the bony architecture to scar and heal.

Primary fusion and open reduction/internal fixation are the most common forms of surgical intervention when warranted. Because of the frequency of reoperation for

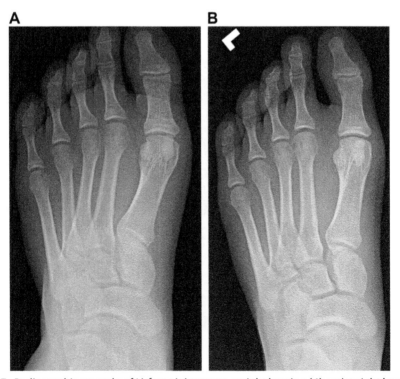

Fig. 7. Radiographic example of Lisfranc injury: non–weight bearing (*A*) and weight bearing (*B*). Note the subtle difference in the space near the base of the first and second metatarsals.

hardware removal and the later need for fusion for posttraumatic arthritis, primary arthrodesis for ligamentous Lisfranc injuries is gaining in popularity[11,12]; this is discussed in detail in articles elsewhere in this issue. Of importance, however, no matter the surgeon's preference, is the use of intraoperative fluoroscopy. This technique has taken the place of most stress radiographs and in difficult ligamentous injuries it can help determine which joints are affected; this is true preoperatively before incisions are made as well as intraoperatively. Joints that are unstable are stabilized sequentially and the complex checked frequently. There must be stability across the entire complex before leaving the operating room (**Fig. 8**).

The last common ligamentous injury to the foot and ankle during sport is the first MTP complex. There are many moving parts and specialized ligaments, which increases the likelihood of injury. In the classic "turf toe" injury, ligaments on the plantar surface are involved. Hyperextension of the MTP can lead to ligament tear in several areas. MTP injury can be a difficult one to treat. First of all, because it involves the foot and a "big toe," many athletes cannot understand why it is so limiting. The constant movement of the joint, the highly specialized nature of the ligaments and anatomy, and the fact it is the largest weight-bearing MTP can make for a long recovery. Treatment consists of rest and immobilization. Stiff-soled shoes or rigid extensions on orthotics may have some benefit, especially in prevention of recurrence. This injury is the third most common causing loss of game time, behind ankle and knee.[13] If symptoms persist, surgery may play a role but one must remember to rule out the associated injuries, including sesamoid fracture, sesamoid avascular necrosis, dislocations, and chondral lesions.

TENDONS

Tendons are composed 30% water and 86% collagen, organized in increasing bundles connecting muscle to bone. The collagen is primarily type I (97%) with the remaining makeup of tendon being elastin, proteoglycans, and some inorganic components. Because of the orientation of the collagen and cross-linking, tendons resist tension and exert the muscle's pulling force. Nerve and vascular components tend to primarily reside in the outer epi- and paratenon layers with a minimal amount of either penetrating deeper. The reasons for this are not exactly known, but may be

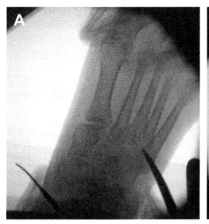
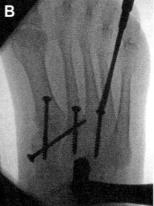

Fig. 8. Intraoperative example of stress view (*A*) for Lisfranc injury and subsequent placement of screws for open reduction/internal fixation (*B*) corresponding to areas of instability.

protective. If these structures were embedded deeper, pain may be associated with every step and use of the tendon. What is known is that this may also be a drawback. The inability to receive feedback about damage while it is occurring, and decreased ability for healing due to vascular insufficiency, may lead to continued play, continued injury, and a more difficult problem when it is noticed.

Tendon, like many tissues when injured, will undergo healing stages of inflammation, repair, and remodeling. Tenocytes lay down a matrix and initially primarily type III collagen. During later stages some type I collagen is laid down and cross-linking occurs. Tendon will continue to remodel for approximately 1 year but never regains the same mechanical properties. Although this does not mean athletes cannot participate or even excel, the scar properties of tendon never match those of preinjury.[14,15]

Another component of tendon injury that must be taken into account is during rupture. Whether this is repaired primarily or allowed to heal secondarily, the length-tension curve is permanently altered. The strength of the muscle-tendon complex relies on a certain length-tension relationship. At a certain length, the complex has its highest strength and power,[14,15] which is never recreated during repair. It is impossible to know the previous length or how the repair will scar and contract. These factors must be kept in mind during discussions with athletes. Athletes should be aware of the possible loss of strength and regarding the calf, a loss in size. Although a majority of Achilles repairs lead to a return to activity, there may be some limitations, and the loss in size due to changes in the length-tension relationship should be discussed.

Looking at specific tendon injuries in the athlete, the Achilles is by far the most commonly affected in the foot and ankle. The Achilles is the largest tendon in the body, measuring approximately 15 cm in length.[16] The function is primarily to plantarflex the foot but also plays a role in inversion. What is forgotten many times is its role in slowing the momentum of the tibia during gait. In the athlete, this function can be extremely important. During the stance phase of gait, the Achilles exerts the gastrosoleal force on the tibia, leg, and body to slow and control momentum, achieved through eccentric loading or slow, controlled elongation as the tibia passes over the foot. For athletes, during running and after the double swing or float phases, this can be a significant stress.

With this increased load the Achilles is at high risk in sports. When combined with the well-known hypovascular properties it is easy to see why this tendon is the frequent cause of office visits. Injection studies have been performed showing the "watershed" area 3 to 4 cm from the insertion.[17] If an athlete has anatomy lacking sufficient vessels in this area, he or she is at high risk for injury, exacerbated by repetitive stress on a tissue that has limited potential for healing.

Other predisposing factors may be weight, foot type, and equinus. Any mechanical issue that would cause limited range of motion to the ankle will stress the Achilles. The most common is the issue of equinus, which has been implicated in these injuries. The lack of dorsiflexion of the ankle requires compensation, putting stress on the Achilles.

Acute tendonitis from overuse or a change in activity can be seen in the Achilles. It is technically a paratenonitis or inflammation of the paratenon, but is commonly referred to generically as tendonitis. One stressful change is running on an incline or uphill. If dorsiflexion is limited to start with, this stresses the Achilles further. Conservative treatments for paratenonitis typically suffice, but more important is prevention of recurrence. Recurrent irritation and acute inflammation to the same area over time may be the etiology of the more typical chronic tendinosis. Scarring and thickening of the Achilles in the watershed area is most likely a sequela of multiple acute attacks. Patients presenting with these "acute-on-chronic" episodes must be watched and educated, as they may be at higher risk for rupture (**Fig. 9**). Studies show 15% of Achilles ruptures had previous "tendonitis" episodes.[18]

Achilles rupture is a common tendon injury in the athletic patient. Injury in males is more common at 2:1, with 75% of all Achilles ruptures during sporting activity occurring in males aged 30 to 40 years.[19] Acute ruptures may not have significant associated pain and may only slightly limit function, which can lead to delayed diagnosis. Achilles ruptures that are delayed longer than 4 weeks are termed "neglected" and may require a difference in treatment. Acute ruptures that are identified in a timely manner should be repaired in healthy active patients. Wound dehiscence has been a concern in years past, but the standard today is primary repair. Changes in incisions and surgical technique, along with changes in postoperative care, seem to have greatly decreased this complication (**Fig. 10**). Primary repair gives the athlete the best chance of returning to full function, and limits or significantly reduces the chance of rerupture (**Fig. 11**). In conservatively treated Achilles ruptures, the rerupture rate has been stated to be as high as 40%.[20]

A majority of other tendon injuries in the foot and ankle during sport are from overuse. As muscle fatigues, increased load is placed on the secondary structures such as ligaments and bony architecture, to maintain form. This theory underlies many acute and chronic sport injuries. During examination of an athletic patient, questions should be geared toward determining if overuse is present. Use may be simple, too much, or too often, but other causes can be less obvious and include biomechanics. For example, an athlete with a flexible flatfoot going for a long run will place stress on the posterior tibial tendon as it tries to maintain the longitudinal arch and achieve a rigid lever for propulsion. This stress may manifest as irritation at the navicular where the tendon inserts, at the medial malleolus in the hypovascular area, or at the origin where the muscle pulls on the tibial periosteum, causing periostitis or "shin splint." This type of overuse may be treated conservatively by addressing the biomechanics, but also includes physical therapy. Therapy serves 2 functions: to strengthen the posterior tibial muscle and to recruit other flexor tendons to slow fatigue.

The posterior tibial tendon, like the Achilles, can manifest overuse in several ways. In patients with an accessory navicular this may decrease the efficiency of the complex

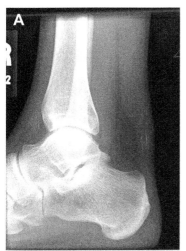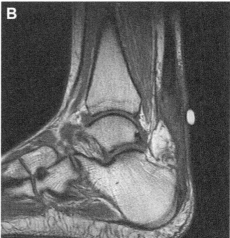

Fig. 9. Example of radiographic (*A*) and MRI (*B*) findings of acute-on-chronic Achilles tendinosis. Note the thickening in the watershed area.

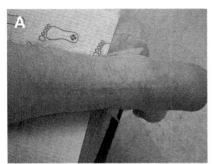
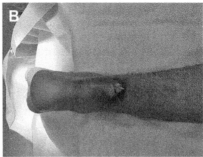

Fig. 10. Clinical pictures of Achilles tendon surgery with (*A*) and without (*B*) wound complications.

as a whole, leading to fatigue and symptoms. Much of this is addressed with orthotics, bracing, and therapy. The posterior tibial tendon does have a hypovascular zone, however, and must be watched.[21] Whether this predisposes to later dysfunction is not known but must be recognized.

The final common tendon issue for foot and ankle in the athlete involves the lateral muscle group. Issues along the peroneal tendons are common, and range from typical insertion tendonitis to tear and tendinosis. As with other tendon disorders, one must examine the biomechanics involved. Many issues with the peroneals stem from mechanical etiology, in particular varus. Varus forces overload the lateral foot, causing overuse of the peroneals as they try to evert the foot and protect against inversion sprains. These forces can be structural, but can also be activity or shoe gear related. Activity on uneven surfaces, forcing constant inversion and eversion, may cause over-use and irritation. Likewise certain shoes may cause inversion, including old shoes. These shoes tend to be worn laterally, causing even further lateral shift and inversion forces, and can be a simple cause of lateral column overload. Many of these problems can be dealt with conservatively with activity and shoe modification.

Unfortunately, if treatment is continued as in other overuse tendon injuries, the pero-neal tendons can become resistant to conservative treatment. Athletes with multiple ankle sprains or a history of instability can progress to a tendinosis. Tenderness poste-rior to the lateral malleolus is a typical site for this pathology, with a few common causes, one of which is overcrowding in the retromalleolar groove (**Fig. 12**). If the groove is too shallow or if space is occupied by a low-lying muscle, the tendons them-selves become vulnerable, which decreases the available volume and places increased pressure on the peroneals. When an athlete adds frequent sprains and

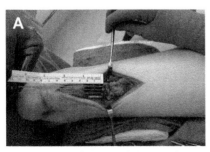
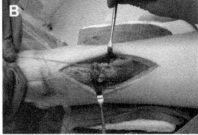

Fig. 11. Example of acute Achilles tendon rupture (*A*) and primary repair (*B*).

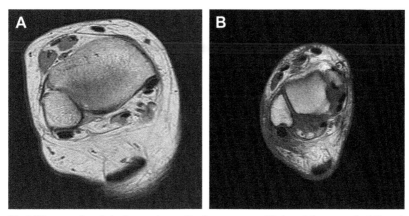

Fig. 12. MRI example of shallow retromalleolar groove with low-lying muscle (*A*) and subsequent deepening procedure (*B*).

instability the peroneal tendons can begin to undergo changes; this is the recurrent theme of an avascular tissue under repetitive stress. Over time the athlete complains of chronic pain. Monitoring ankle function, bracing, and therapy may be of some benefit. Otherwise decompression of the retromalleolar area is required, with primary tendon repair and tubularization. In fewer cases, groove deepening may be warranted.

FRACTURES

Fractures in athletes can be divided roughly into 2 categories, stress and acute. Acute fractures by definition have a specific solitary event and more commonly occur in impact sports. Stress fractures have no specific injury, rather an unusual or repeated stress. Stress fractures have been described in all lower extremity bones and most are benign, simply requiring time to heal. There are those, however, that are termed "high risk" and need to be treated with much more vigilance. High-risk fractures in the lower extremity include femoral neck, patella, proximal anterior tibia, medial malleolus, talar neck, navicular, fifth metatarsal, proximal second metatarsal, and the sesamoids.[22] These stress fractures need to be identified early and treated differently (**Fig. 13**). Talar neck, like femoral neck, is somewhat worrisome, due to possible complete fracture. Complete fractures in these areas could progress to avascular necrosis. The sesamoids act like the patella in the sense that constant pull in multiple directions can interfere with the healing process. The second metatarsal base undergoes significant torque and stress as part of the keystone of the Lisfranc complex. This process can lead to long healing times if not noticed early and weight bearing eliminated. Fifth metatarsal stress fractures are typically seen with chronic instability or varus condition applying tension to the lateral shaft. The continued stresses from altered mechanics may need to be addressed to offload the lateral column and allow healing, especially in recurrent cases (**Fig. 14**).

One of the most important stress fractures to be aware of in the foot of an athlete is the navicular body. Like many of the other high-risk stress fractures mentioned, the navicular body has poor biology under tension. The dorsal mid-portion of the body is an area with limited blood supply. This deficiency under increased stress predisposes the navicular to fatigue and failure. Once failure occurs, the fracture is under constant tension, increasing the probability it will propagate plantarly. Once fractured, the ability to repair is limited by the poor biology that helped initiate the problem.

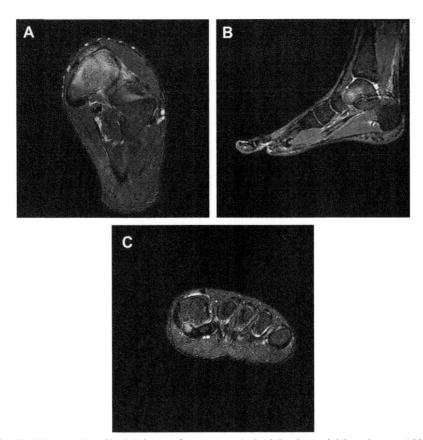

Fig. 13. MRI examples of high risk stress fractures: navicular (*A*), talar neck (*B*), and sesamoid (*C*).

Like most stress fractures, those of the navicular are difficult to identify on initial radiographs and may be diagnosed purely on a clinical basis. A history of repetitive trauma and tenderness at the "N" spot, the most dorsal aspect of the navicular, is a stress fracture until proven otherwise. MRI is much more sensitive, but once the fracture is identified computed tomography (CT) becomes a valuable tool. A CT scan will show cortical integrity and can be used to monitor healing or lack thereof. If the fracture has propagated to mid-body or 50% then it has become high risk for complete fracture and must be treated accordingly. A CT scan may also reveal the sclerosis of nonunion. For athletes, there is some debate as to whether this type of fracture should be treated surgically at initial onset.[23] For all high-risk stress fractures, one must improve both the biology and use fixation that guard against the forces that helped create the injury (**Fig. 15**).

Acute fractures to the lower extremity during athletics take on all shapes and sizes. Some are associated with topics discussed earlier. The most common are those associated with ankle instability. During acute sprain, avulsion fractures of the malleoli as well as chip fractures of the talus and calcaneus should be recognized. Most of these need only conservative treatment. Few may require internal fixation or if too small, fragment excision.

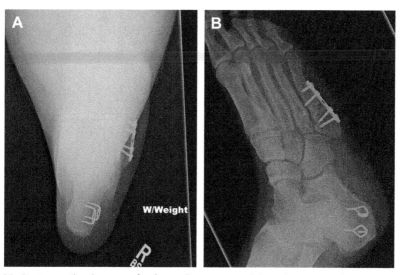

Fig. 14. Postoperative images of calcaneal osteotomy (*A*) and revision of recurrent fifth metatarsal stress fracture (*B*). Calcaneal osteotomy was performed to reduce stress to the lateral column.

Acute fractures of the fifth metatarsal include avulsion, shaft or "dancer" fractures, and the traditional Jones at the metaphyseal-diaphyseal junction. The majority of avulsion and dancer-type fractures need only conservative treatment.[24] When there is significant displacement then internal fixation may be required. One must be careful and remember fixation techniques for these fractures. Avulsion fractures and those distal near the neck can leave small pieces that are difficult to fixate. Small locking plates or tension band techniques may be required and can be tedious.

Jones fractures have been difficult to define over the years, but the consensus seems regard these fractures as starting at the metaphyseal-diaphyseal junction propagating medial toward the fourth to fifth metatarsal base articulation. These fractures

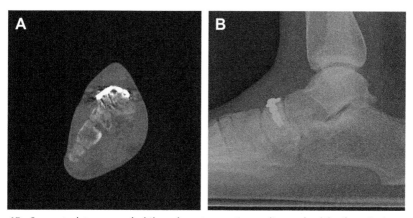

Fig. 15. Computed tomograph (*A*) and postoperative radiographs (*B*) of navicular stress fracture repair. Note the sclerosis and depth of the fracture preoperatively. The repair was made with distal tibial autograft and a dorsal plate to resist further tension.

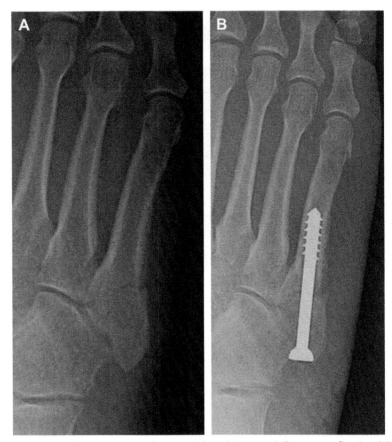

Fig. 16. Example of a typical Jones fracture (A) and intramedullary screw fixation (B).

are typically incomplete but have a negative history of slow or nonhealing. Because of this, Jones fractures in athletes are typically repaired with intramedullary screw fixation (**Fig. 16**). One must be aware of the proximity of the surgery site to branches of the sural nerve.[25] This nerve can be damaged during surgery or chronically irritated by fixation. If irritation occurs, the fixation is left in place at least until the sporting activity or athlete's career is over. Recurrence of those treated conservatively or refractures in those after hardware removal requires a look at the mechanics. As mentioned previously, varus deformities and ankle instability should be recognized and addressed.

SUMMARY

As the number of participants in sporting activities continues to increase, along with the pressure to go faster, become stronger, play longer, and participate in more sports, the number of corresponding injuries will follow. Many sports-related injuries are overuse in nature, affecting all anatomic regions and tissue types. Specialism in the foot and ankle will be on the front line of diagnosis and treatment of these injuries. One must be familiar with the spectrum of injuries and their treatments, and take into account the athlete's age, sport, and level.

REFERENCES

1. Powell JW, Baber-Foss KD. Sex related injury patterns among selected high school sports. Am J Sports Med 2000;28:385–91.
2. Steiner H, McQuivey RW, Pavelski R. Adolescents and sports: risk or benefit? Clin Pediatr 2000;39:161–6.
3. Fernandez WG, Yard EE, Comstock RD. Epidemiology of lower extremity injuries among U.S. high school athletes. Acad Emerg Med 2007;14:641–5.
4. Hootman JM, Dick R, Agel J. Epidemiology of collegiate injuries for 15 sports: summary and recommendations for injury prevention initiatives. J Athl Train 2007;42:311–9.
5. Verhagen E, Vander Beek A, Twisk J, et al. The effect of a proprioceptive balance board training program for the prevention of ankle sprains: a prospective controlled trial. Am J Sports Med 2004;32:1385–93.
6. Cordova ML, Scott BD, Ingersoll CD, et al. Effects of ankle support on lower-extremity functional performance: a meta-analysis. Med Sci Sports Exerc 2005; 37:635–41.
7. Molinari A, Stolley M, Amendola A. High ankle sprains (syndesmotic) in athletes: diagnostic challenges and review of the literature. Iowa Orthop J 2009;29:130–8.
8. Bassett FH, Gates HS, Billys JB, et al. Talar impingement by the anteroinferior tibiofibular ligament. A cause of chronic pain in the ankle after inversion sprain. J Bone Joint Surg Am 1990;72:55–9.
9. Sugimoto K, Takakura Y, Okahashi K, et al. Chondral injuries of the ankle with recurrent lateral instability: an arthroscopic study. J Bone Joint Surg Am 2009; 91:99–106.
10. Nunley JA, Vertullo CJ. Classification, investigation, and management of midfoot sprains: Lisfranc injuries in the athlete. Am J Sports Med 2002;30:871–8.
11. Ly TV, Coetzee C. Treatment of primarily ligamentous Lisfranc joint injuries: primary arthrodesis compared with open reduction and internal fixation. A prospective, randomized study. J Bone Joint Surg Am 2006;88:514–20.
12. Henning JA, Jones CB, Sietsema DL, et al. Open reduction internal fixation versus primary arthrodesis for Lisfranc injuries: a prospective randomized study. Foot Ankle Int 2009;30:913–22.
13. Clanton TO, Ford JJ. Turf toe injury. Clin Sports Med 1994;13:731–41.
14. Benjamin M, Kaiser E, Milz S. Structure-function relationships in tendons: a review. J Anat 2008;212:211–28.
15. James R, Kesturu G, Balian G, et al. Tendon: biology, biomechanics, repair, growth factors, and evolving treatment options. J Hand Surg Am 2008;33A: 102–12.
16. O'Brien M. The anatomy of the Achilles tendon. Foot Ankle Clin N Am 2005;10: 225–38.
17. Langergren C, Lindholm A. Vascular distribution in the Achilles tendon. Acta Chir Scand 1958;19:491–5.
18. Yinger K, Mandelbaum BR, Almekinders LC. Achilles rupture in the athlete; current science and treatment. Clin Podiatr Med Surg 2002;19:231–50.
19. Jozsa L, Kvist M, Balint BJ, et al. The role of recreational sport activity in Achilles tendon rupture: a clinical, pathoanatomical, and sociological study of 292 cases. Am J Sports Med 1989;17:338–43.
20. Nestorson J, Movin T, Moller M, et al. Function after Achilles tendon rupture in the elderly: 25 patients older than 65 years followed for over three years. Acta Orthop Scand 2000;71:64–8.

21. Frey C, Shereff M, Greenridge N. Vascularity of the posterior tibial tendon. J Bone Joint Surg Am 1990;72:884–8.

22. Boden BP, Osbahr DC. High-risk stress fractures: evaluation and treatment. J Am Acad Orthop Surg 2000;8:344–53.

23. Torg JS, Moyer J, Gaughan JP, et al. Management of tarsal navicular stress fractures: conservative versus surgical treatment: a meta-analysis. Am J Sports Med 2010;38(5):1048–53.

24. O'Malley MJ, Hamilton WG, Munyak J. Fractures of the distal shaft of the fifth metatarsal. "Dancer's fracture". Am J Sports Med 1996;24:240–3.

25. Donley BG, McCollum MJ, Murphy GA, et al. Risk of sural nerve injury with intramedullary screw fixation of fifth metatarsal fractures: a cadaver study. Foot Ankle Int 1999;20:182–4.

New Technology and Techniques in the Treatment of Foot and Ankle Injuries

David J. Soomekh, DPM[a,b,c]

KEYWORDS

- Lisfranc dislocation • Achilles rupture • Achilles tendinosis
- TightRope • Extracorporeal shock wave therapy
- Topaz radiofrequency coblation • Platelet-rich plasma

The advancement of new technologies in the treatment of foot and ankle injuries seems exponential over the last several years. As surgeons expand their knowledge of pathology and improve their treatment techniques, they come upon new and different ways to treat the same pathologic conditions. However, the surgeons know that there is always a drive to perfect technique and decrease morbidity and recovery time. Therefore, there are always new and improved techniques and devices to investigate.

SUBTLE LISFRANC DISLOCATION
Anatomy

The stability of the tarsometatarsal (TMT) joint is based on the configuration of the bases of the metatarsals and the cuneiforms and the ligaments that joint them. The TMT joint includes the first, second, and third metatarsals and their corresponding cuneiforms. The metatarsals are joined together by the transverse dorsal and plantar ligaments. The second metatarsal is wedged as a keystone between the medial and lateral cuneiforms, whereas the plantar ligaments stabilize it to the midfoot.[1] The dorsal and plantar ligaments are oriented longitudinally, obliquely, and transversely. The oblique and longitudinal fibers connect the cuneiforms to the proximal aspect of the metatarsals, whereas the transverse fibers are between the bases of the metatarsals. The strongest of the interosseous ligaments that stabilizes the first and second

[a] University Foot and Ankle Institute, 2121 Wilshire Boulevard Suite 101, Santa Monica, CA 90403, USA
[b] Department of Surgery, University of California Los Angeles Medical Center, 17th Street, Los Angeles, CA 90404, USA
[c] Department of Surgery, Cedars-Sinai Medical Center, Beverly Hills, Beverly Boulevard, CA 90048, USA
E-mail address: drsoomekh@footankleinstitute.com

Clin Podiatr Med Surg 28 (2011) 19–41
doi:10.1016/j.cpm.2010.09.004
0891-8422/11/$ – see front matter © 2011 Elsevier Inc. All rights reserved.

metatarsals is often named as the Lisfranc ligament.[2] This ligament is located between the medial cuneiform and the base of the second metatarsal.

Injury

A sprain of the midfoot is a common injury in athletes.[3] The sprain can occur when the foot is placed in a plantar flexed and rotated position when an indirect longitudinal force is applied followed by a forceful abduction. The angle and the intensity of this force determines the degree of injury, whether it is a fracture or ligamentous pathology.[2] It is thought that a torsional force is applied to the midfoot that then unlocks the second metatarsal. This injury is most common in soccer, football, gymnastics, basketball, baseball, ballet, and running. This article presents a discussion of a more subtle dislocation.

Many classification systems have been derived at to describe the level of injury to the ligaments and associated fractures. Hardcastle and colleagues[4] based their classification system on the shift of the midfoot in the transverse plane: type A for total incongruity, type B for partial incongruity, and type C for divergent incongruity. Myerson and colleagues[5] expanded on this system by including subdivisions to the Hardcastle system, ie, B1, B2, C1, and C2, depending on the complexity of the injury.

It was Nunley and Vertullo[6] who presented a classification system for the more subtle injuries from low-impact injuries that are seen in athletes. This system addresses the more-ligamentous injuries to the joint with a possible fleck avulsion fracture. Stage I represents a sprain of the Lisfranc ligament without a measurable diastasis between the base of the second metatarsal and the medial cuneiform or any loss of arch height on weight-bearing radiographs. There is then no measured instability of the Lisfranc joint. Stage II represents a sprain of the ligament with a diastasis of 1 to 5 mm between the base of the second metatarsal and the medial cuneiform. There is still no loss of arch height, but both the dorsal and interosseous ligaments are injured, and the plantar structures are intact. In a stage III injury, there is a diastasis of greater than 5 mm and a loss of arch height.[6]

Diagnosis

When there is a high suspicion for a midfoot sprain, a detailed history and clinical examination can help to confirm the evidence of the injury. The patient usually presents with pain along the first and second rays, with pinpoint palpation pain within the interspace between the bases of the first and second metatarsals and the medial cuneiform. There is often pain in this area with simultaneous medial and lateral compression of the midfoot. The experienced clinician may also appreciate the instability of the medial complex through sagittal and transverse plane range of motions. Weight-bearing radiographic imaging should be used to determine the degree of injury, including stress views. In those cases in which there is a suspicion on plain films, magnetic resonance imaging (MRI) or computed tomography (CT) could be helpful in the final diagnosis of the severity of the sprain (**Fig. 1**).

Treatment

It is well documented that Lisfranc injuries, whether low- or high-grade, must be treated aggressively. There are many reports that early and proper treatment and anatomic reduction leads to better functional results and a reduction in future instability and osteoarthritis.[7–11] Conservative treatments are reserved for those injuries that are classified as Nunley and Vertullo stage I injuries. Treatment includes a period of guarded weight bearing in a pneumatic walker or a non–weight-bearing cast for 6 weeks. Stress views can be reevaluated to determine if a longer course of

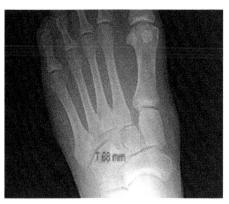

Fig. 1. Isolated Lisfranc rupture dislocation.

non–weight-bearing is indicated. Progressive weight bearing in custom-molded orthotics with physical therapy is recommended for up to 3 months, depending on the severity of the injury.

Nunley and Vertullo stage II and stage III injuries should be treated with open reduction and internal fixation (ORIF). It is important to maintain the stability of the second metatarsal. Traditionally, stability has been achieved with a partially threaded cannulated 3.5-, 4.0-, or 4.5-mm screw. The fixation is placed in a proximal-medial to distal-lateral direction through the central medial aspect of the medial cuneiform into the base of the second metatarsal. There are inherent problems with this type of fixation. The screw needs to be removed after full recovery. This removal requires another surgical setting, with its own inherent risks and complications. It also results in additional recovery time while the void left by the screw fills in. It can be difficult to gain adequate compression with the screw because it does not cross the cortex of the second metatarsal. Attempted compression could cause fracture or pull-out of the screw. Furthermore, there could be disruption of the cartilaginous surfaces by the screw.

In vivo studies have shown that complete immobilization of a ligament could be harmful to its healing and may reduce its mechanical properties.[12,13] This finding indicates that a fixation that could facilitate the dynamic properties of the ligament during healing would be ideal. One way to achieve such a fixation is with the use of a combination suture and button fixation system. The author prefers to use a suture-endobutton combination for fixation to stabilize a stage II or stage III dislocation. The Mini TightRope system (Arthrex, Inc, Naples, FL, USA) is most often used (**Fig. 2**). The TightRope construct is made up of 2 metal buttons connected to one another by 4 strands of No. 2 FiberWire (Arthrex, Inc, Naples, FL, USA). This construct allows for strength from the 4 strands of FiberWire and flexibility that is not achieved by screw fixation. The TightRope is used in the same manner as a screw. However, the advantages of using the TightRope are that removal is not needed, compression can be achieved, dynamic motion of the ligament is restored, and the suture can act as the ligament if the ligament fails to heal. Panchbhavi and colleagues[14] compared the stability provided by a suture-button fixation system with that of the traditional screw fixation for simple diastases of Lisfranc ligament. They used cadaveric specimens with isolated Lisfranc ligament transections, placed the fixation, and applied a 35-kg load. They showed that when a load is applied, the difference between displacement before and after screw fixation and suture-button fixation is significant. They concluded that

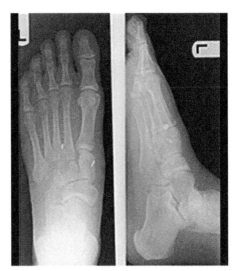

Fig. 2. Repair of Lisfranc injury with TightRope.

stabilization and reduction of the diastases using both methods were not statistically different.

Surgical Technique

An incision is made on the medial aspect of the medial cuneiform. Blunt dissection is performed to the level of the retinaculum. The retinaculum is incised and retracted for later closure. The periosteum over the central aspect of the medial cuneiform is incised and freed with a freer elevator. A second incision is made over the dorsal lateral aspect of the second metatarsal just distal to the base. The muscle tissue and periosteum are reflected off the lateral cortex of the metatarsal. Under fluoroscopy, the guidewire from the set is used to determine the angle of the drill hole and is placed over the dorsum of the foot while obtaining an anteroposterior (AP) view. The wire should be positioned at the center of the medial cuneiform and aimed toward the second metatarsal in a proximal-medial to distal-lateral direction toward the base of the second metatarsal. The guidewire is then driven under fluoroscopic guidance through the cuneiform and out the base of the metatarsal, just exiting at the level where the second interspace is exposed between the second and third metatarsals. It is crucial to exit the center of the width of the metatarsal. Alternatively, the guide pin can be driven from the base of the second metatarsal laterally through the cuneiform medially. The cannulated drill is then placed over the guidewire and driven from medial to lateral, breaking through all 4 cortices; the drill and wire are then removed. The FiberWire with the endobuttons is introduced through the drill hole using the guide pin from the second metatarsal to the cuneiform, which leaves the round button on the lateral aspect of the metatarsal, while the oblong button is brought out from the medial aspect of the cuneiform and placed flush over the cortex. The articulation is reduced by the surgeon's assistant with compression of the midfoot from side to side. The lateral round button is then placed flush over the cortex of the base of the second metatarsal by toggling the 2 free suture ends until the other 2 looped sutures over the button are synched tight. With the button flush over the cortex, the free suture is pulled tight and a knot is made over the button. The assistant's reduction is released, and fluoroscopy is used to confirm that the reduction holds. When the appropriate amount of reduction is achieved, the suture is knotted several more times and then cut. The suture knot is then tucked plantarly and into the musculature to avoid irritation. Some patients have experienced irritation of the nerves in this area because of the knot. Alternatively, the suture can be passed from medial to lateral, leaving the knot on the cuneiform. However, there can be irritation in shoe gear from the large knot placed medially just below the skin. Routine closure is then performed. The foot is placed in a non–weight-bearing cast for 2 weeks and then in a non–weight-bearing pneumatic walker for another 2 to 3 weeks. Light range of motion and physical therapy is started after 2 weeks. The patient is transferred to weight bearing in the walker for another 2 to 3 weeks and then to athletic shoe gear and orthotics. Physical therapy continues with a gradual return to activity.

TIBIOFIBULAR SYNDESMOSIS INJURY

The syndesmotic ligament complex is essential to the function, stability, and support of the ankle joint. Isolated syndesmotic injuries have been shown to occur in about 1% to 18% of ankle sprains. When left untreated, the injuries can be a source of prolonged morbidity, pain, and arthritis in athletes.[15–18] The incidence of injury may be even higher because of the difficulty in diagnosis or missed diagnosis in the absence of frank diastasis or instability in the ankle.[19] In athletes, the syndesmotic injury is most commonly seen in collision sports like rugby, hockey, football, lacrosse, and wrestling.[20–22] With the advent of stiffer ski boots that extend higher above the ankle, there has been an increased prevalence of syndesmotic injuries compared with lateral ankle sprains in skiers.[23]

Anatomy

The ligamentous union between the tibia and the fibula is a complex structure that can be broken down into 3 major parts: the proximal tibiofibular syndesmosis, the aponeurotic interosseous membrane (IOM), and the distal tibiofibular complex. This distal complex is the most important of the 3 and consists of 5 portions: the anterior inferior tibiofibular ligament (AITFL), the posterior inferior tibiofibular ligament (PITFL), the transverse tibiofibular ligament (TTFL), the interosseous tibiofibular ligament (IOL), and the distal portion of the aponeurotic IOM.[19] Studies have shown that serial sectioning of the distal complex increases the tibiofibular diastasis by an average of 2.5 mm. When the entire distal complex is sectioned, a total diastasis of 7.33 mm is appreciated.[24–26]

Injury

An injury to the syndesmosis can occur when there is a forced separation between the distal tibia and fibula. This seperation can happen when there is a forced external rotation of the talus in the ankle mortise. There can also be an internal rotation of the tibia at the same time. Isolated injuries to the syndesmosis without fracture are rare and can occur when there is not enough external rotational force to sustain a fracture.[18,27–29] These injuries are often labeled as high-ankle sprains.

Syndesmotic injuries that are associated with fractures are more common and have been detailed by Lauge-Hansen.[30,31] When the foot is in supination and there is an external rotational force, there can be a rupture of the AITFL, an avulsion at the anterior tubercle of the tibia (Chaput), or an avulsion at the fibular insertion of the ligament (Wagstaffe). When the external rotation continues, there is a spiral fracture of the lateral malleolus. An injury with a supination and external rotation, stage I in the

Lauge-Hansen[30] classification, leads to an isolated rupture of the ligament. When the foot is in pronation with external rotation, the deltoid ligament ruptures first or there is a medial malleolar fracture. With continued external rotation, the AITFL and the IOL rupture, and then there is a spiral or oblique fracture of the fibula or rupture of the IOM with a proximal fibular fracture. The PITFL and the TTFL are avulsed or ruptured in a stage IV injury. When an abduction force is applied to a pronated foot, there is a medial malleolar fracture followed by an avulsion or a rupture of the AITFL and the PITFL and elongation of the IOL and IOM. As this force continues, the fibula fractures at the level of the syndesmosis. The most unstable syndesmotic tears are sustained with a pronation-external rotation stages III and IV.[30]

Diagnosis

The clinical and radiographic examinations are critical when there is a high suspicion for a syndesmotic tear. The patient presents with pain in the anterolateral aspect of the ankle joint, which is increased with forced dorsiflexion. Pain is elicited on palpation in this area. The "squeeze test" can be applied by compression of the tibia to the fibula just above the midpoint of the calf.[32,33] This compression elicits pain at the level of the distal tibiofibular syndesmosis. Frick test can be applied by holding the foot in a neutral position against a fixed lower leg and applying passive external rotation of the foot.[32] This maneuver elicits pain over the area of the syndesmosis. The Frick test has proved to be sensitive and is more reliable than the squeeze test.[34–36]

Plain radiographic examination consists of the standard 3 views of the ankle, including a true AP and mortise view, to rule out fractures. The AP or mortise view aids in the detection of a syndesmotic tear. Proximal radiographs should be obtained to rule out proximal fibular fractures. It is also helpful to obtain contralateral views for comparison. To evaluate the radiograph for a syndesmotic tear without frank diastasis, specific measurements can be obtained. The tibiofibular clear space (ie, espace clair) described by Chaput should measure less than 6 mm, whereas the tibiofibular overlap should measure more than 6 mm and the medial clear space should measure less than 5 mm on the AP radiograph. The tibiofibular overlap should be more than 1 mm on the mortise view.[37–41] Stress radiographs can also be used when there is still a suspicion for a tear that is latent on the regular views.

CT scans can be useful and are more accurate than plain radiographs, mostly in cases of low diastasis that can go undetected on plain films. Bilateral images can be helpful. MRI is specific and sensitive in imaging the syndesmosis and can help determine the degree of the pathologic condition and specifically which ligaments in the complex are torn. There is no clear algorithm for radiographs to determine if surgery is indicated to repair the ligament. It is generally considered that a difference of more than 2 mm when compared with the contralateral side indicates a high suspicion of syndesmotic instability from a rupture of at least 2 or more ligaments and could lead to abnormalities of the ankle joint if not stabilized surgically.[19]

Treatment

Syndesmotic injuries with instability and frank or latent diastasis with or without an associated malleolar fracture that are left untreated can lead to significant joint abnormalities. These injuries should be treated with operative stabilization to heal the ligaments in the correct position to maintain stability to the joint and length to the fibula. Traditionally, surgery is performed with open reduction with 1 or 2 syndesmosis screws.[15,26,29,36,42–46] However, there is debate as to the size of the screws used, the number of cortices to engage, and the distance from the joint the screws should be placed.[19,47–50] Syndesmotic screws may have their disadvantages. There is an inherent motion during regular gait between the tibia and fibula owing to the flexibility of the ligament.[15,51] Rigid screw fixation across the ligament may interfere with the normal motion between the bones. Thornes and colleagues[52] reported that this rigid fixation with screws, where normal movement is needed, can lead to loosening, breakage, or failure of the fixation. Traditionally, screw fixation necessitates removal of the screws later. Soin and colleagues[53] performed a cadaveric study to compare the natural motion of the fibula with screw fixation and suture-endobutton fixation. They found that the fibular motion was similar between the 2 fixation techniques.

The use of interosseous suture and endobuttons to manage a syndesmotic rupture has been increasingly investigated. The technique has been shown to be minimally invasive and provides a semirigid and dynamic fixation across the syndesmosis, which may allow for some of the natural motion between the tibia and fibula. This type of fixation rarely needs to be removed. Klitzman and colleagues[54] performed a study on cadaveric specimens and found that the suture-button fixation maintained reduction when placed under the same loads as an intact syndesmosis. They also found that it allowed for more physiologic movement in the sagittal plane when compared with screw fixation. Seitz and colleagues[55] were able to use the endobutton technique successfully. Thornes and colleagues[56] showed the endobutton to be biomechanically equivalent to a 4.5-mm quadricortical screw. They also reported a decrease in the rehabilitation time.[52] Cottom and colleagues[57] reported a prospective study comparing 25 patients with screw fixation with 25 patients with endobutton fixation. They found no statistical difference between the 2 fixation techniques when measuring age, follow-up duration, time to postoperative weight bearing, or subjective outcomes scores. They found that most of the radiologic measurements had no statistical differences. They offer that the suture endobutton fixation is a valid option compared with traditional AO screw fixation.[57,58]

Surgical Technique

In cases in which ORIF is needed on the fibula or tibia, these procedures should be performed first using standard AO principles. The suture-button complex can be incorporated over a lateral tubular fibular plate through one of its distal holes. The author uses the Syndesmotic TightRope (Arthrex, Inc, Naples, FL, USA). The system comprises a No. 5 FiberWire looped into 4 strands with 2 endobuttons, a 3.5 × 10-mm oblong button for the medial aspect and a 6.5-mm round button for the lateral aspect. The syndesmosis is reduced using a reduction clamp. The guidewire from the set is driven from lateral to medial about 1.5 cm above the tibial plafond aiming about 30° anterior to the coronal plane exiting the medial cortex of the tibia. The cannulated 3.5-mm drill is driven over the guidewire through all 4 cortices. The drill and guidewire are removed. The nitinol needle attached to the suture is passed through the drill hole exiting percutaneously through the medial skin, with care to avoid the saphenous nerve and vein. The pull-through sutures attached to the button are pulled through the skin, bringing the oblong button out of the drill hole and over the cortex. Under fluoroscopy, the button is positioned flush over the medial cortex of the tibia by toggling the 2 pairs of No. 5 FiberWire laterally. The pull-through sutures are cut and removed off the button. The lateral round button is tightened over the lateral cortex of the fibula by pulling the free ends of the suture, with the syndesmosis reduced in internal rotation and mild ankle plantar flexion. The suture is then secured with several knots and tucked over the button to reduce its prominence. In cases of a Maisonneuve fracture or significant syndesmotic instability, a second TightRope can be placed 1 cm above the first with slight axial divergence to increase the rotational stability. Postoperative management depends on the presence of an isolated syndesmotic injury or an associated fracture.

ACHILLES TENDINOSIS AND RUPTURE

Injuries of the Achilles tendon is commonly encountered by the foot and ankle surgeon. Injuries are most often sustained by athletes. However, it also commonly seen in people who play sports regularly. It has been associated with overuse injuries, biomechanical deformity, systemic disease, inflammatory disease, and poor training. The tendon is vital to the proper function and strength in normal gait. Acute or chronic tears or tendinosis can lead to significant loss of function, loss of strength, and pain.

Anatomy

The gastrocnemius muscle merges with the soleus to form the Achilles tendon. It is more round proximally and flattens distally. The tendon fiber is not vertical but rotates 90° before it broadens and inserts into the middle of the posterior calcaneal tuberosity. The tendon does not have a true synovial sheath but has a paratenon comprising a visceral and parietal layer. The tendon receives most of its vascular supply from the paratenon and secondarily from the myotendinous junction and the calcaneal insertion. Vascular studies have shown the watershed area to be about 2 to 6 cm proximal to the insertion. The Achilles tendon works as a spring, storing and releasing elastic strain and energy during gait. In vitro studies have shown the tendon to have a breaking point at about 100 MPa and that it can endure about 70 MPa during maximal eccentric plantar flexions.[59–61]

Tendinosis

Injury

Tendinosis is defined as a chronic degenerative process that lacks an adequate healing response. The tendon shows collagen degeneration, fiber disorientation, scattered vascular in-growth, and the absence of inflammation.[62–66] Leadbetter[65] suggested that tendinosis is a failure of the cell matrix to adapt to repetitive trauma caused by an imbalance between the degeneration and synthesis of the matrix. Tendons heal by scarring instead of by regeneration as normally seen in most tissues.[63,65] Tendinosis of the Achilles tendon often leads to nodular formations within the substance of the tendon, which may or may not be painful. The nodules are thought to be created when there is repetitive microtearing within the tendon, leading to increased scarring and thickness.

The causes of Achilles tendinosis or tendinopathy are still unclear. Theories include overuse, lack of vasculature, decreased flexibility, genetics, and endocrine disorders. Causes may also include tissue hypoxia and free-radical production that can cause changes in the tendon and exercise-induced hyperthermia.[67] A tendon that has been strained repetitively to more than 4% of its original length loses elasticity and has an increased risk of break in the collagen structure.[68]

Diagnosis

Patients present with consistent long-term pain within the tendon, which may have not responded to conservative therapies. It is important to investigate the onset and degree of pain and the aggravating factors. There should be an evaluation of the patient's activities that may be associated with the pathologic condition. The pain is usually located anywhere between 2 and 6 cm proximal to the calcaneal insertion. Some patients present with pain during normal walking, whereas others relate pain only when exercising. Most patients do not have pain at rest.

Clinical examination includes a full lower-extremity evaluation of both legs, including any biomechanical or musculoskeletal deformities. The presence of equinus should be evaluated. The presence and degree of nodules within the tendon should be noted.

The tendon should be palpated to determine the points of maximal tenderness. Crepitation on range of motion should be noted as well.

Imaging modalities include plain radiography, ultrasonography, and MRI. Plain films rule out the presence of a Haglund deformity, spurring at the calcaneal insertion, or calcifications within the substance of the tendon. Ultrasonography can be used in the office setting to evaluate the tendon by evaluating the hypoechoic areas that correlate to nodular, multifocal, or diffuse injury. The hyperechoic areas may represent an accumulation of calcium deposits. MRI is still the best way to image the tendon. It can better differentiate between partial tears and focal degenerative areas of the tendon. MRI shows abnormalities in the tendon as a thickened paratenon, peritendinous fluid, edema in Kager triangle, fusiform thickening of the tendon, focal or diffuse intratendinous intermediate to high signal, or interrupted appearances of the tendon tissue.[69,70]

Treatment

Conservative treatments are more likely to fail in patients with tendinosis than in those with tendonitis. When conservative treatments have failed, more intensive treatments may be warranted. The author uses a protocol that may include a series of options presented to the patient in the form of aggressive conservative treatments to operative treatments. These options include a treatment ladder from extracorporeal shock wave therapy (ESWT), to platelet-rich plasma (PRP) injections, to percutaneous Topaz radiofrequency (RF) coblation, to microtenotomy of the tendon, to open surgical repair.

When injury to the tendon is in a chronic state, there is a lack of blood flow, inflammation, and healing factors. The body has effectively stopped trying to heal the affected area. Theoretically, returning the tendon to an acute state of injury restarts the healing process and allows for healing and recovery. ESWT, PRP, and Topaz RF coblation are based on this theory.

ESWT has been proved to be an effective method for the treatment of Achilles tendonitis over the last several years. Vulpiani and colleagues[71] performed a study with 127 tendons with tendinosis. They used 4 sessions of ESWT treatment at 1500 to 2500 impulses at 0.08 to 0.4 mJ/mm^2. They found satisfactory results in 42.2% of the patients after 2 months, 73.2% after 6 to 12 months, and 76% after 13 to 24 months. Furia[72] studied 34 patients with tendinosis treated with ESWT against a control group of 34 patients treated conservatively. Patients were treated with a single dose of 3000 pulses at 0.21 mJ/mm^2. He found that the percentage of patients with excellent (1) or good (2) Roles and Maudsley scores, that is, successful results, 12 months after treatment was statistically significant in the ESWT group compared with the control group.

Rasmussen and colleagues[73] compared ESWT to placebo in 48 patients. They found improvement in both groups during the follow-up period. However, at 8 and 12 weeks, there was an increased improvement in patients treated with ESWT compared with those receiving placebo. Fridman and colleagues[74] performed ESWT at 21 kV, 2 Hz with 2000 pulses on 23 Achilles tendons followed up for 20 months. They found that 91% of the patients were satisfied or very satisfied, 87% related improvement, 13% related no improvement, and 0% related increased pain. They concluded ESWT to be safe, noninvasive, and effective for Achilles tendinosis. Lohrer and colleagues[75] evaluated 40 Achilles tendons with tendinosis using ESWT, following up the patients for 1 year. Treatments were performed with 2000 impulses at between 0.06 and 0.18 mJ/mm^2, with 5 sessions at weekly intervals. They found significant improvement in pain at rest, tenderness, load-induced pain, pain threshold, and pain-free running time as soon as 1 week after the end of the treatment. At the 1-year follow-up, results were even more improved. They concluded that ESWT seems to be an effective treatment modality for degenerative tendon lesions induced by running and jumping.

The author uses the Swiss DolorClast (Electro Medical Systems, Dallas, TX, USA) to perform ESWT in the office setting (**Fig. 3**). It supplies a low-dose shock wave, which allows it to be a portable device. The machine uses compressed air impulses to accelerate the projectile in the headpiece. The impact of the projectile on the applicator generates the shock wave that is delivered to the tissue through the contact gel. The advantage of shock waves generated with the Swiss DolorClast is that they can produce an extensive analgesic effect to the area because the radiating shock waves extend to the entire area of pain. In most cases, no anesthetic is needed. The patient is positioned prone on the examination table. The machine should be set to deliver between 2000 and 3000 impulses at 5 to 10 impulses a second at 2 bar (0.06 mJ/mm^2) initially. It can be increased to 4 bar (0.18 mJ/mm^2) during the treatment if tolerable to the patient. Ultrasound gel is applied over the treatment area and the handpiece is placed over the tendon at the point of maximal pain. The machine is started using a foot pedal, while the handpiece is gently moved over the tendon. The patient wears a pneumatic walking boot for about 1 to 2 weeks. Most patients require up to 3 treatments 10 days to 2 weeks apart. Once all the treatments have been performed, the patient wears athletics shoes with orthotics and gradually returns to activity by physical therapy. During the initial recovery after each treatment, the patient is restricted from using antiinflammatory medications or modalities.

In recent years there has been an increased interest and use of PRP for chronic injuries of the foot and ankle. Platelets play an essential role in the healing cascade. When activated, they produce cytokines and granules that then produce growth

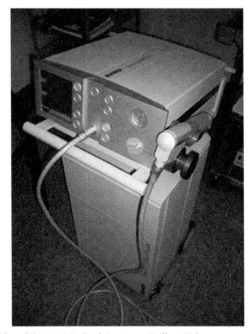

Fig. 3. Swiss DolorClast (Electro Medical Systems, Dallas, TX).

factors that aid in the healing process. In the absence of inflammation in the chronic state, there is a paucity of platelets. The act of injecting a platelet-rich solution into the injured tissue increases the relative concentration of platelets in the tissue, thereby increasing the healing potential. There are an increasing number of studies testing the efficacy of PRP in cases of chronic Achilles tendinosis. PRP is thought to reverse the effects of tendinopathy by stimulating revascularization and improving healing at the microscopic level.[76]

Lyras and colleagues[77] studied the effect of PRP on angiogenesis during tendon healing. The study was performed on the Achilles tendon of rats against a control group injected with saline. They found a significant increase in angiogenesis in the PRP group compared with the control group during the first 2 weeks of the healing process (ie, the inflammatory and proliferative phases), and the number of the newly formed vessels in the PRP group was significantly reduced at 4 weeks compared with the controls, suggesting that the healing process was shortened. They observed that the orientation of collagen fibers in the PRP group was better organized. The investigators concluded that PRP seems to enhance neovascularization, which may accelerate the healing process and promote scar tissue of better histologic quality.

Gaweda and colleagues[78] performed a prospective study on 15 patients with Achilles tendonitis. Patients were followed up for 18 months. They found improvement in pain scores and on ultrasound imaging. The American Orthopaedic Foot and Ankle Score improved from a median of 55 points to 96 points, and the achilles tendon score improved from 24 points to 96 points. They concluded PRP to be a viable treatment alternative for Achilles tendonitis.

Recently, de Vos and colleagues[79] performed a stratified, block-randomized, double-blind, and placebo-controlled study. They included patients between the ages of 18 and 70 years with a diagnosis made clinically with findings of a painful and thickened tendon in relation to activity and on palpation, with symptoms lasting longer than 2 months. The PRP and control groups included 27 patients. They used 54 mL of whole blood to derive the PRP that was mixed with sodium bicarbonate to match the pH of tendon tissue. An undisclosed amount of PRP was injected into 5 sites along the injured tendon under ultrasonographic guidance. Patients were allowed to walk only short distances indoors in the first 48 hours. On days 3 to 7, patients were allowed to walk up to 30 minutes. After 1 week, an exercise routine was started, with 1 week of stretching and 12 weeks of daily eccentric exercise program with heel drops off a step. No weight-bearing sports activities were allowed for 4 weeks followed by a gradual return to activity. The results showed an improvement in 24 weeks by 21.7 points in the PRP group and 20.5 points in the placebo group. They concluded that there was no significant difference between the groups. At present, there are several prospective studies underway, investigating the true efficacy of PRP for Achilles tendinosis. The author's clinical experience with more than 100 injections seems promising. A decrease in pain, size, and number of nodules and an earlier return to activity after PRP use has been observed.

Technique

A local anesthetic block is placed well above the site of injection around the level of the myotendinous junction. From the cubital vein, 60 mL of whole blood is collected. PRP is then prepared using the Magellan Autologous Platelet Separator System (Arterio-cyte Medical Systems Inc, Cleveland, OH, USA). This device allows the operator to choose the amount of PRP desired by the clinician. A volume between 6 and 10 mL was chosen, yielding a concentration of PRP between 5 and 7 more than the baseline, respectively. The PRP is activated by calcium citrate and injected under ultrasonographic guidance within the substance of the tendon, beginning at the site of the pathologic condition (pain and any bulbous mass). The medial or lateral aspect of the tendon is approached with the patient in a prone position. Several pulsed (peppered) doses of about 0.25 mL at a time are injected using a 25-gauge needle, performing fenestrations of the tendon. The patient is restricted from using antiinflammatory medications or modalities for about 1 month after the procedure. Rescue medications such as acetaminophen or narcotics can be used as needed. The patient is placed in a walking boot on crutches (non–weight-bearing) for up to 1 week, then allowed to bear weight in the boot for the next 1 to 3 weeks. The patients are then allowed to wear athletic shoes, with a slow increase in weight-bearing activity over a 4-week period. A significant reduction in pain, a decrease in the size of fibrous nodules within the tendon, and a sooner return to regular and sporting activity after injection of PRP has been observed. Most patients have been able to return to increased exercise and activity within 2 months of the injection. Those patients who had only some improvement in their symptoms have benefited by a second injection about 6 weeks after the first.

Another method to increase angiogenesis and stimulate healing in the avascular, fibrotic, and degenerative Achilles tendon is to use bipolar RF coblation or RF-based microtenotomy. Coblation is a controlled, non–heat-driven process using RF energy to excite the electrolytes in a conductive medium, such as saline solution, creating a precisely focused plasma. The plasma's energized particles have sufficient energy to break the molecular bonds within tissue, causing the tissue to dissolve at relatively low temperatures (typically 40°C–70°C). The result is volumetric removal of target tissue with minimal damage to surrounding tissue. Because RF current does not pass directly through the tissue during the coblation process, tissue heating is minimal. Most of the heat is consumed in the plasma layer, that is, by the ionization process. These ions then bombard the tissues in their path, causing molecular bonds to simply break apart and the tissue to dissolve. RF-based microtenomy was researched early on in the treatment of congestive heart failure to promote angiogenesis.[80–82] The research showed an increase in histologic and clinical outcomes as compared with other procedures. Early research on chronic tendinosis was performed by Tasto and colleagues.[83] Results showed histologic evidence of an early inflammatory response and new blood vessel formation. Further research on human tendons showed improved function and less pain through 1 year by using what they deemed a simple and less-invasive technique.[84,85] Yeap and colleagues[86] prospectively evaluated 15 procedures on chronic tendinosis of the Achilles, posterior tibial, and peroneal tendons using RF-based microtenotomy. They found a marked improvement in pain scores and earlier recovery than was found with other procedures. They concluded that RF-based microtenomy for chronic tendinosis shortens the natural history of disease in the tendon and hastens recovery and that the procedure may be especially useful for young competitive athletes who need a shorter rehabilitation time and quicker recovery.[86] Liu and colleagues[87] evaluated 17 cases of Achilles tendinosis treated with RF-based microtenomy. They performed the procedure using arthroscopy. They found a significant reduction in visual analog scale pain scores from 8.7 to 1.6 about 15 days after the procedure and a marked improvement within 7 to 14 days after the surgery. They also concluded the procedure to be a safe, effective, and minimally invasive to decrease pain and lead to early rehabilitation.

The patient is placed on the operating table in a prone position. The area is anesthetized above the level of the treatment area, and the area is prepared for surgery. The procedure can be performed percutaneously. The author uses the Topaz MicroDebrider (ArthroCare, Sunnyvale, CA, USA) connected to a generator and timer. This technique uses a bipolar, controlled, plasma-mediated RF-based process (coblation). The probe is connected to a saline drip to control the temperature and is set to 1 to 2 drops every 3 seconds. A timer is used to control the amount of microtenotomy at 500 milliseconds. The control unit is set to level 4 (175 V). In a gridlike pattern, percutaneous holes are made through the skin using a Kirschner wire over the pathologic area, while the foot is dorsiflexed to reduce the skin wrinkles. The probe is then inserted through each hole, advancing the wand to the level of resistance against the tendon, and the RF-based microtenomy is performed at about 5-mm intervals at differing depths. The wound is dressed with sterile dressing, and compression is applied. The patient wears a pneumatic walking boot with limited weight bearing for a period of 3 weeks and then wears athletic shoes, and there is a slow increase in activity through physical therapy during the next 3 to 6 weeks. During the first 2 months, the patient should refrain from using antiinflammatory medications or modalities, because inflammation is what the procedure is trying to achieve. Promising results have been seen with several cases using the Topaz RF coblation in both percutaneous and open procedures, with improvement in pain and earlier recovery and return to activities.

Surgical repair of the tendon has been the gold standard in the treatment of recalcitrant Achilles tendinosis when conservative treatments have failed. With the advent of ESWT, RF coblation, and PRP, these techniques should be tried before considering open repair. Open surgery is performed when one or all these therapies have failed. Surgical procedures involve the removal of abnormal tissue and lesions, fenestration of the tendon through multiple longitudinal lacerations, and possibly stripping the paratenon. The goal of open surgery is to remove degenerative nodules, excise fibrotic adhesions, restore vascularity, and stimulate viable cells to initiate an inflammatory response to reinitiate healing.[88–92] The aforementioned techniques can also be used in conjunction with an open surgical technique. The Topaz RF coblation probe can be used in lieu of performing lacerations or perforations within the tendon once opened (**Fig. 4**). Once any abnormal tissue has been removed, RF-based microtenomy can be performed to the tendon in several locations in a grid pattern at several different depths. If the tendon was sectioned sagittally to remove abnormal tissue, RF-based microtenomy can be performed within the substance of the tendon before repairing it. If the surgeon decides that there is no need to remove abnormal tissue, adhesions, or nodules, RF-based microtenomy can be performed percutaneously. PRP can be used during an open surgery as an adjunct to the repair. A layer of concentrated platelets may be sprayed over the tendon before closure of the paratenon. PRP can also be prepared as a gel by adding thrombin to it. This gel can be molded into any

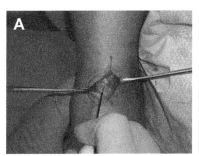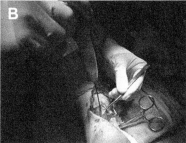

Fig. 4. Open treatment of Achilles tendinosis using Topaz coblation leaving tendon intact (*A*). Open treatment of Achilles tendinosis using Topaz collation after removal of scarred tendon (*B*).

shape to be wrapped around and sutured to the tendon. With either method, the foot is placed in a pneumatic walker or cast and the patient uses crutches for a period of 3 to 5 weeks. Physical therapy is ideal in these cases to begin a slow progression to increased activity and strength.

Rupture

Injury

The Achilles tendon is one of the most commonly ruptured tendons in the human body.[93] Most ruptures are observed in male patients between the ages of 30 and 50 years. About 75% of ruptures have been shown to occur during sports-related activities.[94] Most researchers agree that the precursor is some sort of overuse and that repetitive loading plays a role in the pathophysiology leading to a rupture; however, no direct relationship between physical activity and histopathology has been found.[95] Most agree that patients who have a chronic tendinosis have a higher incidence and chance of rupture.[93,96,97] The rupture usually occurs at the watershed point in the tendon, where it has the least vascularity, approximately 2 to 6 cm proximal to its insertion. A rupture usually occurs when there is an extreme or sudden force on a resting or weakened tendon.

Diagnosis

The diagnosis of an Achilles tendon rupture is usually made based on the patient's history and clinical examination. Patients present describing feeling a sudden pop or snap in the back of the leg and ankle while they were performing an intense physical activity or sudden propulsion. They usually describe the sensation as though they were struck in the back of the ankle and then feeling sudden pain. Most patients relate the pain as subsiding soon after the injury and being able to walk with only a slight limp. For this reason, many ruptures are diagnosed weeks later because the patients think they only sprained their ankle.

Physical examination of the tendon reveals ecchymosis and edema surrounding the posterior ankle and the tendon. A palpable dell or defect can be appreciated at the rupture site. The Thompson-Doherty test can be applied by having the patient in a prone position and squeezing the calf from side to side. If the foot does not plantar flex, the test result is negative. Patients are unable to perform single-heel raises on the affected side. MRI can confirm the diagnosis and help determine the amount of retraction of the proximal portion of the tendon.

Treatment

Open surgical repair is the gold standard for the ruptured Achilles tendon. There have been many procedures described to reapproximate the tendon ends using different suturing techniques and materials. The goal is to have a direct end-to-end anastomosis, usually possible in acute cases. Once the tendon has been exposed, the hematoma removed, and the tendon ends prepared, most surgeons perform some form of the Krackow suture technique, modified Krackow technique, the Bunnell technique, or the modified Kessler stitch. The Krackow stitch has been shown to be stronger than the Bunnell or the modified Kessler stitch.[98]

The author uses a new type of suture material and technique called a FiberLoop (Arthrex, Inc, Naples, FL, USA). FiberWire is a suture made of a nonabsorbable polyethylene core with a braided polyester jacket. FiberLoop is no 2 or 2-0 FiberWire in a continuous loop on a straight nitinol needle. The looped structure of the suture construct allows for a simpler and faster technique for running a whipstitch through the tendon. Botero and Svoboda[99] performed a small study for Arthrex, comparing the Krackow stitch to no 2 FiberLoop, testing their failure load and elongation at failure on porcine tendons. They found that the FiberLoop whipstitch technique provided the best fixation with regard to peak failure load and allowed more elongation than the Krackow Fiber-Wire technique; however, its performance was comparable to the Krackow technique using Ethibond (Ethicon, Somerville, NJ, USA) in resisting elongation with regard to elongation at failure. Cook and colleagues[100] studied 12 cadaveric Achilles tendons comparing the strength of 2-0 FiberLoop to No. 2 Ethibond suture. They found that the smaller-caliber 2-0 FiberLoop maintained a greater load-to-failure strength than No. 2 Ethibond. They concluded that a thicker suture material, as used traditionally in Achilles tendon repair, may be substituted by the thinner and stronger FiberLoop material.

Technique

Once the tendon ends are prepared, the "loop" of the No. 2 or 2-0 (depending on the size of the tendon and the amount of retraction) FiberLoop suture is placed around the proximal aspect of the ruptured tendon about 5 cm from the stump. The suture is oriented so that the needle is posterior and the central aspect of the loop is hugging the tendon on its underside or anterior aspect. An Edna clamp is placed on the end of the tendon for counterpressure. One hand is used to grasp the loop posterior to the tendon, lifting it posterior and proximal, while the other hand drives the nitinol needle into the central posterior aspect of the tendon about 5 mm distal to the loop, exiting the anterior aspect of the tendon. The needle is pulled tight, closing the first loop around the tendon. The next pass is performed by looping the suture over the tendon once again and passing the needle from posterior to anterior through the tendon just distal to the loop and about 5 mm from the previous loop. This looping continues until the suture reaches the distal aspect of the end of the tendon. There should be 5 or more loops around the tendon. The suture is cut at the level of the needle, and each free end of the suture is passed through the tendon from medial to lateral and from lateral to medial, respectively, with the free needle. There should now be a free suture on each side of the proximal stump of the tendon. The same technique is not performed on the distal stump of the tendon with another FiberLoop. Care should be taken to place the first loop as distal as possible to have at least 5 passes through the tendon. With the ankle in maximal plantar flexion, the medial or lateral sutures are sutured together, reapproximating the ends of the tendon with 1 knot to hold it in place. The next suture is then tied several times holding the ends of the tendon tight. Attention is now redirected to the previous knot, and it is tightened again with several more knots. The repair can be augmented at the anastomosis if needed with a 2-0 FiberWire suture. The author has found this suture construct and technique to use less suture material and to be less constrictive on the tendon, more efficient, and simpler to perform than the more traditional types of whipstitch and suture materials.

Now that the tendon ends are repaired, it may be beneficial to augment the repair with some extracellular matrix scaffolding (**Fig. 5**). There has been a great interest in biologic reinforcement and augmentation of soft tissue and tendon repairs with materials that can be wrapped around the tendon to increase strength, decrease healing time, and decrease scar tissue formation within the tendon. Research and advancements have provided numerous materials in the form of allografts and xenografts, which can be easily prepared and applied to the tendon. These acellular regenerative tissue scaffolds are usually allogenic permanent dermal equivalents derived from human cadaveric tissue that is processed in a way that minimizes the destruction of the original human dermis.[101] Vascular pathways in the dermis and extracellular matrix, which contains all collagen types, elastin, proteoglycans, laminins, and tenacin, are preserved in the allograft.[102] These scaffolds are prepared to allow for rapid

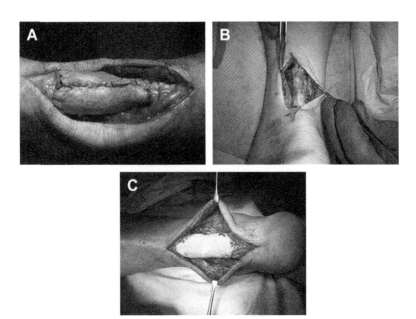

Fig. 5. Achilles tendon rupture repair wrapped with different types of extracellular matrix scaffold (*A, B, C*).

revascularization, cellular repopulation, their ability to maintain tensile strength, and their lack of immunologic host response. These materials do not interfere with healing or become encapsulated like most foreign bodies.

Several studies have shown the effectiveness (increased strength) and histologic incorporation of these acellular scaffolds in both human and animal tendons.[103–107] Barber and colleagues[108] examined the strength and stiffness of 8 pairs of repaired cadaveric Achilles tendon ruptures, comparing suture repair with and without graft augmentation using GraftJacket (Wright Medical Technology, Arlington, TN, USA). They noted a significant increase in the strength (failure load of 217 to 455 N, control vs augmented tendon, respectively) and stiffness (4.3 to 12.99 N/mm, control vs augmented tendon, respectively) of the repaired tendons using the GraftJacket. Liden and Simmons[105] histologically evaluated biopsies taken from Achilles tendon repairs with GraftJacket 6 months after surgery. They concluded that the acellular dermal matrix is biocompatible, supports revascularization and repopulation with noninflammatory host cells, and becomes incorporated by the surrounding tendon tissue.

There are many different materials on the market. Chen and colleagues[109] reviewed 47 articles relating to different types of scaffolds and their effects on ligament and tendon repair augmentation. They found many products being used and both positive and negative reports on each. These products included the Restore Patch (DePuy Orthopedics, Warsaw, IN, USA), GraftJacket, Zimmer Collagen Repair Patch Graft (Zimmer, Warsaw, IN, USA), and TissueMend (Stryker Orthopedics, Mahwah, NJ, USA). The author usually uses GraftJacket for the reinforcement of an acute Achilles tendon rupture repair. Other studies compared these different products with one another to determine the strength and chemical properties and concluded that the chemical and mechanical differences between the materials may be because of the source (dermis or small intestine), species (human, porcine, or bovine), age of donor (fetal or adult), and processing of the extracellular matrix.[110,111]

PRP in the form of a fibrin gel (when combined with thrombin) can also be used as a tendon scaffold. It can be used as a bridge and augmentation within the rupture defect or can be wrapped around the tendon repair. In most cases, PRP is combined with bone marrow aspirate for further enhancement of the PRP matrix. Sarrafian and colleagues[112] performed a study to compare a cross-linked acellular porcine dermal patch (APD) with a PRP fibrin matrix (PRPFM) for repair of acute Achilles tendon rupture in a sheep model. The 2 surgically transected tendon ends were reapproximated in groups 1 and 2, whereas a gap was left between the tendon ends in group 3. APD was used to reinforce the repair in group 2, and autologous PRPFM was used to fill the gap, which was also reinforced with APD, in group 3. Tensile strength testing showed a statistically significant difference in elongation between the operated limb and the unoperated contralateral limb in groups 1 and 3 but not in group 2. In group 1, all surgical separation sites were identifiable, and healing occurred via increasing tendon thickness. In group 2, healing occurred with new tendon fibers across the separation, without increasing tendon thickness in 2 of 6 animals. Group 3 showed complete bridging of the gap, with no change in tendon thickness in 2 of 6 animals. In groups 2 and 3, peripheral integration of the APD to tendon fibers was observed. They concluded that the use of APD, alone or with PRPFM, to augment Achilles tendon repair in a sheep model allowed for a viable and strong repair.

After the tendon ends are repaired and the graft material has been prepared (soaked and trimmed to its proper length), it is wrapped circumferentially around the tendon, with the rupture site central on the graft. The seam of the graft should be centered over the tendon. The dermal side of the graft should be lying over the tendon. The graft is anchored at its proximal lateral corner to the tendon using a 4-0 nonabsorbable suture. The graft is then pulled taut at the distal-lateral corner while the assistant is holding the medial portion of the graft tight, and this corner is anchored to the tendon. The medial portion of the graft is now cut to its proper width to a level where it meets with the opposing lateral aspect of the graft while being taut. The remaining corners are now sutured in the same manner. The central aspect of the tendon is then sutured to itself with every other suture passing through the tendon. Interlocking sutures are not used, so that if the knot slips it does not unravel the repair. If there is available paratenon, it can be reapproximated over the graft. A significant decrease in healing time and increased strength in less time has been observed when using Achilles tendon augmentation. Patients generally have their foot placed in a cast for 3 weeks and are then allowed to begin progressive weight bearing and intensive physical therapy, sooner than those without grafting. There has also been a significant enhancement in the definition of the tendon complex with less edema and thickness to the tendon compared with those repaired without augmentation.

SUMMARY

The number of new technologies and techniques in the treatment of foot and ankle injuries is widespread. In many cases, a surgeon may be introduced to a new technique that is exciting and sound in theory but does not live up to its potential in practice. New technologies that are replacing old ones must have certain criteria. These criteria include less complications, decreased comorbidity, decreased healing time, decreased recovery time, increased patient satisfaction, decreased pain, increased function, and cost effectiveness. It is the responsibility of the clinicians and surgeons to differentiate between those technologies that are fruitful and increase patient care and those that are redundant or harmful. Clinical testing of both in vivo and in vitro studies is critical to best evaluate the efficacy of new technologies. The literature and clinical evidence for the use of the technology and techniques in this review are promising. Yet, more well-designed prospective studies examining these products and techniques are essential to establish them as the gold standard.

REFERENCES

1. Cunningham DJ, Romanes GJ. Cunningham's textbook of anatomy. 11th edition. London: Oxford University Press; 1972.
2. Coetzee JC. Making sense of Lisfranc injuries. Foot Ankle Clin 2008;13(4): 695–704, ix.
3. DeOrio M, Erickson M, Usuelli FG, et al. Lisfranc injuries in sport. Foot Ankle Clin 2009;14(2):169–86.
4. Hardcastle PH, Reschauer R, Kutscha-Lissberg E, et al. Injuries to the tarsometatarsal joint. Incidence, classification and treatment. J Bone Joint Surg Br 1982; 64(3):349–56.
5. Myerson MS, Fisher RT, Burgess AR, et al. Fracture dislocations of the tarsometatarsal joints: end results correlated with pathology and treatment. Foot Ankle 1986;6(5):225–42.
6. Nunley JA, Vertullo CJ. Classification, investigation, and management of midfoot sprains: Lisfranc injuries in the athlete. Am J Sports Med 2002;30(6):871–8.
7. Aitken AP, Poulson D. Dislocations of the tarsometatarsal joint. J Bone Joint Surg Am 1963;45:246–60.
8. Bassett FH 3rd. Dislocations of the tarsometatarsal joints. South Med J 1964;57: 1294–302.
9. Granberry WM, Lipscomb PR. Dislocation of the tarsometatarsal joints. Surg Gynecol Obstet 1962;114:467–9.
10. Hesp WL, van der Werken C, Goris RJ. Lisfranc dislocations: fractures and/or dislocations through the tarso-metatarsal joints. Injury 1984;15(4):261–6.
11. Wilson DW. Injuries of the tarso-metatarsal joints. Etiology, classification and results of treatment. J Bone Joint Surg Br 1972;54(4):677–86.
12. Hart DP, Dahners LE. Healing of the medial collateral ligament in rats. The effects of repair, motion, and secondary stabilizing ligaments. J Bone Joint Surg Am 1987;69(8):1194–9.
13. Walsh S, Frank C, Shrive N, et al. Knee immobilization inhibits biomechanical maturation of the rabbit medial collateral ligament. Clin Orthop Relat Res 1993;297:253–61.
14. Panchbhavi VK, Vallurupalli S, Yang J, et al. Screw fixation compared with suture-button fixation of isolated Lisfranc ligament injuries. J Bone Joint Surg Am 2009;91(5):1143–8.
15. Close JR. Some applications of the functional anatomy of the ankle joint. J Bone Joint Surg Am 1956;38(4):761–81.
16. Fallat L, Grimm DJ, Saracco JA. Sprained ankle syndrome: prevalence and analysis of 639 acute injuries. J Foot Ankle Surg 1998;37(4):280–5.
17. Gerber JP, Williams GN, Scoville CR, et al. Persistent disability associated with ankle sprains: a prospective examination of an athletic population. Foot Ankle Int 1998;19(10):653–60.
18. Hopkinson WJ, St Pierre P, Ryan JB, et al. Syndesmosis sprains of the ankle. Foot Ankle 1990;10(6):325–30.

19. Rammelt S, Zwipp H, Grass R. Injuries to the distal tibiofibular syndesmosis: an evidence-based approach to acute and chronic lesions. Foot Ankle Clin 2008; 13(4):611–33, vii–viii.
20. Nussbaum ED, Hosea TM, Sieler SD, et al. Prospective evaluation of syndesmotic ankle sprains without diastasis. Am J Sports Med 2001;29(1):31–5.
21. Williams GN, Jones MH, Amendola A. Syndesmotic ankle sprains in athletes. Am J Sports Med 2007;35(7):1197–207.
22. Wright RW, Barile RJ, Surprenant DA, et al. Ankle syndesmosis sprains in National Hockey League players. Am J Sports Med 2004;32(8):1941–5.
23. Fritschy D. An unusual ankle injury in top skiers. Am J Sports Med 1989;17(2): 282–5 [discussion: 285–6].
24. Ogilvie-Harris DJ, Reed SC, Hedman TP. Disruption of the ankle syndesmosis: biomechanical study of the ligamentous restraints. Arthroscopy 1994;10(5): 558–60.
25. Sarsam IM, Hughes SP. The role of the anterior tibio-fibular ligament in talar rotation: an anatomical study. Injury 1988;19(2):62–4.
26. Xenos JS, Hopkinson WJ, Mulligan ME, et al. The tibiofibular syndesmosis. Evaluation of the ligamentous structures, methods of fixation, and radiographic assessment. J Bone Joint Surg Am 1995;77(6):847–56.
27. Edwards GS Jr, DeLee JC. Ankle diastasis without fracture. Foot Ankle 1984; 4(6):305–12.
28. Miller CD, Shelton WR, Barrett GR, et al. Deltoid and syndesmosis ligament injury of the ankle without fracture. Am J Sports Med 1995;23(6):746–50.
29. Rose JD, Flanigan KP, Mlodzienski A. Tibiofibular diastasis without ankle fracture: a review and report of two cases. J Foot Ankle Surg 2002;41(1):44–51.
30. Lauge-Hansen N. Fractures of the ankle. II. Combined experimental-surgical and experimental-roentgenologic investigations. Arch Surg 1950;60(5):957–85.
31. Lauge-Hansen N. Fractures of the ankle. IV. Clinical use of genetic roentgen diagnosis and genetic reduction. AMA Arch Surg 1952;64(4):488–500.
32. Frick H. [Diagnosis, therapy and results of acute instability of the syndesmosis of the upper ankle joint (isolated anterior rupture of the syndesmosis)]. Orthopade 1986;15(6):423–6 [in German].
33. Saunders EA. Ligamentous injuries of the ankle. Am Fam Physician 1980;22(2): 132–8.
34. Beumer A, Swierstra BA, Mulder PG. Clinical diagnosis of syndesmotic ankle instability: evaluation of stress tests behind the curtains. Acta Orthop Scand 2002;73(6):667–9.
35. Boytim MJ, Fischer DA, Neumann L. Syndesmotic ankle sprains. Am J Sports Med 1991;19(3):294–8.
36. Grass R, Herzmann K, Biewener A, et al. [Injuries of the inferior tibiofibular syndesmosis]. Unfallchirurg 2000;103(7):520–32 [in German].
37. Clanton TO, Paul P. Syndesmosis injuries in athletes. Foot Ankle Clin 2002;7(3): 529–49.
38. Gardner MJ, Demetrakopoulos D, Briggs SM, et al. Malreduction of the tibiofibular syndesmosis in ankle fractures. Foot Ankle Int 2006;27(10):788–92.
39. Harper MC, Keller TS. A radiographic evaluation of the tibiofibular syndesmosis. Foot Ankle 1989;10(3):156–60.
40. Takao M, Ochi M, Oae K, et al. Diagnosis of a tear of the tibiofibular syndesmosis. The role of arthroscopy of the ankle. J Bone Joint Surg Br 2003;85(3):324–9.
41. Yablon IG, Leach RE. Reconstruction of malunited fractures of the lateral malleolus. J Bone Joint Surg Am 1989;71(4):521–7.

42. Burns WC 2nd, Prakash K, Adelaar R, et al. Tibiotalar joint dynamics: indications for the syndesmotic screw–a cadaver study. Foot Ankle 1993;14(3):153–8.
43. Ebraheim NA, Elgafy H, Padanilam T. Syndesmotic disruption in low fibular fractures associated with deltoid ligament injury. Clin Orthop Relat Res 2003; 409:260–7.
44. McBryde A, Chiasson B, Wilhelm A, et al. Syndesmotic screw placement: a biomechanical analysis. Foot Ankle Int 1997;18(5):262–6.
45. Peter RE, Harrington RM, Henley MB, et al. Biomechanical effects of internal fixation of the distal tibiofibular syndesmotic joint: comparison of two fixation techniques. J Orthop Trauma 1994;8(3):215–9.
46. Zalavras C, Thordarson D. Ankle syndesmotic injury. J Am Acad Orthop Surg 2007;15(6):330–9.
47. Beumer A, Campo MM, Niesing R, et al. Screw fixation of the syndesmosis: a cadaver model comparing stainless steel and titanium screws and three and four cortical fixation. Injury 2005;36(1):60–4.
48. Chissell HR, Jones J. The influence of a diastasis screw on the outcome of Weber type-C ankle fractures. J Bone Joint Surg Br 1995;77(3):435–8.
49. Moore JA Jr, Shank JR, Morgan SJ, et al. Syndesmosis fixation: a comparison of three and four cortices of screw fixation without hardware removal. Foot Ankle Int 2006;27(8):567–72.
50. Reckling FW, McNamara GR, DeSmet AA. Problems in the diagnosis and treatment of ankle injuries. J Trauma 1981;21(11):943–50.
51. Beumer A, Valstar ER, Garling EH, et al. Kinematics of the distal tibiofibular syndesmosis: radiostereometry in 11 normal ankles. Acta Orthop Scand 2003; 74(3):337–43.
52. Thornes B, Shannon F, Guiney AM, et al. Suture-button syndesmosis fixation: accelerated rehabilitation and improved outcomes. Clin Orthop Relat Res 2005;431:207–12.
53. Soin SP, Knight TA, Dinah AF, et al. Suture-button versus screw fixation in a syndesmosis rupture model: a biomechanical comparison. Foot Ankle Int 2009;30(4):346–52.
54. Klitzman R, Zhao H, Zhang LQ, et al. Suture-button versus screw fixation of the syndesmosis: a biomechanical analysis. Foot Ankle Int 2010;31(1):69–75.
55. Seitz WH Jr, Bachner EJ, Abram LJ, et al. Repair of the tibiofibular syndesmosis with a flexible implant. J Orthop Trauma 1991;5(1):78–82.
56. Thornes B, Walsh A, Hislop M, et al. Suture-endobutton fixation of ankle tibio-fibular diastasis: a cadaver study. Foot Ankle Int 2003;24(2):142–6.
57. Cottom JM, Hyer CF, Philbin TM, et al. Transosseous fixation of the distal tibiofibular syndesmosis: comparison of an interosseous suture and endobutton to traditional screw fixation in 50 cases. J Foot Ankle Surg 2009;48(6):620–30.
58. Cottom JM, Hyer CF, Philbin TM, et al. Treatment of syndesmotic disruptions with the Arthrex TightRope: a report of 25 cases. Foot Ankle Int 2008;29(8):773–80.
59. Butler DL, Grood ES, Noyes FR, et al. Effects of structure and strain measurement technique on the material properties of young human tendons and fascia. J Biomech 1984;17(8):579–96.
60. Komi PV, Fukashiro S, Jarvinen M. Biomechanical loading of Achilles tendon during normal locomotion. Clin Sports Med 1992;11(3):521–31.
61. Wren TA, Yerby SA, Beaupre GS, et al. Mechanical properties of the human Achilles tendon. Clin Biomech (Bristol, Avon) 2001;16(3):245–51.
62. Astrom M, Rausing A. Chronic Achilles tendinopathy. A survey of surgical and histopathologic findings. Clin Orthop Relat Res 1995;316:151–64.

63. Jozsa L, Kannus P. Histopathological findings in spontaneous tendon ruptures. Scand J Med Sci Sports 1997;7(2):113–8.
64. Khan KM, Maffulli N. Tendinopathy: an Achilles' heel for athletes and clinicians. Clin J Sport Med 1998;8(3):151–4.
65. Leadbetter WB. Cell-matrix response in tendon injury. Clin Sports Med 1992; 11(3):533–78.
66. Movin T, Gad A, Reinholt FP, et al. Tendon pathology in long-standing achillodynia. Biopsy findings in 40 patients. Acta Orthop Scand 1997;68(2):170–5.
67. Wilson AM, Goodship AE. Exercise-induced hyperthermia as a possible mechanism for tendon degeneration. J Biomech 1994;27(7):899–905.
68. Kader D, Saxena A, Movin T, et al. Achilles tendinopathy: some aspects of basic science and clinical management. Br J Sports Med 2002;36(4):239–49.
69. Karjalainen PT, Soila K, Aronen HJ, et al. MR imaging of overuse injuries of the Achilles tendon. AJR Am J Roentgenol 2000;175(1):251–60.
70. Schweitzer ME, Karasick D. MR imaging of disorders of the Achilles tendon. AJR Am J Roentgenol 2000;175(3):613–25.
71. Vulpiani MC, Trischitta D, Trovato P, et al. Extracorporeal shockwave therapy (ESWT) in Achilles tendinopathy. A long-term follow-up observational study. J Sports Med Phys Fitness 2009;49(2):171–6.
72. Furia JP. High-energy extracorporeal shock wave therapy as a treatment for chronic noninsertional Achilles tendinopathy. Am J Sports Med 2008;36(3): 502–8.
73. Rasmussen S, Christensen M, Mathiesen I, et al. Shockwave therapy for chronic Achilles tendinopathy: a double-blind, randomized clinical trial of efficacy. Acta Orthop 2008;79(2):249–56.
74. Fridman R, Cain JD, Weil L Jr, et al. Extracorporeal shockwave therapy for the treatment of Achilles tendinopathies: a prospective study. J Am Podiatr Med Assoc 2008;98(6):466–8.
75. Lohrer H, Scholl J, Arentz S. [Achilles tendinopathy and patellar tendinopathy. Results of radial shockwave therapy in patients with unsuccessfully treated tendinoses]. Sportverletz Sportschaden 2002;16(3):108–14 [in German].
76. Alfredson H, Lorentzon R. Chronic Achilles tendinosis: recommendations for treatment and prevention. Sports Med 2000;29(2):135–46.
77. Lyras DN, Kazakos K, Verettas D, et al. The influence of platelet-rich plasma on angiogenesis during the early phase of tendon healing. Foot Ankle Int 2009; 30(11):1101–6.
78. Gaweda K, Tarczynska M, Krzyzanowski W. Treatment of Achilles tendinopathy with platelet-rich plasma. Int J Sports Med 2010;31(8):577–83.
79. de Vos RJ, Weir A, van Schie HT, et al. Platelet-rich plasma injection for chronic Achilles tendinopathy: a randomized controlled trial. JAMA 2010; 303(2):144–9.
80. Dietz U, Horstick G, Manke T, et al. Myocardial angiogenesis resulting in functional communications with the left cavity induced by intramyocardial high-frequency ablation: histomorphology of immediate and long-term effects in pigs. Cardiology 2003;99(1):32–8.
81. Fisher PE, Khomoto T, DeRosa CM, et al. Histologic analysis of transmyocardial channels: comparison of CO_2 and holmium:YAG lasers. Ann Thorac Surg 1997; 64(2):466–72.
82. Kwon HM, Hong BK, Jang GJ, et al. Percutaneous transmyocardial revascularization induces angiogenesis: a histologic and 3-dimensional micro computed tomography study. J Korean Med Sci 1999;14(5):502–10.

83. Tasto JP, Cummings J, Medlock V, et al. The tendon treatment center: new horizons in the treatment of tendinosis. Arthroscopy 2003;19(Suppl 1):213–23.

84. Tasto JP. The role of radiofrequency-based devices in shaping the future of orthopedic surgery. Orthopedics 2006;29(10):874–5.

85. Tasto JP, Cummings J, Medlock V, et al. Microtenotomy using a radiofrequency probe to treat lateral epicondylitis. Arthroscopy 2005;21(7):851–60.

86. Yeap EJ, Chong KW, Yeo W, et al. Radiofrequency coblation for chronic foot and ankle tendinosis. J Orthop Surg (Hong Kong) 2009;17(3):325–30.

87. Liu YJ, Wang ZG, Li ZL, et al. [Arthroscopically assisted radiofrequency probe to treat Achilles tendinitis]. Zhonghua Wai Ke Za Zhi 2008;46(2):101–3 [in Chinese].

88. Benazzo F, Maffulli N. An operative approach to Achilles tendinopathy. Sports Med Arthroscopy Rev 2000;8:96–101.

89. Clancy WG. Runners' injuries. Part two. Evaluation and treatment of specific injuries. Am J Sports Med 1980;8(4):287–9.

90. Clancy WG, Heiden EA. Achilles tendinitis treatment in the athletes. Contemporary approaches to the Achilles tendon. Foot Ankle Clin 1997;2:429–38.

91. Clancy WG Jr, Neidhart D, Brand RL. Achilles tendonitis in runners: a report of five cases. Am J Sports Med 1976;4(2):46–57.

92. Rolf C, Movin T. Etiology, histopathology, and outcome of surgery in achillodynia. Foot Ankle Int 1997;18(9):565–9.

93. Jozsa L, Kvist M, Balint BJ, et al. The role of recreational sport activity in Achilles tendon rupture. A clinical, pathoanatomical, and sociological study of 292 cases. Am J Sports Med 1989;17(3):338–43.

94. Cetti R, Christensen SE, Ejsted R, et al. Operative versus nonoperative treatment of Achilles tendon rupture. A prospective randomized study and review of the literature. Am J Sports Med 1993;21(6):791–9.

95. Clain MR, Baxter DE. Achilles tendinitis. Foot Ankle 1992;13(8):482–7.

96. Aroen A, Helgo D, Granlund OG, et al. Contralateral tendon rupture risk is increased in individuals with a previous Achilles tendon rupture. Scand J Med Sci Sports 2004;14(1):30–3.

97. Kannus P, Jozsa L. Histopathological changes preceding spontaneous rupture of a tendon. A controlled study of 891 patients. J Bone Joint Surg Am 1991; 73(10):1507–25.

98. Krackow KA, Thomas SC, Jones LC. A new stitch for ligament-tendon fixation. Brief note. J Bone Joint Surg Am 1986;68(5):764–6.

99. Botero H, Svoboda S. Comparison of the Krackow locking loop stitch to a novel continuous loop suture technique for fixation of free tendon ends. Fort Sam Houston (TX): U.S. Army Institute of Surgical Research and the Brooke Army Medical Center; 2008.

100. Cook KD, Clark G, Lui E, et al. Strength of braided polyblend polyethylene sutures versus braided polyester sutures in Achilles tendon repair: a cadaveric study. J Am Podiatr Med Assoc 2010;100(3):185–8.

101. Callcut RA, Schurr MJ, Sloan M, et al. Clinical experience with alloderm: a one-staged composite dermal/epidermal replacement utilizing processed cadaver dermis and thin autografts. Burns 2006;32(5):583–8.

102. Rubin L, Schweitzer S. The use of acellular biologic tissue patches in foot and ankle surgery. Clin Podiatr Med Surg 2005;22(4):533–52, vi.

103. Valentin JE, Badylak JS, McCabe GP, et al. Extracellular matrix bioscaffolds for orthopaedic applications. A comparative histologic study. J Bone Joint Surg Am 2006;88(12):2673–86.

104. Snyder SJ, Arnoczky SP, Bond JL, et al. Histologic evaluation of a biopsy specimen obtained 3 months after rotator cuff augmentation with GraftJacket matrix. Arthroscopy 2009;25(3):329–33.
105. Liden BA, Simmons M. Histologic evaluation of a 6-month GraftJacket matrix biopsy used for Achilles tendon augmentation. J Am Podiatr Med Assoc 2009;99(2):104–7.
106. Lee DK. A preliminary study on the effects of acellular tissue graft augmentation in acute Achilles tendon ruptures. J Foot Ankle Surg 2008;47(1):8–12.
107. Lee DK. Achilles tendon repair with acellular tissue graft augmentation in neglected ruptures. J Foot Ankle Surg 2007;46(6):451–5.
108. Barber FA, McGarry JE, Herbert MA, et al. A biomechanical study of Achilles tendon repair augmentation using GraftJacket matrix. Foot Ankle Int 2008; 29(3):329–33.
109. Chen J, Xu J, Wang A, et al. Scaffolds for tendon and ligament repair: review of the efficacy of commercial products. Expert Rev Med Devices 2009;6(1):61–73.
110. Derwin KA, Badylak SF, Steinmann SP, et al. Extracellular matrix scaffold devices for rotator cuff repair. J Shoulder Elbow Surg 2010;19(3):467–76.
111. Derwin KA, Baker AR, Spragg RK, et al. Commercial extracellular matrix scaffolds for rotator cuff tendon repair. Biomechanical, biochemical, and cellular properties. J Bone Joint Surg Am 2006;88(12):2665–72.
112. Sarrafian TL, Wang H, Hackett ES, et al. Comparison of Achilles tendon repair techniques in a sheep model using a cross-linked acellular porcine dermal patch and platelet-rich plasma fibrin matrix for augmentation. J Foot Ankle Surg 2010;49(2):128–34.

Hallux, Sesamoid, and First Metatarsal Injuries

Daniel K. Lee, DPM, PhDc[a],*, Gerit D. Mulder, DPM, MS, PhDc, FRCST[b],
Alexandra K. Schwartz, MD[a]

KEYWORDS

• Hallux • Sesamoids • Metatarsal • Fracture • Turf toe

Hallux, sesamoid and first metatarsal injuries are common foot injuries and have important implications in the biomechanical functionality of the first ray and foot.[1,2] The hallux is essential for propulsion in normal gait. As part of the first ray, it is an important contributor to normal locomotion. Any structure disruption or injury can create angular changes or arthritis, which can have biomechanical implications, including pain, disability, compensation, swelling, and reduced range of motion.[3] In a study reviewing amputation and replantation of the hallux,[4] the pedographic studies revealed consistent changes in weight-bearing distribution of the feet with amputated hallux, altering the load distribution of the foot.

ANATOMY

The anatomy of the hallux is different from that of the lesser digits. Besides the consistent two phalanx composition, its anatomy at the base of the hallux, at the first metatarsophalangeal joint (MTPJ), is unique and complex.[5] Understanding of this anatomy is crucial in the diagnosis and treatment of hallux and sesamoids injuries.[6] The first MTPJ inherent stability comes from the complex network of ligamentous and intrinsic muscular structures extending around the base of the proximal phalanx, the head of the metatarsal, and the sesamoids. The sesamoid complex consists of seven muscles, eight ligaments, and two sesamoid bones.[7] In the plantar aspect of the first MTPJ, there is a fibrocartilaginous structure, the plantar plate, which also provides stability to the MTPJ. This extends plantarly from the base of the proximal phalanx into the head of metatarsal. It encompasses the capsule and the sesamoids as well. Medially and laterally, the corresponding collateral ligaments join this network of

[a] Department of Orthopaedic Surgery, School of Medicine, University of California, 350 Dickinson Street, MC 8894, San Diego, CA 92103–8894, USA
[b] Division of Trauma, Department of Surgery, School of Medicine, University of California, 200 West Arbor Drive, San Diego, CA 92103–8896, USA
* Corresponding author.
E-mail address: dklee@ucsd.edu

Clin Podiatr Med Surg 28 (2011) 43–56
doi:10.1016/j.cpm.2010.09.002   podiatric.theclinics.com
0891-8422/11/$ – see front matter. Published by Elsevier Inc.

soft tissue structures, including the abductor hallucis tendon along its medial side, adductor hallucis (transverse/longitudinal) tendons along its plantar side, and flexor hallucis brevis (medial/lateral) tendons along its plantar side. The morphology of the head of the metatarsal varies from round to square shape. A prominent cristae, ridge or crest divides the sesamoid grooves. Some may have absence of this crest.[8] Both the medial and lateral sesamoids are connected via the intersesamoid ligament. In the first MTPJ radiographic study, bipartite sesamoids occurred in 13.5% of 200 feet with a 37% bilaterality.[9] Congenital absence of sesamoids is rare.[10–13] Sesamoids usually ossify at approximately age 10 and usually the medial one is larger than the lateral. Biomechanically, both function to sustain the body's weight/pressure,[14,15] to act as pulley mechanism to the MTPJ, protecting the tendon of the flexor hallucis longus.

HALLUX FRACTURES

Hallux fractures are common injuries of the forefoot usually caused by direct impact or crushing type of mechanism. Depending on the type of injury severity and location, an associated nail injury may occur and complicate the treatment process of the osseous injury. These are treated as open injuries and may require immediate surgical intervention via irrigation and débridement, infection control, and off-loading. In the presence of a subungual hemotoma, decompression or nail removal may be performed. Normally, nail bed injuries/lacerations can be repaired without further consequences, but if the nail matrix is damaged, an abnormal or absent nail growth can be ensured postinjury.

Hallux fractures can occur to the distal phalanx and proximal phalanx with or without intra-articular involvement into the interphalangeal or MTPJs (**Fig. 1**). A direct axial injury to the tip or tuff of the great toe usually can lead to distal phalanx injury, whereas a crushing type of injury can lead to both proximal and distal phalanges injury (**Fig. 2**). The treatment is based on the severity, displacement, and alignment factors of the fracture. When displaced, manipulation, distraction, and reduction maneuvers under sedation or local anesthesia, with or without finger trap devices, can be performed followed by immobilization and digital splinting. Comminuted and displaced

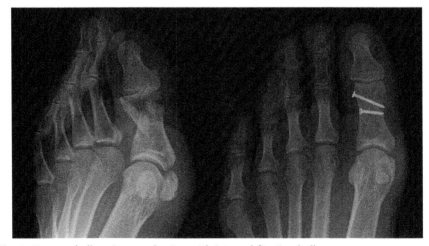

Fig. 1. Fracture hallux. Open reduction with internal fixation hallux.

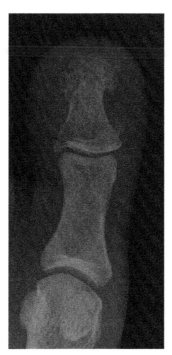

Fig. 2. Distal phalanx fracture, multifragmented.

intra-articular fractures of either phalanx may require surgical fixation. Often, stiffness of the interphalangeal and/or MTPJs remains as residual consequence of the injury.

Stave fractures of the first metatarsal were described by Cooperman. The are equivalent to a Bennett fracture of the thumb metacarpal. These are uncommon injuries. This fracture in the foot occurs from loading of the medial cuneiform into the base of the first metatarsal. The initial report recommended plaster immobilization. Given that this is an intra-articular fracture, however, open reduction with internal fixation is recommended to minimize the risk of post-traumatic arthritis.

TURF TOE INJURIES

Turf toe (TT) injuries are defined as plantar capsular ligament sprain or disruption of the supporting soft tissue structures of the first MTPJ.[9,16,17] The mechanism of injury is usually associated with hyperextension of the MTPJ but can also occur with valgus or varus stress and rarely with hyperflexion (**Fig. 3**).[18–21] With the advent of artificial turf and lighter shoe gear, the incidence of TT in many sports (football, soccer, and dance) and trauma has increased since the late 1960s.[22,23] TT injuries have been reported (eg, soccer, rugby, tennis, track, basketball, wrestling, skydiving, and volleyball).[24]

In a recent National Football League team study, the findings showed that TT injuries are associated with decreased MTPJ motion ($40.6° \pm 15.1°$ vs $48.4° \pm 12.8°$; $P = .04$), increased peak hallucal pressures (535 ± 288 kPa vs 414 ± 202 kPa; $P = .05$), and association of the severity of symptoms or progression to first MTPJ arthritis.[25]

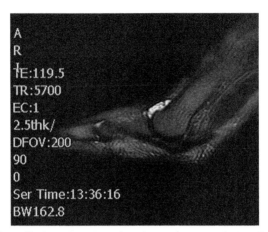

Fig. 3. TT injury, hyperflexion. First MTPJ dorsal capsular tear. T2 MRI view.

Patients often present with acute onset of pain at the first MTP joint. The pain may be somewhat diffuse or more localized. There may be swelling and/or ecchymosis. TT and sesamoids injuries can be unrecognized or undiagnosed. The range of injuries can span from simple sprain/strain/rupture of the plantar structures to dislocation. The more severe injuries may limit athletes' ability to push off, run, and/or pivot. Due to its extensive soft tissue disruption and damage, both TT and sesamoids can lead to chronic disorders, persistent pain, loss of push-off strength, progressive hallux and first MTPJ valgus or varus deformity, and arthritis. The incidence can be as high as 45% of professional football players.[22] Risk factors include advanced age, increased weight, longevity in professional football, pes planus, increased preinjury ankle motion, and decreased preinjury MTPJ range of motion.[22,26]

The treatment options of TT injuries are based on the level of damage/injury incurred, which can range from acute to chronic conditions. A careful and thorough evaluation is essential in maximizing the treatment and successful long-term sequelae. A detailed physical examination of the anatomic structures and advanced imaging studies are essential components of this evaluation. Imaging should include weight-bearing views of the injured foot and comparison films if needed, to assess for possible sesamoid fracture, diastasis of a bipartite sesamoid, and proximal migration of the sesamoid. A lateral stress view of the first MTP joint may identify an occult fracture of the sesamoid or unstable diastasis of a bipartite sesamoid. Capsular avulsion fractures may also be seen. There may be impaction of the metatarsal head with associated intra-articular fragments. Also, when available, continuous live fluoroscopy imaging is useful in visualizing the lack of motion of the sesamoids with ranging of the MTPJ. Using contrast, arthrography can also be performed with a fluoroscopy or plain films. MRI is, however, the most used and provides the highest yield.[27] In most acute cases, capsular disruption can be observed, and in most chronic cases, the associated chronic articular damage and chondrolysis may also be observed.

Initial treatment with anti-inflammatories, rest, ice, compression, elevation, and protection is common in grade 1 injuries with microtears/ruptures. Gentle range of motion can commence less then 1 week post injury. Immobilization and protection consists of digital spica splinting, rocker boot, Morton extension, and modified stiff forefoot sole shoes/orthotics. If the swelling and skin condition allows, taping in the direction opposite to the mechanism of injury can also be useful. Preinjury activities may be returned usually in less then 1 month. In grade 2 injuries with partial soft tissue tears/ruptures, the injury may progress further if not recognized and treated promptly. Pending the level of tear/rupture, MRI findings may or may not reveal fluid uptake or a positive finding. Most injuries can take 1 to 2 months for resuming preinjury activities and a few weeks more for athletic activities. In grade 3 injuries with full tear/ruptures, MRI findings are often positive, and prolonged immobilization and protection are necessary for 3 to 6 months. Preinjury activities are resumed slowly, pending symptoms and physical findings, but athletic activities are not resumed or are carefully performed after many months of recovery. The outcome is not predictive, however, for healing and/or success in the long term; thus, surgical intervention is required.

SESAMOID INJURIES

Hallucal sesamoid injuries have been mainly reported among ballet dancers and in various sports injuries.[28–30] Although the hallux interphalangeal joint may be similar in structure as the other digits, authors have reported specific injuries associated in this location (**Fig. 4**).[31] Sesamoid injuries of the first MTPJ[32] have been described in various forms, including traumatic dislocations,[33–44] TT injuries,[45–47] stress/nonunion fractures/avascular necrosis,[48–51] and open injuries (**Figs. 5** and **6**).[52] Additional symptoms at the first MTPJ can also result from inflammation, chondromalacia, flexor hallucis brevis tendonitis, osteochondritis dissecans, inflamed bursae, intractable keratoses, infection, sesamoiditis, gout arthropathy, and rheumatoid arthritis.[53]

Surgical intervention of TT and sesamoids injuries are indicated once all nonoperative options fail. Recently, the advent of bone stimulation, via pulsed electromagnetic field therapy, has given hope to many patients for salvaging sesamoids from surgical repair attempts or excisions. Most cases seldom require surgery. Medial and lateral

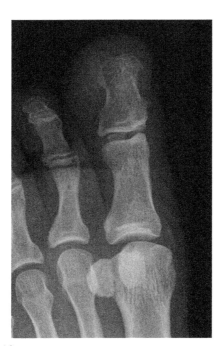

Fig. 4. Hallucal sesamoid.

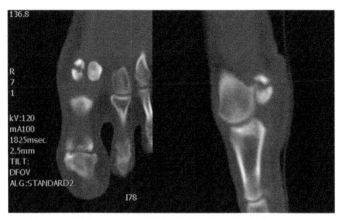

Fig. 5. CT scan of sesamoid fracture, medial, axial and sagittal views.

capsule repair are common in these situations. Proper alignment at the hallux inter-phalangeal joint and MTPJ is crucial for optimal functionality. Articular damage repair and chondroplasty are also performed when indicated. Often, a type of bunionectomy procedure, along with above procedures, is referred. Hallucal or MTPJ sesamoids repair, partial removal, partial resection, or complete removal is also considered in the presence of sesamoids injuries (**Fig. 7**). Adjunctive procedures are also common: abductor/adductor tendon transfer, capsular interposition, osteotomy, and extensor/flexor tendon transfers. It is imperative to discuss the long-term sequelae of these conditions with patients, which may prompt further surgical interventions: sesamoidectomy, hallux interphalangeal joint, and/or first MTPJ arthrodesis, amputation.

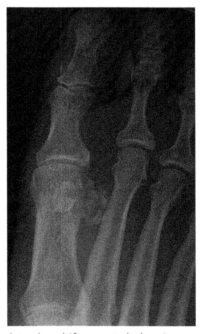

Fig. 6. Sesamoid fracture, lateral, multifragmented, chronic.

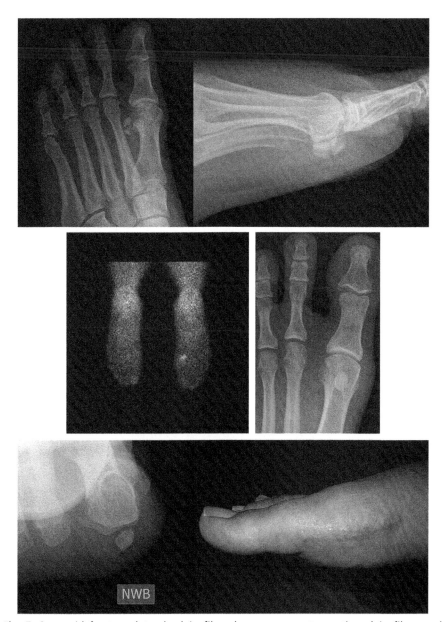

Fig. 7. Sesamoid fracture, lateral, plain films, bone scan, postoperative plain films, and clinical incisional approach.

METATARSAL FRACTURES

Because of the importance of the first metatarsal in the biomechanics of gait and foot function, malreductions of this bone are generally tolerated less than other metatarsals. The first metatarsal is wider, shorter, stronger, and more mobile than the remaining metatarsals. Most of these fractures are due to a direct blow, crush, axial load, or, less often, a twisting mechanism. Due to the frequent direct injury mechanism, it is important to rule out open fractures. Patients present with pain, dorsal swelling, ecchymosis, and, most often, inability to walk. The skin should be carefully evaluated to rule out an open fracture. There is point tenderness over the fracture. Alignment may be abnormal in terms of length and rotation. Initial radiographs should include antero-posterior, oblique, and lateral views of the foot. In cases of suspicion of more severe injuries, for instance, a Lisfranc injury, stress views or weight-bearing views are help-ful. CT scan is not often indicated, except for possible intra-articular fracture assess-ment, including those with impaction. Nonoperative treatment with a short leg cast or removable boot is indicated for nondisplaced, simple fracture patterns without asso-ciated injury. Frequent radiographs should be obtained in the first several weeks to ensure no displacement occurs. Operative treatment is indicated for open fractures, fractures associated with skin tenting, shortened fractures, unstable fracture patterns, intra-articular fractures, or fractures with greater than 10° of plantar angulation.[54] Operative treatment consists of open reduction and stable internal fixation, most often with minifragmentary or small fragmentary screws and/or plates. Low profile plates are helpful to avoid tendon irritation (**Figs. 8–10**).

Stress fractures of the first metatarsal have been reported. The second and third metatarsals are the most common sites of metatarsal stress fractures, but the first metatarsal accounts for approximately 7% to 8% of metatarsal stress fractures.[55] These are injuries as a result of overuse and repetitive injury. They are commonly seen in military recruits, dancers, and runners. Excessive pronation, lower-extremity malalignment, and leg length discrepancy may predispose to first metatarsal stress fractures. Pain occurs with weight bearing and subsides with rest. Initial radiographs may be negative. After 2 to 3 weeks, there may be radiographic evidence of healing and callus formation. An MRI or bone scan is the definitive study if initial radiographs

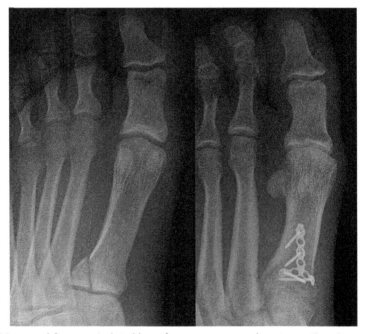

Fig. 8. Metatarsal fracture: isolated base fracture, preop and postoperative views.

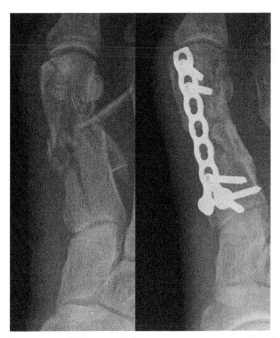

Fig. 9. Metatarsal fracture: multifragmented, preop and postoperative views.

are normal and there is a high suspicion. Treatment is immobilization and nonweight-bearing for 6 to 8 weeks. Patients may then begin low-impact activity but should refrain from any sports until they have has regained pain-free ambulation and full range of motion, strength, and proprioception.

WOUNDS AND LACERATIONS

One of the most common sites of ulceration and laceration on the foot is the hallux. As the largest and perhaps the most biomechanically important of the digits of the foot, the hallux is subject to varying injuries, including ulceration from pressure, lacerations from trauma, and nail-related injuries and/or complications.

Loss of the hallux at the level of the MTPJ may affect propulsion, balance, and weight redistribution, thereby contributing to transfer and other lesions of the foot. A variety of deformities result in the digit becoming more susceptible to tissue breakdown. Ambulation on a severely plantarflexed hallux may result in a distal tip or distal plantar lesion. Shoe modification or specialized walkers provide minimal pressure relief, particularly when a rigid deformity is present. Off-loading through the use of crutches or a wheelchair is impractical. Contact casting may have little to no effect on such a deformity. These types of wounds are best addressed through surgical selection with flexible deformities corrected through tendon releases and rigid deformities modified through bone excision or positional modification. Once the pressure has been relieved, wounds respond, in the absence of infection, to most topical dressings without the need for advanced therapies. Even after addressing the underlying anatomy and physiology, selection of appropriate shoe-gear is imperative.

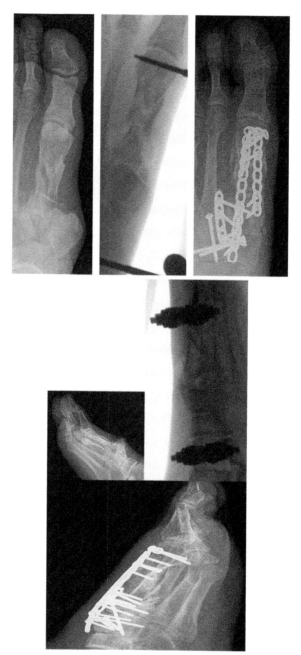

Fig. 10. Tarsometatarsal fracture/dislocation: preoperative, intraoperative, and postoperative views.

Hallux deviation, when present with hallux valgus or other MTPJ anomalies, is a significant contributor to medial and distal hallux ulcer development. In scenarios where the metatarsal is involved, the clinician must determine the relevant biomechanical forces and type of anatomic abnormality before attempting to correct the problem.

Surgical intervention, when not contraindicated, provides the most rapid means of correcting and permanently addressing the problem. Splints and positional devices are only temporary measures and may be rendered ineffective unless a patient is wearing the device at all times. Wounds occurring at the medial MTPJ are commonly found in the presence of hallux valgus deformities. Determining the depth of the wound and involvement of underlying structures assists with dressing selection. When tendon or bone involvement is present, osteomyelitis must be ruled out. Amputation of the hallux may be necessary yet may not significantly affect gate if the metatarsal head is left intact.

The nail and nail bed may become ingrown and infected as a result of poor nail care and/or poorly fitted shoes. When ingrown, the nail border should be excised down to the level of the matrix. A matrixectomy may be considered for recurrent ingrowth of the nail. Determining adequate vascular flow to the digit as well as a patient's medical status and ability to heal must be established before nail removal. Patients should be forewarned of the high risk of amputation in cases where re-establishing the blood flow is not an option. Amputation should be limited to the hallux whenever the metatarsal is not involved.

Trauma to the hallux may result in deep tissue damage, infection, and fractures. Standard radiographs are recommended during the initial examination with possible MRI or labeled white blood cell scan radiography when osteomyelitis is suspected. Fractures of the hallux, when nondisplaced, heal well with splinting. Major displacement may require surgical intervention. When the joint capsule has been compromised, surgical intervention is usually the only treatment option.

SUMMARY

In summary, the hallux is a source of many injuries. Hallux fractures, TT injuries, and sesamoid injuries are common yet challenging because of the myriad possible etiologies and complex anatomy. Unstable, displaced, open, and intra-articular fractures of the first metatarsal should be treated operatively, most often with open reduction and internal fixation to restore proper anatomy and function. A high suspicion should be had for athletes with first metatarsal pain to rule out stress fracture. An MRI or bone scan is diagnostic if plain radiographs are negative. A few of the causes of wounds and lacerations have been discussed; however, clinicians must develop a comprehensive differential diagnosis that may include other lesions, including, but not limited to, melanoma of the skin (and occasionally below the nail bed), tinea, skin carcinomas, hyperkeratosis diseases, and other dermatologic conditions. Biopsies should also be considered when lesions do not respond to traditional approaches to care, in the presence of abnormal tissue, or when wounds have been open for greater than 3 months without response to appropriate care. As discussed previously, a thorough examination and evaluation and advanced imaging techniques are essential. When nonoperative measures fail, surgical interventions are indicated. When addressing athletes, the return to nonathletic and athletic activities needs to be discussed and custom tailored based on the sports and/or condition of the athlete, due to the possible long-term sequelae associated with these conditions.

REFERENCES

1. Perlman MD. Fractures of the proximal phalanx of the hallux: the use of plates with displaced multifragment fractures. J Foot Surg 1992;31(3):260–7.
2. Mittlmeier T, Haar P. Sesamoid and toe fractures. Injury 2004;35(Suppl 2): SB87–97.

3. Christensen JC, Jennings MM. Normal and abnormal function of the first ray. Clin Podiatr Med Surg 2009;26(3):355–71.

4. Ademoğlu Y, Ada S, Kaplan I. Should the amputations of the great toe be replanted? Foot Ankle Int 2000;21(8):673–9.

5. Sarrafian SK. Anatomy of the Foot and Ankle: descriptive, topographic, functional. 2nd edition. Philadelphia (PA): Lippincott Williams & Wilkins; 1993.

6. Oloff LM, Schulhofer SD. Sesamoid complex disorders. Clin Podiatr Med Surg 1996;13(3):497–513.

7. Alvarez R, Haddad RJ, Gould N, et al. The simple bunion: anatomy at the metatarsophalangeal joint of the great toe. Foot Ankle 1984;4(5):229–40.

8. Brenner E, Gruber H, Fritsch H. Fetal development of the first metatarsophalangeal joint complex with special reference to the intersesamoidal ridge. Ann Anat 2002;184(5):481–7.

9. Prieskorn D, Graves SC, Smith RA. Morphometric analysis of the plantar plate apparatus of the first metatarsophalangeal joint. Foot Ankle 1993;14(4):204–7.

10. Kanatli U, Ozturk AM, Ercan NG, et al. Absence of the medial sesamoid bone associated with metatarsophalangeal pain. Clin Anat 2006;19(7):634–9.

11. Le Minor JM. Congenital absence of the lateral metatarso-phalangeal sesamoid bone of the human hallux: a case report. Surg Radiol Anat 1999;21:225–7.

12. Leventen EO. Sesamoid disorders and treatment. An update. Clin Orthop Relat Res 1991;269:236–40.

13. Hubay CA. Sesamoid bones of the hands and feet. Am J Roentgenol 1949;61:493–505.

14. Stokes IA, Hutton WC, Stott JR, et al. Forces under the hallux valgus foot before and after surgery. Clin Orthop Relat Res 1979;142:64–72.

15. Nigg BM. Biomechanical aspects of running. In: Nigg BM, editor. Biomechanics of running shoes. Champaign (IL): Human Kinetics Publishers; 1986. p. 1–25.

16. Bowers KD Jr, Martin RB. Turf-toe: a shoe-surface related football injury. Med Sci Sports 1976;8(2):81–3.

17. Tewes DP, Fischer DA, Fritts HM, et al. MRI findings of acute turf toe. Clin Orthop Relat Res 1994;304:200–3.

18. Coker TP, Arnold JA, Weber DL. Traumatic lesions of the metatarsophalangeal joint of the great toe in athletes. J Ark Med Soc 1978;74(8):309–17.

19. Clanton TO, Butler JE, Eggert A. Injuries to the metatarsophalangeal joints in athletes. Foot Ankle 1986;7(3):162–76.

20. Watson TS, Anderson RB, Davis WH. Periarticular injuries to the hallux metatarsophalangeal joint in athletes. Foot Ankle Clin 2000;5(3):687–713.

21. Douglas DP, Davidson DM, Robinson JE, et al. Rupture of the medial collateral ligament of the first metatarsophalangeal joint in a professional soccer player. J Foot Ankle Surg 1997;36(5):388–90.

22. Rodeo SA, O'Brien S, Warren RF, et al. Turf-toe: an analysis of metatarsophalangeal joint sprains in professional football players. Am J Sports Med 1990;18(3):280–5.

23. Allen LR, Flemming D, Sanders TG. Turf toe: ligamentous injury of the first metatarsophalangeal joint. Mil Med 2004;169(11):xix–xxiv.

24. Coughlin M. Med Chir Pied 2005;21:65–72.

25. Brophy RH, Gamradt SC, Ellis SJ, et al. Effect of turf toe on foot contact pressures in professional American football players. Foot Ankle Int 2009;30(5):405–9.

26. Clanton TO, Ford JJ. Turf toe injury. Clin Sports Med 1994;13(4):731–41.

27. Tewes DP, Fischer DA, Fritts HM, et al. MRI findings of acute turf toe. A case report and review of anatomy. Clin Orthop Relat Res 1994;304:200–3.

28. Burton EM, Amaker BH. Stress fracture of the great toe sesamoid in a ballerina: MRI appearance. Pediatr Radiol 1994;24:37–8.
29. Lo SL, Zoga AC, Elias I, et al. Stress fracture of the distal phalanx of the great toe in a professional ballet dancer: a case report. Am J Sports Med 2007;35(9):1564–6.
30. Khan K, Brown J, Way S, et al. Overuse injuries in classical ballet. Sports Med 1995;19(5):341–57.
31. Gong HS, Kim YH, Park MS. Varus instability of the hallux interphalangeal joint in a taekwondo athlete. Br J Sports Med 2007;41(12):917–9.
32. Vanore JV, Christensen JC, Kravitz SR, et al, Clinical Practice Guideline First Metatarsal Joint Disorders Panel of the American College of Foot and Ankle Surgeons. Diagnosis and treatment of first metatarsophalangeal joint disorders. Section 4: sesamoid disorders. J Foot Ankle Surg 2003;42(3):143–7.
33. Tosun B, Akansel G, Sarlak AY. Traumatic dislocation of the first metatarsophalangeal joint with entrapment of the flexor hallucis longus tendon. J Foot Ankle Surg 2008;47(4):357–61.
34. Maskill M, Mendicino R, Saltrick K, et al. Traumatic dislocation of the first metatarsophalangeal joint with tibial sesamoid fracture: a case report of a type III B dislocation. J Am Podiatr Med Assoc 2008;98(2):149–52.
35. Isefuku S, Hatori M, Kurata Y. Traumatic dislocation of the first metatarsophalangeal joint with tibial sesamoid fracture: a case report. Foot Ankle Int 2004;25(9):674–9.
36. Ozkoç G, Hersekli MA, Akpinar S, et al. Iatrogenic medial dislocation of hallucal sesamoids with hallux varus in an adolescent. Arch Orthop Trauma Surg 2004;124(8):568–70.
37. Ando Y, Yasuda M, Okuda H, et al. Irreducible dorsal subluxation of the first metatarsophalangeal joint: a case report. J Orthop Trauma 2002;16(2):134–6.
38. Good JJ, Weinfeld GD, Yu GV. Fracture-dislocation of the first metatarsophalangeal joint: open reduction through a medial incisional approach. J Foot Ankle Surg 2001;40(5):311–7.
39. Hussain A. Dislocation of the first metatarsophalangeal joint with fracture of fibular sesamoid. A case report. Clin Orthop Relat Res 1999;359:209–12.
40. Massari L, Ventre T, Iirillo A. Atypical medial dislocation of the first metatarsophalangeal joint. Foot Ankle Int 1998;19(9):624–6.
41. Iian FJ, Carpenter BB, Mostone E. Dorsal dislocation of the first metatarsophalangeal joint. J Foot Ankle Surg 1997;36(2):131–5.
42. Brunet JA. Pathomechanics of complex dislocations of the first metatarsophalangeal joint. Clin Orthop Relat Res 1996;332:126–31.
43. Garcia Mata S, Hidalgo A, Martinez Grande M. Dorsal dislocation of the first metatarsophalangeal joint. Int Orthop 1994;18(4):236–9.
44. Jahss MH. Traumatic dislocations of the first metatarsophalangeal joint. Foot Ankle 1980;1(1):15–21.
45. Rodeo SA, Warren RF, O'Brien SJ, et al. Diastasis of bipartite sesamoids of the first metatarsophalangeal joint. Foot Ankle 1993;14(8):425–34.
46. Hall RL, Saxby T, Vandemark RM. A new type of dislocation of the first metatarsophalangeal joint: a case report. Foot Ankle 1992;13(9):540–5.
47. Graves SC, Prieskorn D, Mann RA. Posttraumatic proximal migration of the first metatarsophalangeal joint sesamoids: a report of four cases. Foot Ankle 1991;12(2):117–22.
48. Hulkko A, Orava S, Pellinen P, et al. Stress fractures of the sesamoid bones of the first metatarsophalangeal joint in athletes. Arch Orthop Trauma Surg 1985;104(2):113–7.

49. Saxena A, Krisdakumtorn T. Return to activity after sesamoidectomy in athletically active individuals. Foot Ankle Int 2003;24(5):415–9.
50. Biedert R, Hintermann B. Stress fractures of the medial great toe sesamoids in athletes. Foot Ankle Int 2003;24:137–41.
51. Karasick D, Schweitzer ME. Disorders of the hallux sesamoid complex: MR features. Skeletal Radiol 1998;27(8):411–8.
52. Van Pelt M, Brown D, Doyle J, et al. First metatarsophalangeal joint dislocation with open fracture of tibial and fibular sesamoids. J Foot Ankle Surg 2007; 46(2):124–9.
53. Richardson EG. Hallucal sesamoid pain: causes and surgical treatment. J Am Acad Orthop Surg 1999;7:270–8.
54. Greene WB. Essentials of musculoskeletal care. 2nd edition. Rosemont (IL): AAOS; 2001. 453–5.
55. Levy JM. Stress fractures of the first metatarsal. AJR Am J Roentgenol 1978;130: 679–81.

Plantar Plate Tears: A Review of the Modified Flexor Tendon Transfer Repair for Stabilization

Bob Baravarian, DPM[a,b,c,*], Jonathan Thompson, DPM[c,d],
Doron Nazarian, DPM[c]

KEYWORDS

- Plantar plate tear • Metatarsal-phalangeal joints • Forefoot
- Flexor tendon • Dislocation toe • Flexor tendon transfer
- Girdlestone procedure • Hammertoe

Forefoot pain is one of the most common presenting problems in a foot and ankle practice. One of the most common presenting problems, yet most commonly missed problems, is a plantar plate tear. Often the problem is considered to be potential neuroma, fat pad atrophy, or a generalized diagnosis of metatarsalgia or metatarsal head overload. Unfortunately, not enough attention is placed on the plantar and medial/lateral ligamentous structures of the metatarsal-phalangeal joints (MPJ). This lack of attention results in poor diagnosis, lack of care, treatment for the wrong condition, and ultimate frustration for the patients and doctor.

ANATOMY OF THE PLANTAR PLATE AND CAUSE OF INJURY

The plantar plate is a thick, rectangular to trapezoidal structure mostly made up of collagen type I that proximally attaches just distal to the metatarsal flare and distally attaches to the plantar surface of the proximal phalanx, which turns out to be the stronger of the two attachments.[1–3] It gets thicker and broader under the metatarsal head as it provides attachments for collateral ligaments, deep transverse metatarsal

[a] Santa Monica/UCLA and Orthopedic Hospital, 1250 Sixteenth Street, Santa Monica, CA, USA
[b] David Geffen UCLA School of Medicine, CA, USA
[c] University Foot and Ankle Institute, CA, USA
[d] VA Medical Center, West Los Angeles, Los Angeles, CA, USA
* Corresponding author. Santa Monica/UCLA and Orthopedic Hospital, 1250 Sixteenth Street, Santa Monica, CA.
E-mail address: BBaravarian@mednet.ucla.edu

Clin Podiatr Med Surg 28 (2011) 57–68
doi:10.1016/j.cpm.2010.11.002
0891-8422/11/$ – see front matter © 2011 Published by Elsevier Inc.

ligaments, intraosseous tendons, and the fibers from the plantar aponeurosis. It provides a smooth gliding surface for the metatarsal head and flexor tendons. Accordingly, it is one of the primary stabilizers of the MPJs[1] and also plays an important role in the windlass mechanism.[4,5] The plantar plate is therefore the most important stabilizer to prevent hyperextension at the MPJ with its ligamentous and muscle-tendinous attachments.[1,2,4,6]

Although the actual cause of plantar plate injury may be from multiple reasons, the most common causes are associated with chronic repetitive mild overload or acute traumatic overload. Deland and colleagues performed cadaveric studies and determined that transverse deviation or crossover toes were associated with an abnormal position of the long and short flexor tendons on the involved foot versus central position of the flexor tendons in the uninvolved foot.[5,7] Although any MPJ can be injured, the most common injury is associated with the second MPJ. The frequency of second MPJ plantar plate injury may be caused by inflammation and pain from overload secondary to first ray hypermobility and hallux abducto valgus causing overload of the second MPJ. A long second metatarsal, short first metatarsal, forefoot varus, forefoot overload secondary to equinus deformity, neuromuscular imbalance, and systemic or inflammatory arthritidies have also been common sources for plantar plate injury. Although all of the previously mentioned sources have been found by the authors, it is still unclear why the problem occurs in some patients and not others with similar conditional findings.

PATIENT WORKUP

Subsecond metatarsal pain can be difficult to diagnose. Common findings that must be ruled out include capsulitis, synovitis, lesser metatarsal stress fracture, Freiberg's infarction, second interspace neuromas, inflammatory arthropathy, degenerative joint disease, or simple joint overload. Commonly, patients will present with a generalized forefoot swelling and most local pain in the associated joint. If the treating physician is not careful, they may confuse the pain in the MPJ with interspace pain. In the second MPJ, the pain is most commonly plantar and lateral, which can easily be confused with a neuroma. There may be an associated hammertoe deformity that is caused by the weakness of the plantar ligamentous structures resulting in a flexor and extensor imbalance. It is essential to not get confused with the cause of MPJ pain being from the hammertoe contracture as missing the plantar plate tear and just correcting the hammertoe is destined for failure. A keratotic lesion under the associated metatarsal is rare in plantar plate tear cases and is more commonly associated with a hammertoe contracture that is causing symptomatic retrograde metatarsal head pressure. Probing patients for type of pain and associated timing of pain is critical for differential. Most patients with plantar plate pain do not complain of sharp shooting or tingling pain. The pain is commonly a dull ache with ambulation, chronic in nature, and better with a stiff shoe and cushioning. Patients will also suggest that the pain is fairly consistent and not different with differing activity. As the plantar plate tear advances, patients will suggest a medial shift in their toe position and gapping from the lateral toes. This finding is most common on the second toe, which moves medial and dorsal toward the great toe (**Fig. 1**).

Clinically you can evaluate second MPJ sagittal plane instability with the modified Lachman test, or the anterior/dorsal drawer test, originally described by Thompson and Hamilton and Thompson and Deland (**Fig. 2**).[8–10] Although difficult to judge, a noted sign of plantar plate tear in the literature has been a dorsal drawer of more than 2 mm or 50% or greater dorsal displacement.[4,11] It should be noted that false positives can result in patients with ligamentous laxity. Another widely accepted

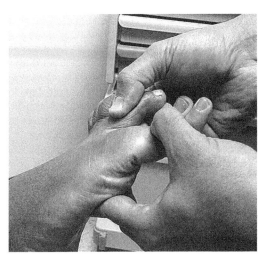

Fig. 1. Dorsal drawer test of the second MPJ. With dorsal pull of the toe, there is pain in the plantar capsule and laxity of the associated toe is noted.

maneuver evaluating the integrity of the MPJ is the Kelikian push-up test that evaluates the relative reducibility of the deformity by pushing or loading the plantar metatarsal head to see if the toe will reduce or straighten out. In cases of a normal to slight hammertoe deformity with a torn, plantar plate, there is medial deviation of the toe with a Kelikian push-up test. Patients will also complain of pain with plantar pressure on the region of plantar plate tear.

Radiographs are important to rule out other osseous etiologies, such as acute fractures, stress fractures, Friedberg's infarction, arthritic changes, appropriate evaluation

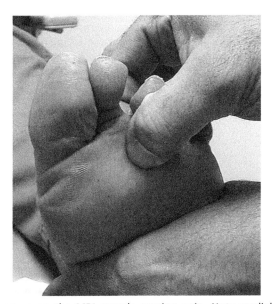

Fig. 2. Plantar pressure on the MPJ capsule causing pain. Note medial shift of the toe commonly associated with lateral plantar plate and ligament tear.

of the metatarsal parabola, and overall MPJ alignment. Furthermore, a combination of mostly plantar soft-tissue pain, with possible instability on physical examination, and radiographs negative for gross osseous pathology can be sufficient for plantar plate injuries. However, further imaging studies can help confirm diagnosis and also rule out other etiologies. The two most common imaging studies are arthrography and MRI (**Fig. 3**). Because the plantar plate is continuous with the flexor sheath, some investigators considered arthrography as the gold standard and diagnosis is confirmed with extravasation of the dye from the joint into flexor sheath.[4]

A study by Yao and collogues[1] in 1996 demonstrated that all 5 subjects diagnosed with plantar plate tears by MRI were confirmed by intraoperative findings. They diagnosed plantar plate tears that demonstrated "increased signal intensity in the plantar plate that extended beyond the immediate area of plantar attachment on the proximal phalangeal base...on the gradient-recalled images."[1]

The use of ultrasound can also aid in the diagnosis, but the availability and user dependence can make the procedure difficult. One advantage of ultrasound is that it can a dynamic and the operator can move the toe, as well as compare with other toe plantar plates for difference.[12] An abnormal plantar plate demonstrates a loss of homogenicity with focal areas of hypoechoic defects.

Conservative Measures

Each practitioner will try different conservative modalities but should attempt a variety of conservative measures before surgical procedures. Common conservative treatments include but are not limited to the following: shoe gear modification, accommodative or functional orthotics with appropriate metatarsal pad or metatarsal head cut, soft insoles, elimination of high-heeled shoes and sandals, activity modifications, taping and strapping of toe, ice, physical therapy with antiinflammatory modalities, oral nonsteroidal antiinflammatory drugs (NSAIDS) or steroids, and possibly steroid injections. If conservative measures fail to relieve symptoms, then there has been a variety of surgical procedures described in the literature.

What the authors have found to work on a conservative basis includes a stiff-soled rocker-sole shoe that decreases the roll-off phase of push off. Taping the toe in a plantar position has also been found to decrease dorsal movement of the toe and relieve pressure on the plantar metatarsal head. Orthotic use can be an excellent

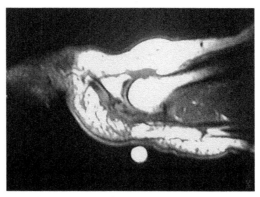

Fig. 3. MRI of MPJ joint showing tear of the plantar plate off the base of the proximal phalanx.

source of pain relief and also may be used after surgical care to control pressure distribution. In most cases, a metatarsal head cutout is performed. The second metatarsal head is the most commonly affected and therefore a second metatarsal head cutout is the most commonly performed. If the second metatarsal head is affected because of hypermobility of the first ray or hallux valgus deformity, a stiff extension under the first ray to the distal toe is used to improve pressure distribution under the first metatarsal area. A metatarsal pad can also be used to relieve generalized forefoot pressure and move some of the weight to the mid metatarsal area. If high heels are necessary in the patients' lifestyle, it is recommended that they wear a wedge-type shoe that has a stiff sole and thick forefoot. This type of shoe decreases forefoot pressure and also decreases the heel height as the forefoot also has height. Physical therapy and NSAIDS can be useful to calm the inflammation, but control of MPJ overload is the critical portion of conservative measures.

Of interest is the idea of the potential use of materials, such as platelet rich plasma (PRP) and short-term cast immobilization, to decrease stress on the MPJ and increase local inflammation in an attempt to allow the ligament to heal. This method has been attempted at the authors' institute several times on older patients with little high-stress use on the MPJ region with moderate relief. Combined with orthotic use, these patients have been able to perform their normal life activity with little to no pain. To date, the authors have not tried PRP therapy of plantar plate tears in active patients. In cases that do not improve with conservative care, surgical reconstruction is attempted.

DISCUSSION

It is important to understand the underlying causes of plantar plate injury when dealing with any deformity to address the primary and secondary deforming forces. This article focuses on repair of an isolated pathology of plantar plate injury and toe deformity. Accordingly, if there are concomitant pathologies, such as severe hallux valgus, laxity at the metatarsocuneiform joint causing abnormal peak pressures of lesser MPJs, or equinus deformity, they must be addressed conservatively or surgically to prevent recurrence.

There have been a variety of ways to surgically correct the deformity presented in the literature and are briefly described. In 1938 Lambrunidi advocated straightening the toe by performing a proximal interphalangeal (IPJ) arthrodesis to allow the long flexors to only act at the MPJ.[13] Over time, a flexor-to-extensor transfer procedure was added to secondarily stabilize the torn plantar plate and associated MPJ. Flexor tendon transfers were first described in the literature in 1947 by Girdlestone in which he transferred the long and short flexor tendons into dorsal expansions of extensor tendons for claw-toe deformities.[14] The objective of this procedure was twofold: (1) to allow the long flexors to substitute for intrinsic muscle weakness by providing plantar-flexion of the toes at the MPJ, and (2) to release the plantar contracture at the distal toe allowing extension of the toes at the IPJs. This finding was also supported by Taylor[15] in 1951 when he evaluated the benefit of transferring the flexor tendon into the extensor tendons as well as extensor digitorum longus lengthening and dorsal capsulotomies at the MPJ, and plantar capsulotomies at the IPJs in the treatment of claw toes. Taylor[15] described that with toe deformity/contracture, the intrinsic muscles lost the function of flexing the toes at the MPJ level and now the forces were increased at the plantar metatarsal heads. Furthermore, he found that the integrity of the intrinsic muscles were mostly found to be intact and have normal-appearing anatomy.

In 1951, Pyper[16] did a follow-up study and compared the Lambrunidi and Taylor procedures and found only subtle differences between the two procedures. In 1973 Parrish described flexor tendon transfer for the reducible claw-toe deformity by harvesting the long flexor tendon that was split longitudinally at the level of the MPJ and then the each half of the tendon is wrapped around the midportion of the proximal phalanx and the ends are sutured together underneath the extensor tendons. Parrish[17] found good-to-excellent results in 20 out of 23 subjects. In 1980, Kuwada and Dockery[18] described a modification to eliminate the MPJ and IPJ capsulotomies procedures in which they transferred the long flexor tendon to the dorsal side at the anatomic neck of the proximal phalanx through a drill hole and sutured into the dorsal capsule and soft tissue. In 1984, Barbari and Brevig,[19] reevaluated the success of the flexor-extensor transfer procedure for claw-toe deformities, in which they harvested the long flexor tendon and then sutured it end-to-side to the extensor tendon. They found good-to-excellent outcomes with the procedure. Ross and Faux[8] described good-to-excellent results in 96% of subjects undergoing a dorsal approach using a combined long extensor Z lengthening, proximal phalanx arthroplasty, and a long flexor tendon transfer.

One of the main problems with these procedures is the well-known and accepted postoperative stiffness. In 1993, Thompson and Deland evaluated this and found that no subject that could perform at least 20° of dorsiflexion experienced postoperative stiffness. They emphasized removal of the stabilizing k-wire at about 2 to 3 weeks and encouraged toe range of motion equal to adjacent toes.[10]

A cadaveric study by Ford and colleagues[20] in 1998 demonstrated that primary anatomic direct repair of plantar plate is as viable as flexor tendon transfer for transected plantar plate. Some investigators advocate that only isolated plantar plate repairs are indicated for reducible MPJ contractures, and that only nonreducible deformities require additional procedures.

In 2005, Shurnas and Sanders[2] described a combination of procedures, including oblique osteotomy of metatarsal, extensor lengthening with hammer toe repair, as well as flexor tendon transfer to the dorsal aspect of proximal phalanx fixated with a bio-tenodesis screw. They found excellent outcomes and minimal stiffness associated with this combination of procedures.

UNIVERSITY FOOT AND ANKLE INSTITUTE SURGICAL PROCEDURE SELECTION AND OUTCOMES

Plantar plate treatments have become one of the most presenting problems in the authors' institutes. The authors have performed several hundred cases of plantar plate tear and noted that each case is different and requires different treatments. In general, the factors causing pain may differ and all of the factors must be considered for an excellent outcome. As noted earlier, hallux valgus problems, equinus and secondary causes of pain must be addressed and treated but will not be further discussed in this article. This article concentrates on the plantar plate tear and associated ray in explaining the authors' surgical techniques.

The first problem to consider is whether there is a hammertoe associated with the deformity. If there is a hammertoe, the type of plantar plate transfer differs. If we perform a hammertoe correction, we will attempt a proximal IPJ fusion with a cup and cone technique. We will try to remove minimal bone from the proximal IPJ region to avoid shortening of the toe and allow better bone contact for the IPJ fusion. The type of tendon transfer performed in association with a hammertoe correction is a split flexor to extensor transfer around the base of the proximal phalanx and k-wire fixation of the fusion and MPJ joint. If there is minimal hammertoe deformity, patients are given the option of if they would like the toe corrected and if the toe bothers them in shoes. If no hammertoe is associated with the plantar plate tear, the flexor-to-extensor transfer is performed with an interference-screw technique through the proximal phalanx base. In such a case, a dorsal-MPJ incision is made extending to the dorsal base of the proximal phalanx. The long flexor tendon is harvested through a small plantar incision at the distal IPJ. The tendon is then passed through a drill hole from plantar to dorsal in the proximal phalanx base with the use of a suture passer and tensioned. Once proper toe position and flexor tension is achieved, an interference screw is used to stabilize the transferred tendon. In both cases, the dorsally transferred tendon can be used to tie into the lateral ligamentous structures to perform a plication of the loose ligaments resulting in medial deviation of the toe. Primary repair of the plantar plate is not performed at the authors' institute and has been noted to not stand up over time and to be difficult to perform when cadaveric studies have been attempted by the surgeons at the authors' institute. However, the MPJ joint is opened and the plantar plate is inspected. If the tear is visible, which is common, a Topaz probe is used to fenestrate the plantar plate in an attempt to stimulate scar formation and added stability during the recovery period.

Ligament plication techniques of the lateral collaterals have also proven to be helpful for toe positioning. This technique is either performed by a pants-over-vest plication with nonabsorbable suture or with an anchor. The decision of suture versus anchor is made based on whether the soft tissue is torn off bone or centrally. If there is adequate soft tissue for pants-over-vest plication, an anchor is not deemed necessary. If the soft tissue is torn off bone, a small anchor is used to pull the soft tissue back to bone with a nonabsorbable suture.

The final consideration of surgery is whether or not to perform a metatarsal head shortening. This procedure may be simple and the idea of decreasing pressure on the second metatarsal head seems legitimate, but care must be taken to avoid shortening the ray and causing transfer lesions or pain. The decision is based on whether there is overload of the ray from a primary or secondary cause. For example, if there is a hallux valgus deformity causing second metatarsal overload, the hallux valgus deformity is corrected and then second metatarsal length is checked. We will not correct the second ray length without correct the hallux valgus deformity, which is considered the primary source of overload. That said, there is commonly a problem with a long metatarsal associated with plantar plate injury and shortening may be necessary. The second metatarsal is the most commonly affected ray and is shortened, leaving it just slightly longer than the third metatarsal. Overshortening of the second metatarsal will cause continued forefoot pain and transfer metatarsalgia under the surrounding metatarsals. The preferred type of metatarsal osteotomy we prefer to perform is a Weil-type osteotomy. This osteotomy allows for proper control of metatarsal shortening and length and is adjustable for proper positioning during surgery and is also simple and stable to fixate. For example, the metatarsal length is checked under fluoroscopy and can be adjusted to the desired position and readjusted as necessary before permanent fixation. The metatarsal can also be translated medially to move the phalanx laterally if there is a medial deviation of the ray. A metatarsal osteotomy is performed before flexor tendon transfer to avoid a slack tendon transfer (**Figs. 4–7**).

Once correction is achieved, patients are placed in a protective postoperative boot and heel weight is allowed. If a k-wire is not used and hammertoe correction is not necessary, the toe is splinted in a plantar position with the dressings to avoid dorsal stress and potential flexor tendon pullout. Pullout of the flexor tendon has not been seen with

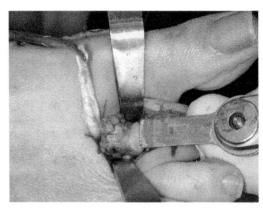

Fig. 4. Angle for proper Weil osteotomy. Note the need to skive the dorsal articular surface to shorten the metatarsal with minimal plantar flexion.

interference-screw fixation. The k-wire is left intact for 6 weeks and then pulled. We have not found stiffness of the metatarsal to be a common complaint and think it is essential to avoid overtightening of the flexor tendon transfer to avoid MPJ stiffness. If no k-wire is used, therapy is started at 4 weeks with passive range of motion and toe strengthening. If a k-wire is used, patients are referred to therapy after wire removal.

It is critical to use therapy to strengthen the transferred tendon and get the surgical toe to purchase the ground. Patients not treated with home therapy or physical therapy often end up with toe purchase weakness, which is a common source of complaint. Range of motion of the MPJ is also performed in therapy as is gait work to avoid abnormal ambulation patterns after surgery.

Our outcomes with this combination of surgical procedures have been excellent. The rate of complication is low and no nerve issues have been noted with tendon flexor tendon transfer in 268 cases in the past 7 years involving more than 300 toes. The most common procedure performed is a proximal phalanx IPJ fusion with side-to-side flexor tendon transfer and capsule plication. A metatarsal osteotomy was performed in 87% of subjects in association with tendon transfer. Only 7% of subjects had secondary plantar plate repair with interference screw fixation. The most common

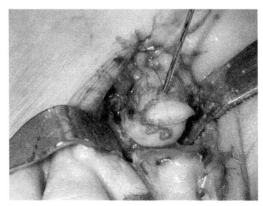

Fig. 5. Shift of the metatarsal after osteotomy in transverse plane for angular correction of the toe.

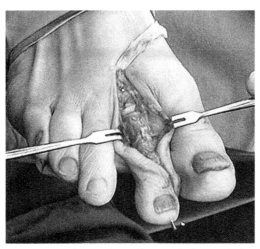

Fig. 6. Split flexor tendon transfer performed around the medial and lateral proximal phalanx and tied to the dorsal base of the toe. Note the proximal positioning of the transfer to better support the MPJ.

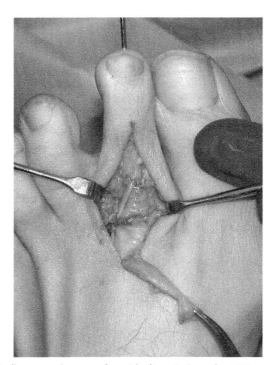

Fig. 7. Dorsal split flexor tendon transfer with sling tie into the MPJ capsule after capsular reefing for added correction of the medial toe deviation.

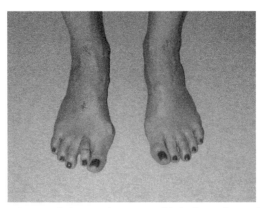

Fig. 8. Preoperative picture of plantar plate tear with hallux valgus, elevated second toe, hammertoe deformity, and medial shift of the second toe.

postoperative complaint was a nonpurchasing toe in 6% of subjects. All such cases involved a metatarsal osteotomy and hammertoe correction. These cases required a dorsal soft-tissue release in 3% of subjects, which resolved complaints in all cases. The other 3% of subjects improved with time and therapy. With time, the flexor tendon transfer with made slightly tighter in cases of metatarsal osteotomy and the case of toe purchase was found to be significantly improved. No cases of MPJ stiffness were noted as a subject complaint. Plantar plate pain was present after pin removal for about 4 months after surgery but resolved in 98% of subjects. Revision surgery was not necessary in any subject. Postoperative pressure control was performed with an orthotic in most subjects to avoid further trauma to the forefoot and protect the surgical site. Subjects were told to use the orthotic device for a minimum of 1 wear with stiff shoes and then to use the orthotic device as much as possible in the long term. Women requiring high-heel use were allowed high heels at 3 months after surgery but were told to use a stiff wedge-type shoe with a back strap for 6 months after surgery (**Figs. 8** and **9**).

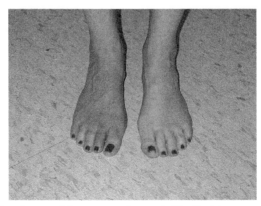

Fig. 9. Postoperative picture of the same patient as in **Fig. 8** with osteotomy bunionectomy, hammertoe correction with arthrodesis, flexor tendon transfer, and capsular reefing of the MPJ.

SUMMARY

Plantar plate tears are a far more common problem than noted. Often this problem is confused with a neuroma or hammertoe deformity and commonly mistreated. A dorsal drawer test, medial shift of the toe, and plantar capsular pain are the most indicative diagnostic signs. MRI and ultrasound diagnosis are commonly used to confirm a suspected problem. Strapping of the toe and stiff shoes with orthotics are common conservative treatments but offer limited improvement. Surgical procedures include flexor tendon transfer, hammertoe correction, ligament plication, and metatarsal osteotomy; each case must be judged separately for best outcome. Postoperative protection is necessary for 4 to 8 weeks in a below-the-knee walking boot followed by aggressive physical therapy. Toe purchase issues are more common in cases of hammertoe correction and metatarsal osteotomy; this issue is improved with a slight increased tightening of the flexor tendon transfer.

It is essential to consider this problem as part of the differential diagnosis in cases of suspected second interspace neuroma and in any case of hammertoe formation without MPJ keratoma. With proper patient selection, adequate workup, and surgical planning, this common problem is fairly easy to treat with excellent outcomes. The authors' results showed patient satisfaction in more than 95% of cases and minimal operative complications.

REFERENCES

1. Yao L, Cracchiolo A, Farahani K, et al. Magnetic resonance imaging of plantar plate ruptures. Foot Ankle Int 1996;17:33–6.
2. Shurnas P, Sanders A. Second MTP joint capsular instability with clawing deformity: metatarsal osteotomy, flexor transfer with biotenodesis, hammer toe repair, and MTP arthroplasty without the need for plantar incisions. Tech Foot Ankle Surg 2005;4(3):196–201.
3. Marks RM. Anatomy and pathophysiology of lesser toes deformities. Foot Ankle Clin 1998;3:199–213.
4. Blitz N, Ford L, Christensen J. Plantar plate repair of the second metatarsophalangeal joint: technique and tips. J Foot Ankle Surg 2004;43(4):266–70.
5. Deland JT, Lee KT, Sobel M, et al. Anatomy of the plantar plate and its attachments in the lesser metatarsal phalangeal joint. Foot Ankle Int 1995;16(8):480–6.
6. Johnston R, Smith J, Daniels T. The plantar plate of the lesser toes: an anatomical study in humans. Foot Ankle Int 1994;15(5):276–82.
7. Deland JT, Sung IH. The medial crossover toe: a cadaveric dissection. Foot Ankle Int 2000;21(5):375–8.
8. Ross SD, Faux JR. Surgical treatment of the unstable lesser metatarsophalangeal joint. Tech Foot Ankle Surg 2004;3(2):106–12.
9. Thompson FM, Hamilton WG. Problems of the second metatarsophalangeal joint. Orthopedics 1987;10:83–9.
10. Thompson FM, Deland JT. Flexor tendon transfer for metatarsophalangeal instability of the second toe. Foot Ankle 1993;14:385–8.
11. Bouche RT, Heit EJ. Combined plantar plate and hammertoe repair with flexor digitorum longus tendon transfer for chronic, severe sagittal plane instability of the lesser metatarsophalangeal joints: preliminary results. J Foot Ankle Surg 2008;47(2):125–37.
12. Simmons DN. Imaging of the painful forefoot. Tech Foot Ankle Surg 2008;7(4): 238–49.

13. Lambrunidi C. The feet of the industrial worker. Functional aspect: action of the foot muscles. Lancet 1938;II(1):480.
14. Kirchner JS, Wagner E. Girdlestone-Taylor extensor tendon transfer. Tech Foot Ankle Surg 2004;3(2):91–9.
15. Taylor RG. The treatment of claw toes by multiple transfers of flexor to extensor tendons. J Bone Joint Surg Br 1951;3(2):539–42.
16. Pyper JB. The flexor-extensor transplant operation for claw toes. J Bone Joint Surg Br 1958;40:528–33.
17. Parrish TF. Dynamic correction of claw toes. Orthop Clin North Am 1973;4: 97–102.
18. Kuwada GT, Dockery GL. Modification of the flexor tendon transfer procedure for the correction of flexible hammertoes. J Foot Surg 1980;19:38–40.
19. Barbari SG, Brevig K. Correction of claw toes by the Girdlestone-Taylor flexor-extensor transfer procedure. Foot Ankle 1984;5:38–40.
20. Ford LA, Collins KB, Christensen JC. Stabilization of the subluxed second metatarsophalangeal joint: flexor tendon transfer versus primary repair of the plantar plate. J Foot Ankle Surg 1998;37(3):217–22.

Lisfranc Injury and Jones Fracture in Sports

Bora Rhim, DPM[a],*, Joshua C. Hunt, BA[b]

KEYWORDS

- Midfoot sprain • Lisfranc ligament • Jones metatarsal fracture
- Sports injuries

LISFRANC INJURIES

With an incidence rate of 1 in 55,000 people in the United States, the Lisfranc injury is not very common.[1,2] Most injuries to the tarsometatarsal (TMT) joint/tarsometatarsal complex (TMC) are acquired through high-velocity trauma such as motor vehicle accidents or a fall from a height.[2,3] More than 50% of the high-velocity cases involve polytrauma.[2,3] Of the cases with polytrauma, around 20% of the Lisfranc injuries were misdiagnosed and 40% were completely missed.[2,3] Another, less-common method of injury to the TMC is low-velocity trauma, which only accounts for about 30%.[2,3] Low-velocity trauma of Lisfranc injury has been reported to occur to participants of soccer, football, baseball, running, basketball, wind surfing, horseback riding, and ballet.[1] Lisfranc injuries are difficult to diagnose on field because of mild edema and other distracting injuries at the ankle.[4] The athlete typically tries to walk it off and grossly underestimates the gravity of the injury. A Lisfranc injury is severe and has the potential to end an athlete's career; thus, a timely diagnosis and correct treatment are imperative.[3,4]

Mechanism of Injury

Midfoot injuries are the second most common foot injury experienced by an athlete.[3] The mechanism of injuries to the midfoot can be direct and indirect.[2] The direct mechanism of injury involves crushing trauma directly to the midfoot,[2] which is usually from a falling object.[2,5] The indirect mechanism of injury involves an axial load applied to a plantar-flexed and slightly rotated foot followed by an abrupt abduction or twisting.[2,5]

The authors have nothing to disclose.
[a] Department of Podiatric Medicine, Surgery, and Biomechanics, College of Podiatric Medicine, Western University of Health Sciences, 309 East Second Street, Pomona, CA 91766-1854, USA
[b] College of Podiatric Medicine, Western University of Health Sciences, 309 East Second Street, Pomona, CA 91766-1854, USA
* Corresponding author. Foot and Ankle Center, 309 East Second Street, Suite 7, Pomona, CA 91766–1854.
E-mail address: brhim@westernu.edu

Clin Podiatr Med Surg 28 (2011) 69–86
doi:10.1016/j.cpm.2010.09.003
0891-8422/11/$ – see front matter Crown Copyright © 2011 Published by Elsevier Inc. All rights reserved.

This mechanism of injury happens when a football player falls on the heel of another player's plantar-flexed foot while the metatarsophalangeal joints are maximally dorsiflexed.[5] The indirect mechanism also occurs when a windsurfer falls backward and the foot remains in the strap causing it to be forced into a hyper–plantar-flexed position.[1,5] Although it is common to fracture the cuneiform, the second metatarsal base is the most commonly fractured component of the TMC.[2,3,5,6] The less common fractures of TMC are of the navicular, cuboid, and other metatarsals.[2,3,5,6]

Anatomy

To fully understand how an injury can occur at the TMT joint, an understanding of the anatomy involved with the joint is necessary. The TMC is stabilized by both osseous and ligamentous structures, providing primary and indirect stability, respectively.[1,2,6,7] The osseous structures involved distally are the metatarsals 1 to 5, which articulate proximally with the medial, middle, and lateral cuneiforms and the cuboid. The cuboid articulates with metatarsals 4 and 5. The medial, middle, and lateral cuneiforms articulate with metatarsals 1 to 3, respectively. The middle cuneiform is more proximal than the medial and lateral cuneiforms, creating a mortise and allowing the second metatarsal to articulate with all the 3 cuneiforms, thus creating more osseous stability.[1,2,6,7] The depth of this mortise has a direct correlation with injury to the Lisfranc joint.[1,2,6,7] This osseous confirmation allows the base of the second metatarsal to be the keystone in the transverse arch of the foot, enhancing coronal plane stability.[1,2]

The indirect ligamentous stability is organized by its location: dorsal, plantar, and interosseous.[1,2,6] Without these ligaments the medial longitudinal arch would collapse.[1,2,6] The dorsal and plantar ligaments have 3 components: longitudinal, transverse, and oblique. The longitudinal and oblique fibers connect the tarsals to the base of the metatarsals. The transverse fibers interconnect the bases of the metatarsals. There are dorsal and plantar interosseous ligaments for the metatarsals, cuneiforms, and cuboid. The dorsal ligaments are weaker than the plantar ligaments and this weakness is thought to be a reason for the dorsal dislocation at this joint. The interosseous ligaments are the strongest, yet there is no interosseous ligament between the first and second metatarsals. The first metatarsal is stabilized by the plantar attachment of the peroneus longus and the dorsal attachment of the tibialis anterior. The second metatarsal is stabilized by its osseous surroundings and the Lisfranc ligament. The Lisfranc ligament spans from the lateral aspect of the medial cuneiform, attaching to the base of the medial aspect of the second metatarsal. The Lisfranc ligament measures 1 cm in height and 0.5 cm in width, making it the largest and strongest interosseous ligament.[1,2]

Normal motion of each component of the TMC varies because of the involvement of different osseous and ligamentous structures at each TMT joint.[1,2] The least amount of motion is found at the base of the second metatarsal, with only 0.6° of dorsiflexion–plantar flexion arch. The first TMT joint has a dorsiflexion–plantar flexion arch of 3.5°. The most mobile joint of the TMC is the most lateral fourth and fifth TMT joints, with an average of 10° dorsiflexion and plantar flexion.

Anatomy not directly involved with the TMC but still of great concern are the perforating branches of the dorsalis pedis artery and the deep peroneal nerve that courses between the bases of the first and second metatarsals.[1] Injuries to this nerve and artery can happen in concord with Lisfranc fractures and dislocations. Complications with these neurovascular structures serve as the main necessity for immediate reduction and diagnosis of a Lisfranc injury. The anterior tibial tendon has been proven to prevent proper reduction of a lateral dislocation in a Lisfranc injury.[1]

Classification

The first classification system was created by Quenu and Kuss in 1909, which was later modified by Hardcastle and colleagues[8] and ultimately adapted by Myerson and colleagues in 1986.[9] The Myerson classification system divides Lisfranc injuries into 3 classes: type A, type B, and type C.[2,3] These classes are based on the congruency of the TMT joints and the direction of displacement of the metatarsals. Type A involves a complete TMT joint incongruity, with all metatarsals displaced in the same direction or plane. Type B involves a partial TMT joint incongruity, with 1 or more displaced metatarsals. Type B1 is a medial displacement of the metatarsals, whereas type B2 is a lateral displacement of the metatarsals. Type C1 involves a divergent pattern of the TMC, with the first metatarsal displaced medially and the lateral 4 metatarsals displaced with partial incongruity. Type C2 involves a divergent pattern of the TMC, with total incongruity.

Nunley and Vertullo[3] created a classification system that addresses the low-velocity injuries. This classification system is based on clinical findings, bilateral weight-bearing radiographs, and bone scans. The Lisfranc injury is classified into 3 stages: stage 1, stage 2, and stage 3. A stage 1 Lisfranc injury is a ligament sprain with no diastasis at the base of the second metatarsal and medial cuneiform. The Lisfranc complex is stable. Bone scintigrams are used to show increased uptake at the site of the injury because radiographs, computed tomographic (CT) scans, and magnetic resonance images would likely provide negative results.[3] The stage 2 Lisfranc injury has a ruptured Lisfranc ligament, a diastasis between 2 and 5 mm at the base of the second metatarsal and medial cuneiform, and no decrease in arch height. The stage 3 Lisfranc injury has a ruptured Lisfranc ligament, diastasis between 2 and 5 mm at the base of the second metatarsal and medial cuneiform, and loss of longitudinal arch height.[3]

Diagnosis and Imaging

Diagnosis of a high-velocity injury such as an automobile accident, crushing injury, or a fall from a height is fairly straightforward. This injury presents with significant edema to the foot accompanied by severe pain and midfoot instability (**Fig. 1A**).[1–3,6,7] The injured foot may seem wider or flatter on bilateral comparison to the uninjured foot. A delayed, yet still diagnostic, presentation of a Lisfranc injury is plantar ecchymosis, either in high- or low-velocity injury (see **Fig. 1B**).

Depending on the amount of edema present, palpation of the dorsalis pedis pulse may prove difficult.[1–3,6,7] In cases of severe edema, compartment syndrome should be suspected.[1–3,6,7] Significant pain on passive dorsiflexion of the toes in a tensely swollen foot indicates compartment syndrome, and pressures should be measured. A pressure of greater than 40 mm Hg indicates emergent compartment release.[7] In a hypotensive patient, a compartment pressure within 30 mm Hg of the diastolic pressure indicates compartment release.[7]

Diagnosis of a low-velocity injury is more difficult. Athletes may underestimate the severity of the injury, especially if they are still weight bearing.[4] It is imperative to rule out a Lisfranc injury with any complaint of pain in the foot or ankle.[1–3] The low-velocity injuries are not as visually obvious as high-velocity injuries and do not present with as much edema.[1–3,6] The patient may or may not be weight bearing with a complaint of slight to severe pain.[1–3,6,7] The following bony landmarks should be palpated for tenderness: navicular, medial and middle cuneiforms, bases of metatarsals 1 to 5, and the first intermetatarsal space. Passive pronation and supination of the forefoot can assess the stability of the Lisfranc row, and if this maneuver produces

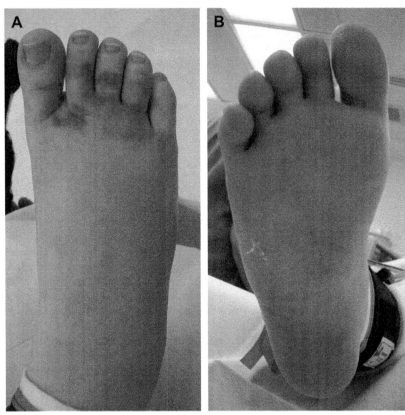

Fig. 1. (*A*) Significant swelling and ecchymosis shown dorsally from midfoot spain. (*B*) Plantar medial ecchymosis commonly observed in Lisfranc injury.

pain, it indicates Lisfranc injury.[1–3] If the patient is manifesting more subtle symptoms of a Lisfranc injury, provocation may be achieved by holding the hindfoot fixed in one hand and passively abducting and pronating the forefoot with the other hand.[1–3]

The initial radiographic evaluation should consist of anteroposterior (beam 15° off vertical), lateral, and 30° oblique views of the foot. The radiograph should be weight bearing to prevent any false-negative results and to clearly see any diastasis from ligamentous injury.[1–6] If the injury is mild, it may be necessary to do a bilateral comparison to identify any subtle differences. In an uninjured foot, the anteroposterior radiograph shows the medial side of the second metatarsal base line up with the medial side of the middle cuneiform and the first intermetatarsal space line up with the intertarsal space.[5] In the lateral view of an uninjured foot, the dorsal surface of the first and second metatarsal bases align with their respective cuneiforms. In the 30° oblique view of an uninjured foot, the medial border of the fourth metatarsal is aligned with that of the cuboid.[5] The most consistent finding in a Lisfranc injury is when the medial base of the second metatarsal does not line up with the medial aspect of the middle cuneiform.[5] The presence of a fleck sign on the radiograph is diagnostic of Lisfranc injury.[1–3,5,6] On a radiograph, a fleck of bone caused by an avulsion fracture from the Lisfranc ligament can be seen between the first and second metatarsal bases.

If Lisfranc injury is suspected and radiographic results are negative, some investigators suggest CT, magnetic resonance imaging (MRI), and/or bone scan. MRI is most helpful when a sprain or tear of the Lisfranc ligament is suspected. Bone scan has proved to be the most useful technique when all others produce negative results.[3,5] Bone scan shows slight increases of uptake in the injured region for up to 1 year after the injury.[3,5] CT scan is most useful when plain film radiography produces negative results or the injury is too acute to perform weight-bearing imaging.[2,3,5] CT scan may show small avulsions not seen by plain film radiography and is the best means for preoperative planning (**Figs. 2** and **3**).[2,5]

Stress radiography has been recommended for both acute and nonacute injuries.[1–3] Abduction stress radiography allows a better view between the second metatarsal and medial cuneiform.[3] However, if the diastasis is too subtle, abduction stress radiography cannot detect much separation because the x-ray is too oblique to capture the joint of interest.

Treatment

Nonsurgical treatment

Nonoperative treatment can be used on Nunley and Vertullo[3] stage 1 Lisfranc injuries. An important concept to help the patient understand is the amount of time this injury takes to heal.[1,2] The patient needs to realize that a foot sprain does not heal like an

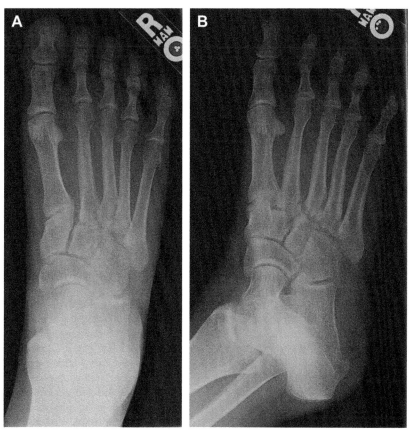

Fig. 2. (A) AP non-weight bearing foot radiograph, there is diastasis observed between 1st and 2nd metatarsals. (B) Oblique foot radiograph shows 2nd, 3rd, 4th metatarsal base fractures.

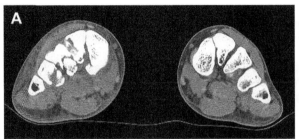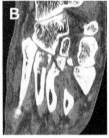

Fig. 3. (A, B) Axial and coronal views of CT scan confirming TMT injury.

ankle sprain. If the patient understands this concept, compliance is much more likely. Radiographic results of weight bearing must be negative for both displacement and fracture at the TMC.[2,3] The TMT joint must be stable in stress radiographs.[2] Although not highly recommended, immediate weight bearing with custom orthotics is appropriate in some cases. Cast immobilization with limited, or no, weight bearing for 6 weeks is the standard nonoperative treatment. A follow-up appointment after 2 weeks for radiographic evaluation of possible diastasis at the base of the second metatarsal and the medial cuneiform is recommended.[5] If the patient is still point tender after 2 weeks, cast immobilization must be continued for a minimum of 4 more weeks. If the patient is not point tender, weight bearing can be resumed without cast immobilization with or without custom orthotics.[5] After the patient has completed a minimum of 6 weeks of cast immobilization, weight bearing can be resumed in a walking cast for a minimum of 6 more weeks with range of motion exercises.[1–3,5–7] After 3 months, progressive weight bearing can be allowed along with physical therapy, as needed.[5,6] Between 3 and 4 months, from initial treatment, unrestricted activity may be permitted. Closed reduction of Nunley and Vertullo[3] stage 2 or stage 3 Lisfranc injury has had highly varied outcomes with an increased incidence for poor results. The most common complication after a Lisfranc injury is posttraumatic arthritis.[1–3,5–7] This complication, and other complications arising from TMT joint injury, is reduced when anatomic joint reduction is achieved quickly after an initial injury.[2]

Surgical treatment
Surgical treatment is preferred in any Lisfranc injury more severe than Nunley and Vertullo[3] stage 1 injury.[2,5,6] Soft tissue and osseous structures can prevent TMT joint reduction.[2] Open reduction with internal fixation (ORIF) and arthrodesis are the 2 most common operative treatments. Regardless of the operative procedure chosen, it is imperative to allow at least 48 hours, from the time of initial injury, for decrease in edema. ORIF can use partially or fully threaded 3.5- to 4.5-mm cannulated or solid screws.[2,3,6] There does not seem to be a preferred screw. Screw fixation provides greater biomechanical stability than pinning except in TMT joints 4 and 5 where more motion is required during gait. When the patient has a Myerson type B1 Lisfranc injury, a screw is placed from the medial cuneiform to the base of the second metatarsal. Another screw is placed from the medial to the intermediate cuneiform **(Fig. 4)**.[5] If the patient has a Myerson type B2 Lisfranc injury, a percutaneous screw can be placed from the medial cuneiform to the base of the second metatarsal.[5] The disadvantages of using screws are potential hardware breakage, articular damage to the affected joint, and postsurgical hardware removal. A few solutions to these disadvantages are use of absorbable hardware and dorsal plate and tightrope fixation. Thordarson and Hurvitz[10] used polylactide screws in 14 patients with Lisfranc injury none of whom required screw removal and had no reports of local tissue

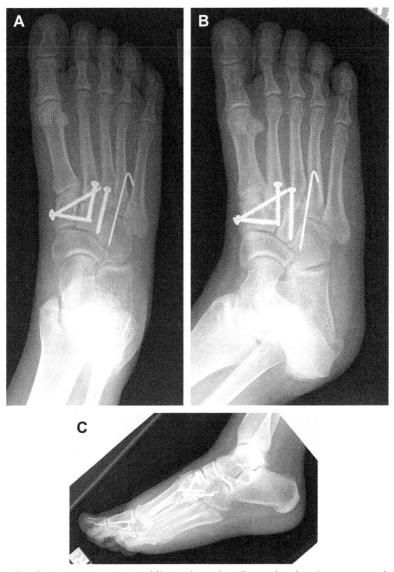

Fig. 4. (A–C) Post-operative AP, oblique, lateral radiographs showing open reduction internal fixation of TMT using solid screws and percutaneous K-wire.

reaction to the screws. The dorsal plate eliminated articular damage to the affected joint. A biomechanical study on dorsal plate versus screws showed minimal difference in stability and the dorsal plate allowed for earlier postoperative range of motion.[2]

Typically, arthrodesis is used as a salvage procedure after a failed ORIF, after a delayed and/or missed diagnosis, or for a comminuted fracture in the TMC.[1–3,5,6] Many recommend arthrodesis of the Lisfranc joint to be the first choice, with a primary ligamentous injury caused by poor healing at the ligament-osseous structure interface.[2,3,6] However, among the athletic population, this treatment option is in question for primary ligamentous Lisfranc injury.

After operative treatment, the patient should be placed in a non–weight-bearing cast for a minimum of 8 weeks.[1–3,6] Between 8 and 12 weeks, partial weight bearing is permitted.[1–3,6] After 12 weeks, the patient can begin progressive weight bearing with custom orthotics.[1–3,6] There is much debate whether to remove the screws or not after ORIF of TMT joints. Lattermann[5] recommends hardware to be removed between 12 and 16 weeks after surgery in athletes weighing less than 200 pounds. In athletes weighing more than 200 pounds, hardware is to be removed after 24 weeks.[5]

There is a lot of controversy as to which surgical procedure should be performed to maximize patient outcomes. The largest study to date, performed retrospectively by Myerson and colleagues[9] consisted of 76 fractures-dislocations of the Lisfranc ligament. Arntz and colleagues[11] reported on 41 Lisfranc injuries in 1988. In both of these studies, ORIF was performed with outcomes reported as good to excellent in about 50% of the patients.[9,11] There is not much literature on the criteria used to determine the status of good to excellent outcomes. Kuo and colleagues[12] did a retrospective review of 48 patients with a Lisfranc injury initially corrected by ORIF. They reported that 25% of the patients developed polytraumatic arthritis and 50% underwent arthrodesis. For the 48 patients, the average American Orthopaedic Foot & Ankle Society (AOFAS) midfoot score was 77. In 2001, Richter and colleagues[13] retrospectively reviewed 49 Lisfranc fracture-dislocations with an average AOFAS midfoot score of 71; the best results were from patients who underwent ORIF. There is no reported literature on the percentage of athletes who return to their respective sports after ORIF of the Lisfranc joint.

Ly and Coetzee[14] proposed that most TMT joint dislocations treated with temporary fixation eventually develop degenerative joint disease at the TMT joint. The investigators reviewed 41 patients with Lisfranc injury who underwent ORIF. Patients who underwent ORIF had an average AOFAS midfoot score of 68.6, whereas patients who underwent primary arthrodesis had an average AOFAS midfoot score of 88.[6] After 6 months, patients who underwent primary arthrodesis were at 62% compared with preinjury status, whereas patients who underwent ORIF were at 44% compared with preinjury status. After 1 year, patients who underwent primary arthrodesis were at 86% compared with preinjury status, whereas patients who underwent ORIF were at 61% compared with preinjury status. After 2 years, patients who underwent primary arthrodesis were at 92% compared with preinjury status, whereas patients who underwent ORIF were at 65% compared with preinjury status.[6] Ly and Coetzee[14] reported a reoperation rate of 75% in patients with an initial Lisfranc injury correction by ORIF. The patients with fusion at the Lisfranc joint had a reoperation rate of 20%. It was found that people who underwent ORIF had difficulty doing single-leg heel raises, whereas patients with fusion had no problem performing single-leg heel raises.

According to Coetzee,[6] the indications for primary fusions of Lisfranc fractures and dislocations are (1) major ligamentous disruptions with multidirectional instability/dislocation of the Lisfranc joints, (2) comminuted intra-articular fractures at the base of the first or second metatarsal, and (3) crush injuries of the midfoot with intra-articular fracture dislocation. The contraindications for primary fusions of Lisfranc injuries are (1) Lisfranc injuries in children with open physes, (2) unidirectional Lisfranc instability, and (3) unstable extra-articular metatarsal base fractures with questionable ligamentous disruption. Anderson and colleagues[15] showed similar results in a prospective randomized study and showed reoperative rates of 79% in the ORIF group and 17% in the fusion group. Nunley and Vertullo[3] reported on 5 professional athletes who underwent TMT joint fusion. Of the 5 athletes, 2 played football in the National Football League and both returned to their sport after treatment.[3] Despite this report, there is no prospective study published on the percentage of athletes returning to their respective sports after an arthrodesis of the Lisfranc joints.

Summary

Lisfranc fractures account for 0.2% of all fractures, with an incidence of about 1 in 55,000 people yearly. The Lisfranc injury is often misdiagnosed or completely missed because of its subtle symptoms and its usual involvement with polytrauma. Because a Lisfranc injury can often compromise important anatomic structures in its vicinity, long-term effects of a missed diagnosis can end an athlete's career. The typical mechanism of injury is hyper–plantar flexion of the Lisfranc joint. Examination findings of the Lisfranc injury are pain and tenderness at the metatarsal bases and medial/middle cuneiform, pain with rotational stress of forefoot, and ecchymosis on the plantar aspect of the midfoot. If a Lisfranc injury is suspected, compartment syndrome should not be overlooked. The Lisfranc injury is confirmed with weight-bearing radiographs. If the weight-bearing radiographs show negative results while the patient has positive symptoms, MRI can be used for diagnosis. Nunley and Vertullo classification of the Lisfranc injury involves the amount of diastasis present. Stage 1 injury has diastasis greater than 2 mm and is considered a sprain of the Lisfranc ligament. Conservative treatment involves applying a non–weight-bearing cast for 4 to 6 weeks, with a 2-week follow-up to check for further diastasis with weight-bearing radiographs. Stages 2 to 3 involve a diastasis greater than 2 mm and require surgical reduction of the Lisfranc joint. The Lisfranc injury can be treated by multiple surgical methods, but there is not enough research to determine which method has the best outcome. Reduction of the Lisfranc joint is imperative and must be achieved rapidly after the injury to avoid serious complications.

JONES FRACTURE

In 1902, Robert Jones,[16] an English surgeon, sustained a foot injury while dancing around a tent pole at a military party. Radiographic examination of his foot later revealed a fracture about three-fourths of an inch from the base of the fifth metatarsal. In the same year, Jones[16] published a report on his fracture as well as 6 other similar cases of fifth metatarsal fracture caused by an indirect injury. As a result, this type of fracture has been referred to as Jones fracture or dancer's fracture.

There are 3 types of fracture that can occur at the base of the fifth metatarsal.[17] The first fracture is an acute fracture involving the fifth metatarsal tuberosity, which is either an avulsion or comminuted type fracture. The second fracture is the true Jones fracture. The definition of Jones fracture is a transverse fracture located at the diaphyseal and metaphyseal junction, which involves the fourth and fifth intermetatarsal facets on the medial side. The third fracture occurs in the proximal diaphysis of the fifth metatarsal.[17] The third type is a stress fracture, also known as proximal diaphyseal stress fracture.

Anatomy

A thorough understanding of the regional anatomy of the fifth metatarsal is essential in distinguishing the various fractures in this region of the foot. The fifth metatarsal bone is composed of the base, styloid process or tuberosity, diaphysis, neck, and head. The base of the fifth metatarsal mainly articulates with the cuboid bone and medially with the fourth metatarsal. The soft tissue structure includes the dorsal and plantar cuboideometatarsal ligaments, an intermetatarsal ligament, and the joint capsule. These structures provide stability to the lateral tarsometatarsal joint complex. The peroneus brevis tendon inserts to the dorsolateral aspect of the fifth metatarsal tuberosity, and the peroneus tertius inserts to the dorsal shaft of the fifth metatarsal. Another structure that inserts to the tip of the tuberosity is a lateral band of the plantar aponeurosis that links the tuberosity to the lateral margin of the medial calcaneal tubercle. The flexor digiti minimi brevis muscle originates from the plantar surface of the base of the fifth metatarsal, and the dorsal and plantar interosseous muscles originate from the diaphysis of the fifth metatarsal.

Historically, when the Jones fractures were treated conservatively, numerous delayed unions or nonunions have been reported due to the watershed area at the junction between the diaphysis and tuberosity.[18,19] Carp[20] was the first to report 21 proximal fifth metatarsal fractures with a series of delayed unions. He suspected vascular insufficiency as a potential cause for the high incidence of delayed unions in his patients. Shereff and colleagues[18] and Smith and colleagues[19] reported the intraosseous and extraosseous vascular anatomy of the fifth metatarsal from cadaver models. The dorsal metatarsal artery, the plantar metatarsal artery, and the branch of the lateral plantar artery or the fibular plantar marginal artery have been found to make up the extraosseous circulation of the fifth metatarsal. The blood supply of the fifth metatarsal is similar to that of the long bones. The intraosseous circulation to the fifth metatarsal consists of 3 systems of vessels: the metaphyseal arteries, the periosteal arteries, and the nutrient artery. The periosteal arteries run parallel to the metatarsal shaft and lie within the periosteum. The metaphyseal arteries are derived from the surrounding soft tissues and are found in the head and neck region of the fifth metatarsal as well as the base of the fifth metatarsal. At the junction of the middle and proximal third of the diaphysis, the nutrient artery enters and bifurcates into a short proximal branch and a longer distal branch. The study by Smith and colleagues[19] reported evidence of different arterial sources for the tuberosity and the proximal diaphysis, thus creating a relative avascular zone between these 2 distributions. The zone of relative avascularity corresponds to the site of Jones fracture, which correlates to the region of poor fracture healing.

Mechanism of Injury

About 70% to 90% of Jones fractures occur in active age groups, from ages 15 to 22 years. According to many reports, those at the greatest risk of suffering Jones fracture are younger athletes with a high level of activity in a running and/or jumping sport.[21–24] This type of injury occurs when an adduction force is applied to the forefoot with the ankle plantar flexed.[25,26] For example, misstepping on the lateral border of the foot, pivoting, or shifting/cutting in sports such as soccer, basketball, or football, with the heel off the ground.[25,27] Owing to the ligamentous attachments at the fifth metatarsal, with enough bending motion created from the fifth metatarsal head, the bone fractures before it dislocates.[28] As a result, a short oblique or transverse fracture at the junction of the metaphysis and diaphysis results, entering the fourth-fifth intermetatarsal joint.

Classification

There are several classification systems that describe the proximal fifth metatarsal fracture. Stewart[27] was the first to classify fractures at the base of the fifth metatarsal. Stewart[27] devised a classification system based on the location of the fracture, the potential for avascular necrosis, and/or the joint involvement of the fifth metatarsal. He defined Jones fracture as an extra-articular fracture between the metatarsal base and diaphysis. Jones fracture was then categorized as type I fracture under Stewart classification.[27] The rest of the Stewart classification system includes Type II, intra-articular fracture of the metatarsal base; type III, avulsion fracture of the base;

type IV, comminuted fracture with intra-articular extension; and type V, partial avulsion of the metatarsal base with or without a fracture.[27]

The proximal fifth metatarsal fractures are classified into 3 subanatomic fracture zones.[21,29,30] Zone 1 is the most proximal avulsion fracture that extends intra-articularly through the metatarsocuboid articulation (**Fig. 5**A). Zone 2 is a Jones fracture at the metaphyseal-diaphyseal junction (see **Fig. 5**B). Even though Stewart defined Jones fracture as an extra-articular fracture, the fracture is now considered to begin laterally at the distal portion of the fifth metatarsal tuberosity and extend transversely or obliquely into the area of the medial cortex where the fifth metatarsal articulates with the fourth metatarsal.[21,30,31] Zone 3, a stress fracture that occurs at the proximal 1.5 cm of the diaphysis (see **Fig. 5**C). Owing to the close proximity, on a radiograph, the distinction between Jones and proximal diaphyseal fractures is often difficult to make. Chuckpaiwong and colleagues[32] determined that differentiation between Jones and proximal diaphyseal stress fractures is not necessary because regardless of the treatment type, the clinical outcomes were not different between the 2 fracture locations.[33]

Torg and colleagues[23] published a classification system to distinguish the healing potential of proximal diaphyseal fifth metatarsal fractures. This classification system is widely used and has become the standard treatment strategy for the Jones and proximal diaphyseal fractures. Torg classification consists of 3 types of fractures based on radiographic findings. Acute type I fracture is defined radiographically by sharp fracture margins, minimal or no periosteal reaction, and minimal cortical hypertrophy. Type I fractures are clinically acute. Type II fractures are characterized radiographically by some periosteal reaction, widened fracture margins, and some intramedullary sclerosis. This injury is characterized by a history of previous injury or fracture. Type II fracture is considered a delayed union. Type III fractures are nonunion fractures that are characterized by a clinical history of repetitive trauma or recurrent symptoms and are characterized radiographically by sclerosis obliterating the medullary canal and blunt fracture edges.

Diagnosis and Imaging

Obtaining a proper history from the patient along with a complete leg-ankle-foot examination is required to make a proper diagnosis. It is vital to rule out other associated injuries, including lateral column Lisfranc sprain and peroneus brevis tendon tear or strain, and to perform stress inversion test for displacement or stability of the foot, subtalar joint, and ankle joint.[28]

There are a few predisposing factors that have been reported to indicate a higher likelihood of Jones fracture. These predisposing factors can be addressed during surgery to prevent chances of delayed union or nonunion or possible recurrence of the Jones fracture. Often, it is imperative that the examiner observes for these predisposing factors when examining a patient[28]:

- Hindfoot varus can be assessed clinically by observing posteriorly at the Achilles-calcaneal axis, calcaneal axial radiograph, or looking for the peekaboo heel sign.[34] Normally, the axis is in a slight valgus position instead of a varus position. In hindfoot varus, one should be able to visualize the medial heel pad when the patient is standing with the feet aligned straight ahead.
- The examination of peroneal tendon weakness by comparing with the posterior tibial tendon strength. This weakness is often present, especially with a history of ankle sprain and is a common predisposing factor in lateral foot overload.[28]

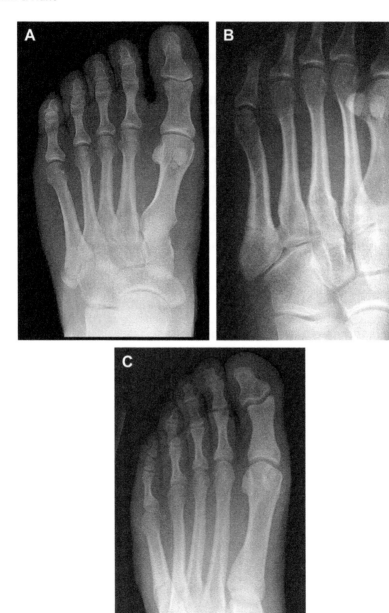

Fig. 5. Three subanatomic fracture zones of proximal fifth metatarsal fractures. (*A*) Zone 1: Avulsion fracture. (*B*) Zone 2: Jones fracture. (*C*) Zone 3: Diaphyseal stress fracture.

For initial evaluation, 3 views of weight-bearing foot radiograph is recommended. Bilateral standing radiographs are rarely required to make the diagnosis. Other ancillary studies such as CT scan, MRI, and bone scan are helpful in diagnosing the injury and suspected associated injury and in the later stages of treatment and management when dealing with possible delayed union or nonunion.

Treatment

Nonsurgical treatment

A nondisplaced Jones fracture and Torg type I (acute) fractures can be treated in a non–weight-bearing ambulation in a short leg cast for 6 to 8 weeks followed by a weight-bearing cast or walking boot for an additional 6 weeks.[21,29,30] However, the exceptions to this treatment option include the high-performance athlete or an informed patient who refuses surgical treatment. When there is no tenderness at the fifth metatarsal and imaging evidence of healing is present, the athlete can resume to play or return to leg-based activities, such as soccer, basketball, or running.

In the literature, there is some question about the success of closed treatment with immobilization in Jones fracture. Even in Jones fracture, immobilization improves the likelihood of union.[35] Torg and colleagues[23] reported a series of 46 patients with fractures of the fifth metatarsal base, which were treated nonoperatively and operatively. In this study, 15 patients with acute Jones fractures were cast and immobilized with protected weight bearing. At an average of 6.5 weeks, 93% of the patients healed and 1 patient developed a symptomatic nonunion that required operative management. Only 4 of the 10 patients who followed a partial weight-bearing protocol progressed to union. Therefore, Torg and colleagues[23] stressed the importance of non–weight bearing in a short leg cast with immobilization.

The biggest disadvantage of the non–weight-bearing cast is that the time to union is often prolonged. Especially, in athletes with prolonged immobilization, the onset of cast disease is of concern. Zogby and Baker[35] reported a radiographic healing of 21 to 22 weeks on average for acute and subacute Jones fractures treated conservatively. Clapper and colleagues[36] reported a 72% union rate in a series of 25 acute Jones fractures, whereas 28% had clinical and radiographic evidence of nonunion at 25 weeks since the initial injury. From those 25 patients, 7 were then treated with intramedullary screw fixation and a 100% union rate was achieved at an average of 12.1 weeks.[36] Quill[30] reported 1 in 3 conservatively treated fractures as refractured and therefore recommended early surgical treatment. Mologne and colleagues[37] reported a nearly 50% reduction in both the time to clinical union and the time to return to sports when Jones fractures were randomized to 8 weeks of non–weight-bearing cast or early intramedullary screw fixation. However, discussion continues regarding treatments for athletes versus nonathletes. Konkel and colleagues[38] recommend nonoperative treatment of fifth metatarsal fracture for patients in whom the time to return to full activities is not critical. As a result, a more aggressive approach of intramedullary fixation has evolved for the athletic population to avoid prolonged healing.

Presently, bone stimulation can be used as an adjunct primary therapy to accelerate fracture healing. Various bone stimulators are available that work by electromagnetic fields, high-frequency low-magnitude mechanical stimuli, or ultrasound.[39] In Jones fracture, because of the nature of the injury and the documented prolonged time it takes to union, bone stimulators can be readily used. Bone stimulators are painless, can be placed outside the cast, and can be applied on a daily basis in the patient's home. With this treatment, if union occurs, there can be an earlier return to play and avoidance of surgery without the risks of developing postoperative complications.

Surgical treatment

The goal of the operative treatment is to minimize the risk of delayed union, nonunion, and refracture. Most importantly, the goal is to decrease the time to return to athletic activity and allow athletes or even recreational athletes to return to their sports activities more quickly.[21,23,30,31] The indication for operative treatment includes acute displaced fractures, Torg type II and III diaphyseal stress fractures, and failed nonoperative management.[40] There are several surgical treatment options available: a percutaneous approach with intramedullary screw, intercalated corticocancellous bone graft, ORIF with minifragment plate and screws, tension band construct, or closed reduction, and Kirschner wire fixation.[21–23,28,41] Especially, in treating nonunions, bone grafts can be added for biologic supplementation.

With reports of increased union rates and rapid recovery, intramedullary screw fixation of the proximal fifth metatarsal has become first-line treatment option in acute fractures. The intramedullary screws provide compression across the fracture, and the technique allows the placement of the screw in a percutaneous fashion without having to open the fracture site or strip the periosteum, which increases the rate of healing. There are numerous articles reporting increased union rates with using the intramedullary screw approach in athletes. DeLee and colleagues[40] demonstrated a 100% union rate (11 patients) without complications by using a 4.5-mm malleolar screw. Porter and colleagues[42] reported a 100% union rate with high satisfaction rates with 2 refractures by using a cannulated 4.5-mm stainless steel screw. Kavanaugh and colleagues[22] reported on 13 proximal fifth metatarsal fractures treated with a 4.5-mm

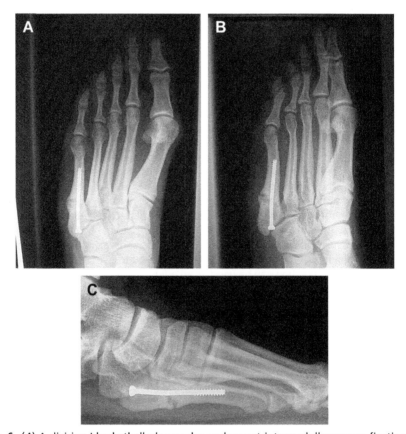

Fig. 6. (A) A division I basketball player who underwent intermedullary screw fixation for acute Jones fracture using a 4.0 mm cannulated screw. Patient developed nonunion 8 months after returning to his sport. (B, C) With the development of nonunion, oblique and lateral views showed bent intermedullary screw.

malleolar screw and demonstrated a 100% union rate with no refractures. Even though all 3 studies have small study groups, average mean time for healing clinically and radiographically was 6.2 weeks and 7.4 weeks, respectively.

The most common complication reported in intramedullary fixation is the recurrence of Jones fracture with screw failure. In this case, the screw size ranges from 4.0 to 5.0 mm after 2.5 to 4.5 months of return to sports activity (**Fig. 6**).[43,44] Larson[44] also reported a case of 4 refractures and 2 symptomatic nonunions, using 4.0- to 6.5-mm screws. It was recommended that athletes returning to full activity before complete radiographic union was predictive of failure. To counter the higher amount of torsional stress placed on the fracture site, Wright and colleagues[43] recommended using a larger solid screw in competitive athletes (**Fig. 7**). During surgery, it has been recommended that the dissection to the fifth metatarsal tuberosity be achieved via blunt dissection to minimize damage to the sural nerve. It is also recommended to always use a fluoroscope when placing the guide wires and screw and to use the largest possible screw to maximize pullout strength.[28,42]

On reviewing numerous published data, the authors recommend using either cannulated or solid screw systems in fixating Jones fractures.[20–22,31,40,43,44] The lag screw length is important to consider; the intramedullary screw should be inserted perpendicular to the fracture. Normally, a screw diameter of less than 4 mm is not recommended except in certain instances. Athletes with large body mass require a larger screw (5.5 or 6.5 mm) and a protected early return to activity. These screws, when inserted properly within the medullary canal, provide for bending and tension stability. Studies reveal these screws to be less resistant to torsional stress. In case of comminution, small plates can be used, but the plates can destroy extraosseous blood supply. This consequence is important because the injury damages the intraosseous blood supply.

Postoperative care includes placement of the foot in a cast or a boot, and weight bearing should not occur (at the earliest) until 3 weeks after injury. Even then, there must be partial weight bearing if full weight bearing is painful. Patients should be allowed to return to their respective sports when there is no tenderness with imaging evidence of complete union. If plain radiographs are difficult to interpret for complete radiographic union, CT scan of the foot can be used to assess the level of bony healing (**Fig. 8**).[40]

Once union is observed, physical therapy is essential for a proper course of rehabilitation, involving regaining of strength through eccentric and concentric open chain

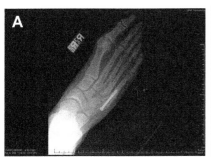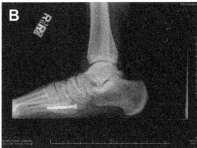

Fig. 7. (*A*) Post-operative radiograph demonstrating revision surgery to the nonunion site with 6.5 mm solid screw with bone graft. (*B*) Post-operative lateral radiograph showing good alignment of the screw.

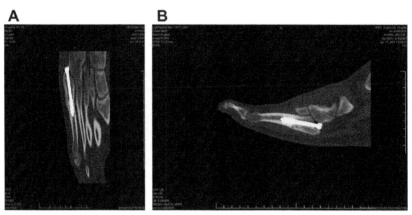

Fig. 8. (*A*) Prior to allowing the athlete to return to playing basketball, CT scan was ordered. CT scan confirmed complete fusion at the nonunion site. (*B*) Sagittal view of CT scan demonstrating complete union.

exercises or muscle-specific work.[28] Closed chain nonimpact activities such as cycling, working out in an elliptical trainer or similar equipments, or deep-water running can be helpful. A graduated return to impact loading and sport-specific agility work is required. The reported pain level from the patient should dictate the activity level and progression during rehabilitation. Especially, in patients with varus of the hindfoot, custom orthotics with significant arch support and the lateral hindfoot wedge extending to the lateral forefoot may decrease the incidence of refractures. Raikin and colleagues[25] reported 20 patients with 0% refracture rate when the hindfoot varus was corrected with an orthotic.

Summary

Numerous treatment options have been reported for the fifth metatarsal base fractures. For the general population, use of a short leg cast with immobilization seems to be a viable and accepted option; however, for the active population, particularly in competitive athletes who require a faster return to play, surgical treatment is recommended. Owing to numerous reports of early healing and return to play, the treatment options for Jones fracture has changed from nonoperative approach to a more aggressive and operative framework in athletes. Surgically, intramedullary screw fixation has been the technique of choice. Intramedullary fixation is a relatively straightforward procedure that offers a predictable union rate and a minimal period of immobilization, with return to weight bearing in 3 weeks. Immediate intramedullary fixation for Jones fracture is recommended for acute Jones fracture or Torg types II and III fractures. If surgery is chosen, careful dissection with the use of a fluoroscope is must and a cannulated screw with the largest diameter should be used, which increases pull out strength to prevent recurrence or screw failure. Most importantly, complete union should be observed using radiographs or CT scans, before releasing the patient to physical activity.

REFERENCES

1. DeOrio M, Erickson M, Giuseppe F, et al. Lisfranc injuries in sport. Foot Ankle Clin 2009;14:169–86.

2. Desmond EA, Chou LB. Current concepts review: Lisfranc injuries. Foot Ankle Int 2006;27(8):653–60.

3. Nunley JA, Vertullo CJ. Classification, investigation, and management of midfoot sprains: Lisfranc injuries in the athlete. Am J Sports Med 2002;30(2):871–8.

4. Sauers RJ, Dilorio EJ, Weiss CB. A Lisfranc's fracture-dislocation in a collegiate football player. J Athl Train 1992;27(1):25–6.

5. Lattermann C, Goldstein JL, Wukich DK, et al. Practical management of Lisfranc injuries in athletes. Clin J Sport Med 2007;17(4):311–5.

6. Coetzee C. Making sense of Lisfranc injuries. Foot Ankle Clin 2008;13:695–704.

7. Thompson MC, Matthew MA. Injury to the tarsometatarsal joint complex. J Am Acad Orthop Surg 2003;11(4):260–7.

8. Hardcastle PH, Reschauer R, Kutscha-Lissberg E, et al. Injuries to the tarsome-tatarsal joint. Incidence, classification and treatment. J Bone Joint Surg Br 1982; 64(3):349–56.

9. Myerson MS, Fisher RT, Burgess AR, et al. Fracture dislocations of the tarsome-tatarsal joints: end results correlated with pathology and treatment. Foot Ankle 1986;6:225–42.

10. Thordarson DB, Hurvitz G. PLA screw fixation of Lisfranc injuries. Foot Ankle Int 2002;23:1003–7.

11. Arntz CR, Veith RG, Hansen ST. Fractures and fracture-dislocations of the tarso-metatarsal joint. J Bone Joint Surg Am 1988;70:173–81.

12. Kuo RS, Tejwani NC, Digiovanni CW, et al. Outcome after open reduction and internal fixation of Lisfranc joint injuries. J Bone Joint Surg Am 2000;82(A):1609–18.

13. Richter M, Wippermann B, Krettek C, et al. Fractures and fracture dislocations of the midfoot: occurrence, causes and long-term results. Foot Ankle Int 2001;22:392–8.

14. Ly TV, Coetzee JC. Treatment of primarily ligamentous Lisfranc joint injuries: primary arthrodesis compared with open reduction and internal fixation. A prospective, randomized study. J Bone Joint Surg Am 2006;88(3):514–20.

15. Henning JA, Jones CB, Sietsema DL, et al. Open reduction internal fixation versus primary arthrodesis for Lisfranc injuries: a prospective randomized study. Foot and Ankle Int 2009;30:913–22.

16. Jones R. Fracture of the base of the fifth metatarsal bone by indirect violence. Ann Surg 1902;35(6):697–700.

17. Dameron TB. Fracture and anatomic variations of the proximal portion of the fifth metatarsal. J Bone Joint Surg Am 1975;57(6):788–92.

18. Shereff MJ, Yang QM, Kummer FJ, et al. Vascular anatomy of the fifth metatarsal. Foot Ankle 1991;11:350–3.

19. Smith JW, Arnoczky SP, Hersch A. The intraosseous blood supply of the fifth meta-tarsal: implications for proximal fracture healing. Foot Ankle 1992;13:143–52.

20. Carp L. Fracture of the fifth metatarsal bone with special reference to delayed union. Ann Surg 1927;86:308–20.

21. Dameron TB. Fractures of the proximal fifth metatarsal: selecting the best treat-ment options. J Am Acad Orthop Surg 1995;3(2):110–4.

22. Kavanaugh JH, Brower TD, Mann RV. The joins fracture revisited. J Bone Joint Surg Am 1978;60(6):776–82.

23. Torg JS, Balduini FC, Zelko RR, et al. Fractures of the base of the fifth metatarsal distal to the tuberosity. Classification and guidelines for non-surgical and surgical management. J Bone Joint Surg Am 1984;66(2):209–14.

24. Zelko RR, Torg J, Rachun A. Proximal diaphyseal fracture of the fifth metatarsal—treatment of the fractures and their complications in athletes. Am J Sports Med 1979;7:95–101.

25. Raikin SM, Slenker N, Ratigan B. The association of a varus hindfoot and fracture of the fifth metatarsal metaphyseal-diaphyseal junction: the Jones fracture. Am J Sports Med 2008;36(7):1367–72.
26. Vertullo CJ, Glisson RR, Nunley JA. Torsional strains in the proximal fifth metatarsal: implications for Jones and stress fracture management. Foot Ankle 2004;25(9):650–6.
27. Stewart IM. Jones's fracture: fracture of base of fifth metatarsal. Clin Orthop 1960; 16:190–8.
28. McBryde AM. The complicated Jones fracture, including revision and malalignment. Foot Ankle Clin 2009;14(2):151–68.
29. Lawrence SJ, Botte MJ. Jones' fractures and related fractures of the proximal fifth metatarsal. Foot Ankle 1993;14:358–65.
30. Quill GE. Fractures of the proximal fifth metatarsal. Orthop Clin North Am 1995; 26:353–61.
31. Rosenberg GA, Sferra JJ. Treatment strategies for acute fractures and nonunions of the proximal fifth metatarsal. J Am Acad Orthop Surg 2000;8(5):332–8.
32. Chuckpaiwong B, Queen RM, Easley ME, et al. Distinguishing Jones and proximal diaphyseal fractures of the fifth metatarsal. Clin Orthop Relat Res 2008; 466:1966–70.
33. Acker JH, Drez D. Nonoperative treatment of stress fractures of the proximal shaft of the fifth metatarsal (Jones' fracture). Foot Ankle 1986;7(3):152–5.
34. Manoli A II, Graham B. The subtle cavus foot, "the underpronator": a review. Foot Ankle Int 2005;26(3):256–63.
35. Zogby RG, Baker BE. A review of nonoperative treatment of Jones' fracture. Am J Sports Med 1987;15(4):304–7.
36. Clapper MF, O'Brien TJ, Lyons PM. Fractures of the fifth metatarsal. Analysis of a fracture registry. Clin Orthop Relat Res 1995;315:238–41.
37. Mologne TS, Lundeen JM, Clapper MF, et al. Early screw fixation versus casting in the treatment of acute Jones fractures. Am J Sports Med 2005;33:970–5.
38. Konkel KF, Ag Menger, Retzlaff SA. Nonoperative treatment of fifth metatarsal fractures in an orthopaedic suburban private multispecialty practice. Foot Ankle Int 2005;26:704–7.
39. Siska PA, Gruen GS, Pape HC. External adjuncts to enhance fracture healing: what is the role of ultrasound? Injury 2008;39:1095–105.
40. DeLee JC, Evans JP, Julian J. Stress fracture of the fifth metatarsal. Am J Sports Med 1983;11:349–53.
41. Fetzer GB, Wright RW. Metatarsal shaft fractures and fractures of the proximal fifth metatarsal. Clin Sports Med 2006;25:139–50.
42. Porter DA, Duncan M, Meyer SJ. Fifth metatarsal Jones fracture fixation with a 4.5-mm annulated stainless steel screw in the competitive and recreational athlete. A clinical and radiographic evaluation. Am J Sports Med 2005;33(5):1–8.
43. Wright RW, Fischer DA, Schively C, et al. Refracture of proximal fifth metatarsal (Jones) fracture after intramedullary screw fixation in athletes. Am J Sports Med 2000;28(5):732–6.
44. Larson CM, Almekinders LC, Taft TN, et al. Intramedullary screw fixation of Jones fractures. Analysis of failure. Am J Sports Med 2002;30(1):55–60.

Chronic Ankle and Subtalar Joint Instability in the Athlete

Matthew J. Hentges, BA[a,b], Michael S. Lee, DPM[c,d,*]

KEYWORDS

• Ankle • Subtalar joint • Instability • Athlete

Ankle sprains represent one of the most common ailments in the athletic population, accounting for more than 40% of all athletic injuries.[1] Sports in which ankle injuries most commonly occur include volleyball, basketball, and football; however, many other athletic activities can cause injury to the ankle.[2] Because there has been an increase in the awareness of healthy lifestyles and an increase in physical activity is promoted for all age groups, the number of ankle injuries related to sport seen by the foot and ankle specialist is likely to increase. Functional instability is the most common complication of injury of the lateral ankle ligaments and is because of the interruption of proprioceptive mechanoreceptors in the ankle joint.[3] As many as 20% of all ankle sprains result in functional instability.[3,4] Although early functional rehabilitation is the mainstay for acute lateral ankle injuries, 10% to 30% of injuries ultimately result in chronic instability.[5]

Chronic lateral ankle instability is frequently accompanied by subtalar joint (STJ) instability. About 10% to 15% of patients with ankle instability have associated STJ instability.[6] STJ instability can also occur as an isolated problem and was first described by Rubin and Witten.[7] Chronic ankle instability and subtalar instability are debilitating problems for the competitive athlete. A proper diagnosis of the condition must be made in a timely manner and the correct treatment initiated. The foot and ankle surgeon must balance treatment goals with the expectations of the athlete, parents, and/or coaches.

The authors have nothing to disclose.

[a] College of Podiatric Medicine and Surgery, Des Moines University, Des Moines, 3000 Grand Avenue, IA, USA

[b] 5054 EP True Pkwy #208, West Des Moines, IA 50265, USA

[c] Capital Orthopaedics and Sports Medicine, P.C., 12499 University Avenue, Suite 210, Des Moines, IA 50325, USA

[d] Des Moines University, Des Moines, 3000 Grand Avenue, IA, USA

* Corresponding author. Capital Orthopaedics and Sports Medicine, P.C., 12499 University Avenue, Suite 210, Des Moines, IA 50325.

E-mail address: mlee@dsmcapitalortho.com

Clin Podiatr Med Surg 28 (2011) 87–104

doi:10.1016/j.cpm.2010.10.001

0891-8422/11/$ – see front matter © 2011 Elsevier Inc. All rights reserved.

podiatric.theclinics.com

ANATOMY AND PATHOMECHANICS

The ankle joint and STJ are complex anatomic structures that derive their stability from bony apposition, ligamentous support, gravity, muscular activity, and ground reactive forces.[8,9] Disruption of the static or dynamic support of these structures can result in instability if not properly managed.

Ankle Joint

The ankle joint consists of the body of the talus, lateral malleolus, medial malleolus, inferior tibiofibular syndesmosis, deltoid ligaments, and lateral collateral ligaments. The lateral ankle ligamentous complex consists of the anterior talofibular ligament (ATFL), calcaneofibular ligament (CFL), and posterior talofibular ligament (PTFL). These ligaments make up the static support of the ankle joint.[8] The ATFL is a fan-shaped intracapsular structure that originates at the anterior border of the lateral malleolus and inserts into the lateral talar body. The ATFL is the primary stabilizer of the lateral ankle, despite being the shortest and weakest of the lateral ligaments.[9] The CFL is a cordlike extracapsular ligament that originates from the inferior border of the lateral malleolus and inserts on a small tubercle located on the posterior aspect of the lateral calcaneal surface (**Fig. 1**). The peroneal tendons pass superficially to the CFL as they course anteriorly from the lateral malleolous.[9] The PTFL is a very strong and intracapsular ligament originating on the medial surface of the lateral malleolus and inserts on the lateral tubercle of the posterior process of the talus.[9]

The ankle is most unstable in plantar flexion as the narrow posterior surface of the talus rotates into the mortise. The ATFL is subjected to higher amounts of strain than

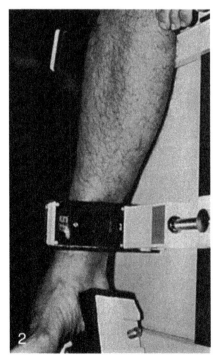

Fig. 1. The Telos apparatus used for talar tilt examination. (*From* Lee MS, Hofbauer MH. Evaluation and management of lateral ankle injuries. Clin Podiatr Med Surg 1999;16: 659–78; with permission.)

the other lateral collateral ligaments when the ankle is plantar flexed and is thus subjected to a great deal of injury.[10] The CFL becomes taught as the ankle moves from plantar flexion to dorsiflexion.[10] Broström noted that the ATFL was injured in 66% of lateral ankle injuries versus the CFL becoming injured in only 20% of cases.[11]

The mechanism of injury of lateral ankle sprains has been described as an inversion force applied to the foot while the ankle is in plantar flexion. The ATFL is the first ligament to rupture, followed by the CFL, and in severe cases, the PTFL may rupture, causing dislocation of the ankle joint.[9,11] Deficits in peroneal strength and muscle action have also been associated with instability of the ankle.[12]

STJ

The STJ consists of 3 articular facets between the inferior surface of the talus and the dorsal surface of the calcaneus. The posterior facet of the STJ makes up the largest articulation between the talus and calcaneus. This facet is separated from the middle and anterior facets by the tarsal canal medially and the tarsal sinus laterally.[9] Typically, the anterior and middle facets are described individually; however, a study by Hyer and colleagues[13] revealed that the anterior and middle facets are conjoined in 56% of cases. The middle and anterior facets are supported by the sustentaculum tali and anterior process of the calcaneus, respectively.[9]

The articulating surfaces are stabilized by the CFL, interosseous talocalcaneal ligament (ITCL), cervical ligament, and lateral root of the inferior extensor retinaculum.[14] The CFL, described earlier, is nearly perpendicular to the posterior facet of the STJ and is responsible for the maintenance of congruity between the articular surfaces.[15] The CFL is the main stabilizer of the STJ complex. Disruption of this ligament results in a significant increase in joint motion in all 3 cardinal planes and resultant instability.[16,17] The ITCL is a fundiform ligament that lies in the sinus tarsi and tarsal canal and is also important for subtalar stability.[16,18] Pisani[19] describes the ITCL as being located at the pivot point of the STJ and stresses the importance of reconstructing the ITCL in reestablishing stability in the STJ. The cervical ligament is located along the anterolateral portion of the STJ and is the strongest ligament connecting the talus and the calcaneus.[9]

The mechanism of injury in subtalar instability is described as an inversion force applied to the foot while the ankle is in dorsiflexion. This force places stress directly on the CFL, causing disruption and subsequent instability.[20] If the deforming forces continue, the ITCL and cervical ligament can also be injured.[18] Pisani[19] also describes a whiplash injury responsible for disrupting the ITCL. This injury is common in basketball and volleyball players and is seen when the player comes to an abrupt stop. The talus continues to move anteriorly on the planted calcaneus because of the body's inertia, thus rupturing the ITCL. Because both lateral ankle instability and subtalar instability are inversion injuries, they can often occur concomitantly. As many as 10% to 75% of individuals with ankle instability also have STJ instability.[6,21,22]

CLINICAL HISTORY AND PATIENT EXAMINATION

Obtaining a clear and accurate history of the athlete's injury is vital to proper treatment. The athlete with chronic ankle and/or STJ instabilities presents with a history of recurrent lateral ankle sprains and may present to the office with an acute-on-chronic injury.[23] The patient should be asked to provide a visual description of the injury, including the position of the foot or ankle at the time of the injury. The athlete should also be questioned about the subjective stability of the ankle and the presence of functional instability.[24] A feeling of "giving way" with a normal physical examination is a common finding in the patient with functional instability. Mechanical instability is appreciated objectively during physical examination of the ankle joint. The patient may relate a popping or tearing sensation during the injury. It is important to inquire about the number of times that the ipsilateral ankle has been injured as well as the number of injuries to the contralateral side. In addition, chronic or low-grade pain in between acute events may indicate other concurrent lesions, such as peroneal tendon pathology or osteochondral lesions of the talus. Previous treatment plans should also be elucidated. The type of the athlete who is being treated is important in surgical decision making and should not be overlooked.[25]

Examination of the injured foot and ankle begins with inspection. The amount of edema, presence of ecchymosis, and presence of gross deformities should be noted by the clinician. Palpation of the ankle joint and surrounding structures for the point of maximal tenderness is important and has been shown to have some clinical reliability in the acute injury.[26] This point of tenderness may not be as specific an indicator in the chronically injured ankle as the amount of scar tissue increases and concomitant injuries may be present. Sensory and motor function should also be evaluated. Range of motion (ROM) of the ankle and STJ should be evaluated and compared with the uninjured extremity. Muscle strength and tendon integrity should be evaluated as well. Peroneal weakness is a common finding.[12,27] Hindfoot varus, plantar-flexed first ray, or a cavus foot type should be identified because these may contribute to chronic instability of the ankle and/or STJ.[23,27,28]

The presence of associated pathologic condition must be ruled out when the foot and ankle surgeon is evaluating chronic ankle and/or subtalar instability. DiGiovanni and colleagues[29] and Strauss and colleagues[30] recognized a high percentage of patients who had concomitant peroneal tendon injury. Other pathologic conditions that must be ruled out include os trigonum lesions, lateral gutter ossicles, hindfoot varus alignment, anterior tibial spurs, tarsal coalitions, attenuated peroneal retinaculum, ankle synovitis, osteochondral fracture, anterior calcaneal process fracture, high fibular fracture, Lisfranc fracture dislocation, first metatarsal base fracture due to peroneus longus avulsion, medial malleolar fracture, deltoid ligament injury, and syndesmosis injury.[23,25,28–30] Failure to identify any of the associated injuries listed earlier leads to inappropriate treatment, recurrence of symptoms, and prolonged recovery for the athlete.

Evaluation of chronic lateral ankle instability continues with anterior drawer and talar tilt tests. A suction sign or sulcus sign over the anterolateral ankle joint during the anterior drawer test has been described as evidence of ATFL rupture.[26] STJ instability can be evaluated by attempting to displace the calcaneus anteriorly on the talus.[31] Thermann and colleagues[32] describe a rotational component in addition to the tilt in subtalar instability. The investigators use the term "chronic anterolateral rotator instability of the ankle and subtalar joint." The examination includes holding the heel and forefoot rigid with the foot in 10° dorsiflexion while an inversion and internal rotation stress is applied to the heel. An adduction stress is then applied to the forefoot. Comparison with the contralateral limb may provide information regarding the extent of the injury. These clinical maneuvers are also used for stress radiography. Standard radiographs should be obtained before any stress maneuvers if there is concern for fracture.

RADIOGRAPHIC EVALUATION

Radiographic assessment begins with the evaluation of standard weight-bearing anteroposterior, lateral, and mortise views of the ankle to evaluate alignment and rule out associated injuries. Stress radiography using the anterior drawer and talar tilt tests, either manually or mechanically with a Telos device (Telos Medical, Austin, TX, USA), can be helpful in identifying mechanical instability of the ankle joint (see **Fig. 1**).[23,33] Stress Broden views and anterior displacement of the calcaneus on the talus can be used to identify instability in the STJ.[15,31] However, these examinations are highly examiner dependent and their results have been questioned. Frost and Amendola[34] state that the large variability in the reported measurements of anterior drawer and talar tilt precludes their clinical use. The use of a local anesthetic block can often help in the evaluation of the affected and painful joint. The results of stress radiography are often used to verify the diagnosis based on clinical history taking and physical examination of the patient.

The integrity of the ATFL is examined using the anterior drawer test. The anterior movement of the talus is measured on the lateral radiograph. Greater than 10 mm of anterior translation of the talus in the ankle mortise is generally accepted as a significant finding.[35] When comparing extremities, the injured ankle should present an anterior drawer test result of 3 mm or greater to be considered significant (**Fig. 2**).[35]

The integrity of the CFL is examined with talar tilt stress radiography measured on an anteroposterior view of the ankle joint (**Fig. 3**). Many values are described in the literature regarding normal or abnormal talar tilt. Cox and Hewes[36] measured 404 ankles of 202 midshipmen in the United States Naval Academy using stress radiographs and determined that a talar tilt greater than 5° indicates significant injury to the lateral ankle ligamentous complex. Karlsson and colleagues[35] recommended abnormal values for talar tilt to be greater than 9° absolute or 3° or greater when compared with the uninjured contralateral ankle. The investigators found a predictive value of 90% for mechanical instability when using the values of anterior translation of 10 mm absolute (or 3 mm compared with contralateral ankle) and talar tilt of 9° absolute (or 3° compared with contralateral ankle).[35]

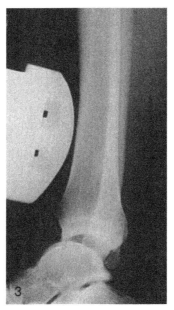

Fig. 2. Anterior drawer test with the Telos apparatus showing significant anterior subluxation of the talus in the ankle joint. (*From* Lee MS, Hofbauer MH. Evaluation and management of lateral ankle injuries. Clin Podiatr Med Surg 1999;16:659–78; with permission.)

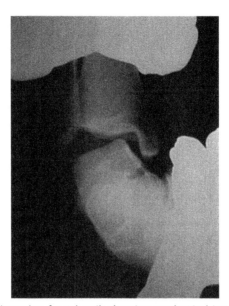

Fig. 3. Manual stress inversion for talar tilt showing mechanical instability. (*From* Lee MS, Hofbauer MH. Evaluation and management of lateral ankle injuries. Clin Podiatr Med Surg 1999;16:659–78; with permission.)

Radiographic examination of STJ instability historically involves stress Broden views.[37] To perform the stress Broden view, the examiner internally rotates the foot 40°, the beam is centered on the talonavicular joint, and the tube is angled from 20° to 50° cephalad. This positioning allows the surgeon to view different portions of the posterior facet of the STJ.[38] In 1990, Heilman and colleagues[15] published an anatomic study showing that sectioning of the CFL produced a 5-mm opening of the STJ. Thus, a lack of parallelism is demonstrated between the articular surfaces of the posterior facet. This study was consistent with the work of Laurin and colleagues[39] who sequentially sectioned the lateral ligaments in cadaveric hindfeet to show that a lack of parallelism in the posterior facet was present on inversion stress Broden views. However, the effectiveness of the stress Broden view in the diagnosis of subtalar instability has been called into question by some investigators. van Hellemondt and colleagues[40] and Sijbrandij and colleagues[41] do not support the use of stress inversion views of the STJ in the evaluation of instability. These respective studies show that when patients with suspected subtalar instability are assessed by helical computed tomography (CT), there is no evidence of subtalar tilt, although increased amounts of subtalar tilt was observed on stress radiographs. This difficulty in diagnostic imaging is thought to be in part because of the translation and rotation of the facets on one another, curvature of the articular facets, and inconsistency in the stress applied to the hindfoot during examination.[14] The surgeon must obtain a complete history of the athlete's injury, and the physical examination and radiographic examination, with or without stress radiographs, aid in the definitive diagnosis.

Other diagnostic imaging techniques for chronic ankle and STJ instability include magnetic resonance imaging (MRI), CT, arthroscopy, and arthrography. MRI can be useful in identifying which ligaments of the ankle or STJ are injured.[42,43] In the chronically unstable ankle or STJ, MRI can be useful in evaluating the joint surfaces for osteochondral defects and identifying peroneal tendon injury. O'Neill and colleagues[44] have shown that MRI results are variable and dependent on whether or not the radiologist is a specialist in identifying musculoskeletal pathologic conditions. The investigators report that the sensitivity of radiologists in identifying secondary lesions with MRI was 45%, whereas the sensitivity of surgeons was 63% when reading the MRI. O'Neill and colleagues also report that chondral lesions and peroneus brevis tears were the most commonly identified secondary pathologic condition. These results agree with the results of other investigators reporting secondary pathology.[29,30] It is therefore reasonable to obtain a preoperative MRI to rule out concomitant talar osteochondral defect and peroneal tear, which may be partially responsible for the athlete's instability.

CT has been used by some investigators to identify the presence of STJ instability. Some investigators have recommended its use because of the inaccuracies of stress radiographs.[40,41] Pearce and Buckley[45] developed a method of measuring STJ motion with CT scan. Their series of patients showed that clinical evaluation of STJ ROM was overestimated by threefold. This large discrepancy is thought to be because of the influence of soft tissues, talocrural motion, and examiner error. Beimers and colleagues[46] reported their results for the evaluation of STJ ROM. These investigators sought to quantify the extremes in ROM using multidetector CT imaging, which could then be used for the clinical evaluation of the pathologic condition. Their results revealed that the greatest relative motion in the STJ is from extreme eversion to extreme inversion. Although this result is helpful in establishing normal STJ ROM, quantification of STJ instability is still not possible using CT scan.

Arthrography of the ankle and STJs can also be used for the evaluation of ruptured ligaments and associated pathologic condition. Standard arthrography includes intra-articular injection of contrast media and the use of fluoroscopic imaging. Arthrography is typically used in the acute ankle injury to identify rupture of the ATFL, CFL, PTFL, deltoid ligaments, and tibiofibular syndesmosis.[47,48] Sugimoto and colleagues[49] stated that STJ arthrography has a sensitivity of 92% and a specificity of 87% for the diagnosis of CFL rupture in patients with recurrent ankle instability. Arthrography, although seldom used at present, can aid the surgeon in determining whether repair is required of the ATFL or of the ATFL and CFL when planning for delayed anatomic reconstruction.

Arthroscopic evaluation of the ankle or STJ can also be used for the evaluation of the pathologic condition. Although there is a learning curve associated with arthroscopy, its use allows for direct visualization of intra-articular pathologic condition. Ferkel and Chams[50] found that 95% of their patients undergoing modified Broström procedure for lateral ankle instability had associated intra-articular pathologic condition visible on arthroscopy. These investigators also report that only 20% of the intra-articular findings would have been noted at the time of the open ligament repair. They believe the addition of an arthroscopic evaluation and treatment of the associated intra-articular pathologic condition to be an important adjunct procedure to the modified Broström repair. The use of arthroscopic evaluation is not a new approach, and the findings of Ferkel and Charms are supported by others in the literature.[51,52]

It is often useful to obtain some type of diagnostic imaging when evaluating the athlete presenting with instability of the ankle and/or STJ. However, imaging does not take the place of a well-documented history taking and physical examination. Often the diagnosis of ankle and/or STJ instability can be made from the presenting symptoms and history of inversion ankle injury. Imaging studies are often most helpful in ruling out concurrent pathologic conditions.

CONSERVATIVE MANAGEMENT

The goal of treatment of lateral ankle injuries is to prevent the development of chronic functional or mechanical instability. Although most investigators agree on functional rehabilitation methods, 10% to 30% of acute injuries develop chronic lateral ankle instability.[5] Initial conservative treatment of chronic instability includes treating the acute event with which the athlete presents. This treatment includes protection, rest, ice, compression, elevation (PRICE), and physical therapy. Physical therapy typically includes strengthening peroneal musculature and improving ankle proprioceptive deficits.[23,33,53] Chronic functional instability often responds well to a functional rehabilitation program.[54,55] However, chronic mechanical instability often requires surgical intervention.

SURGICAL MANAGEMENT

The literature is replete with reports of the surgical treatment of chronic lateral ankle instability. The management of chronic subtalar instability is addressed to a much lesser degree. However, the concepts are virtually the same, establishing stability of the affected joint, allowing normal physiologic motion in adjacent joints, and preventing recurrence. These principles are made even more important in the competitive athlete.

Surgical repair of chronic ankle instability is divided into 2 types: (1) delayed primary anatomic repair and (2) nonanatomic tenodesis procedures.[56] Identification of associated STJ instability is important and can often change the surgical approach. Surgical procedures are performed only after conservative therapy has failed to relieve symptoms.

Anatomic Repair

Broström[57] first described his surgical technique for anatomic repair of chronic ligament ruptures in 1966. This involved a midsubstance repair of the ruptured ATFL, and CFL when indicated. In 1980, Gould and colleagues[58] modified the Broström technique by incorporating the inferior extensor retinaculum into the repair for added stability. The primary indication for the Broström-Gould procedure is mild to moderate mechanical instability. A review by Baumhauer and O'Brien[59] highlighted the success that this procedure has had in treating chronic lateral ankle instability. These investigators report a success rate of 85% to 95% with minimal complications. More recently, Li and colleagues[60] presented their results in the high-demand athletic population. Their results were significant in that 94% (49/52) of patients returned to their preinjury functional level after a modified Broström repair of the lateral ankle ligaments using suture anchors. Krips and colleagues[61] found that anatomic reconstruction (Broström procedure) was superior to tenodesis (Evans or Watson-Jones procedure) in all outcome measures used to evaluate functional outcome and sports activity level in 77 patients.

It is the opinion of the senior author Lee MS that patients should undergo a Broström-Gould anatomic reconstruction before a tenodesis procedure.

Broström-Gould Surgical Technique

Routinely, the senior author advocates arthroscopic inspection and debridement before the lateral ankle procedure. These procedures are often completed with the patient in the supine position with subsequent turning of the patient before initiating the Broström-Gould procedure. The Broström-Gould procedure is performed with the patient supine with a bump under the ipsilateral hip or in the lateral decubitus position. Most often, a high thigh tourniquet is used and the patient is under general or spinal anesthesia.

A curved incision is made from just anterior to the lateral malleolus and passing inferiorly to the tip of the fibula and ending just posterior to the lateral malleolus

(**Fig. 4**A). A linear incision over the lateral malleolus toward the sinus tarsi can also be used (see **Fig. 4**B). The intermediate dorsal cutaneous nerve is often encountered and must be protected. The deep fascia and peroneal tendon sheath are incised and the peroneal tendons are retracted inferiorly, allowing access to the CFL. The inferior extensor retinaculum is identified and tagged for future use in the repair. The antero-lateral capsule of the ankle joint is identified and incised exposing the ruptured ATFL. This incision is carefully placed anterior to the anterior border of the fibula to leave a cuff of tissue for proper repair of the ruptured ligaments. The proximal cuff is then slightly elevated off the distal fibula, exposing the anterior margin of the distal fibula (**Fig. 5**). Two small anchors are placed into the anterior distal fibula. The distal cuff of the ATFL is then repaired and approximated to the distal fibula using these 2 soft tissue anchors (**Fig. 6**). The proximal and distal cuffs of ATFL are then repaired in a "vest-over-pants" manner, typically using a nonabsorbable suture of the surgeons' choice (**Fig. 7**).

Attention is then turned to the repair of the CFL. In many cases, the CFL is attenu-ated and inserted into the distal fibula more in the lateral gutter. Rarely does the CFL demonstrate a midsubstance tear. When attenuation is apparent, the CFL is detached from the distal fibula and reinserted more proximally under greater tension using another anchor device. It should be noted that the foot is placed in neutral dorsiflexion and slight eversion throughout the reconstruction.

The inferior extensor retinaculum is then advanced proximally to the anterior border of the fibula or the proximal cuff of anterior talofibular tissue using an absorbable suture (**Fig. 8**). Buried knots are used during imbrication of the ligaments to prevent postoperative knot prominence and skin irritation. The ankle and STJ are checked

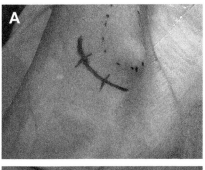
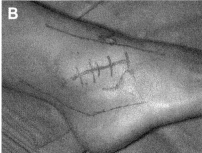

Fig. 4. (*A*) Curvilinear incision for Broström-Gould repair. (*B*) Linear incision for Broström-Gould stabilization.

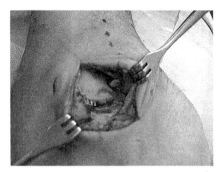

Fig. 5. Exposure of the anterior margin of the distal fibula.

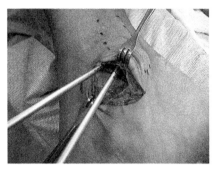

Fig. 6. Insertion of 2 corkscrew anchors in the distal fibula used to attach the distal cuff of tissue.

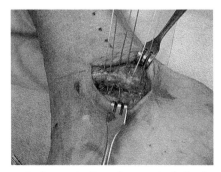

Fig. 7. Vest-over-pants repair, demonstrating placement of all sutures before tying off each throw.

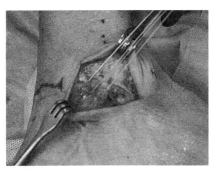

Fig. 8. Incorporation of the inferior extensor retinaculum into the repair (Gould modification).

to verify stability and normal physiologic motion. The wound is closed in layers according to the surgeon's preference.

The patient is kept non–weight-bearing for 4 weeks at which time weight bearing is initiated as tolerated. Physical therapy is used for strengthening and gait training. A recent systematic review has shown that early functional rehabilitation after surgery is superior to immobilization for 6 weeks regarding the time to return to work and sports.[62]

Tenodesing Procedures

When delayed anatomic repair fails or there are contraindications to the Broström procedure, such as significant mechanical instability or morbid obesity, the surgeon must elect for one of the tenodesing procedures.[23] There is an abundance of tenodesis procedures noted in the literature, however the 3 (1) Watson-Jones, (2) Evans, and (3) Chrisman-Snook.[4,22,33,63] These procedures use the entire peroneus brevis tendon or a portion of the brevis tendon to complete the repair. The major disadvantage of the tenodesing procedures is that it significantly reduces the postoperative hindfoot motion.[64] However, in the presence of STJ instability, this reduction of hindfoot motion may be considered advantageous. This advantage has led the Chrisman-Snook procedure to become the procedure of choice for patients with isolated STJ instability.[32]

The Chrisman-Snook tenodesis procedure reconstructs both the ATFL and CFL using a split peroneus brevis tendon transfer and passing the proximal part of the tendon graft through the fibula in an anterior to posterior direction and securing the tendon to the calcaneus near the original insertion of the CFL.[22] Colville and colleagues[65] showed that the split graft did not result in a loss of eversion strength and that its position is considered more anatomic than other tenodesis procedures. Overall results of the Chrisman-Snook procedure show more than 80% good to excellent results.[22,32,66–70] Although stiffness is a common result of tenodesis procedures, it is often a necessary tradeoff to gain stability of both the ankle joint and STJ.[28,70] However, this loss of motion does not necessarily cause a poor result as is reflected in the high percentage of good to excellent results.[28] It is evident that tenodesis procedures have their place in the treatment of chronic lateral ankle joint instability. It is important that the patient understands and accepts the loss of hindfoot motion before undergoing a tenodesis procedure.

STJ Instability Procedures

The surgical treatment of STJ instability is limited to tenodesis procedures and ligamentous reconstruction with autogenous tendon grafts. Thermann and colleagues[32] evaluated their results of treating 223 patients with chronic ankle and subtalar joint instability. Of these patients, 42 were treated with the Chrisman-Snook tenodesis procedure for isolated or combined subtalar instability. Of the 34 procedures reviewed, 31 had good to excellent results. The investigators concluded that the Chrisman-Snook tenodesis is the procedure of choice in cases of isolated subtalar joint instability. In the event of combined ankle and subtalar joint instability, the investigators recommend reinforcement of the anterolateral ankle joint complex by including the talus in the tenodesis sling. Other procedures addressed in the literature include ITCL reconstruction, ligamentous reconstruction using the entire peroneus brevis tendon to recreate the ATFL and CFL, and triligamentous reconstruction procedures to address the ruptured ATFL, CFL, ITCL, and cervical ligament.[18,19,38,71] Good results have been seen with the various procedures presented here, and careful examination of the athlete and proper planning of the surgical procedure ensure a positive outcome for the patient as well as the foot and ankle surgeon.

Chrisman-Snook Surgical Technique

The patient is placed in the lateral decubitus position. The authors prefer a 3 incisional approach as opposed to a single "hockey stick" incision. The first incision is placed over the peroneal tendons posterior to the distal fibula, a second over the sinus tarsi extending distally toward the peroneal brevis at the base of the first metatarsal, and the third laterally over the posterior tuber of the calcaneus (**Fig. 9**). The peroneal brevis tendon is identified posterior to the fibula and split in half and umbilical tape is placed through the midsubtance split. The anterior-most incision is then carried deep and distal to identify the peroneal brevis tendon sheath. A hemostat is passed distally to proximally, whereby the umbilical tape is then reversed down through the sheath. Splitting the brevis tendon is then easily completed by pulling the umbilical tape distal to the base of the fifth metatarsal. Once the tendon is split, half of it is transected proximally, so the distal half may be pulled into the anterior incision (**Fig. 10**).

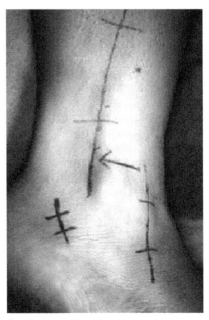

Fig. 9. Incision approach for Chrisman-Snook.

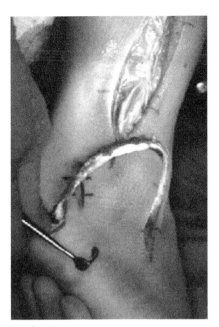

Fig. 10. Peroneal tendon graft.

A drill hole is placed anteriorly to posteriorly through the distal fibula. The tendon graft is passed subcutaneously from the base of the fifth metatarsal to superiorly to the sinus tarsi region. It is then passed anteriorly to posteriorly through the distal fibular using a tendon passer (**Fig. 11**). With the foot held in an ankle-neutral STJ-everted position, the anterior aspect of the fibular periosteum and the peroneal brevis tendon are sutured under appropriate tension using a nonabsorbable suture.

A second subcutaneous tunnel is developed from the posterior lateral malleolus to the lateral wall of the calcaneus. Orientation of the tendon should be as vertical as possible. The third incision is carried to bone and the tendon is inserted into the calcaneus using either an interference screw, stable or an anchoring device (**Fig. 12**).

Postoperatively, the patient's foot is place in a non–weight-bearing cast or boot for 4 weeks. Protective weight bearing is initiated for an additional 4 weeks, and activities and weight bearing are progressed from that point.

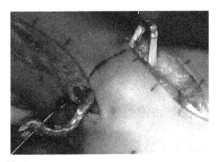

Fig. 11. Brevis through fibula.

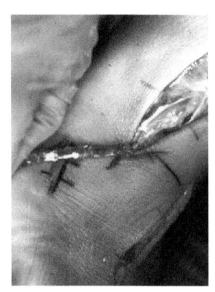

Fig. 12. Brevis into calcaneus.

Free Tendon Graft Alternative

With recent advancements in biologics, free tendon allografts have become increasingly available. The senior author now prefers to use a free semitendinosus allograft rather than half of the peroneal brevis tendon. This technique allows for the reconstruction of the ATFL and/or CFL ligaments. The graft is initially placed in the lateral talar neck using an interference screw. The tendon is then passed through the distal

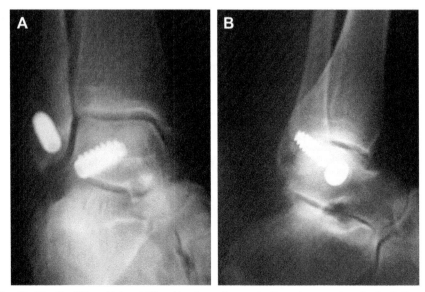

Fig. 13. Mortise (*A*) and lateral (*B*) ankle views demonstrating placement and orientation of interference screws used for a semitendinosus allograft.

fibula anteriorly to posteriorly. The foot and ankle can be positioned appropriately in a neutral dorsiflexion and STJ eversion, and then a second interference screw locks the graft in the distal fibula (**Fig. 13**). If reconstruction of the CFL is also desired, the graft can be passed distally and anchored into the lateral wall of the calcaneus using a similar technique as described in the Chrisman-Snook procedure. The postoperative technique is again similar to that described previously.

SUMMARY

Chronic ankle and STJ instability is a common clinical entity and the physician must be able to determine the exact pathologic condition for proper treatment. There are many diagnostic techniques that can be used to evaluate the ankle joint and STJ. These diagnostic techniques do not take the place of a proper patient history taking. Appropriate and aggressive rehabilitation should be attempted in all cases of chronic ankle and subtalar instability before electing surgical reconstruction. The Broström-Gould procedure is favored by the senior author in most primary cases of chronic ankle instability and has been shown to be highly successful. Tenodesing procedures of the ankle and STJs are effective, although they may hinder the athletes return to prior level of competition.

REFERENCES

1. Balduini FC, Vegzo JJ, Torg JS, et al. Management and rehabilitation of ligamentous injuries to the ankle. Am J Sports Med 1987;4:364–80.
2. Garrick JG, Requa RK. The epidemiology of foot and ankle injuries in sports. Clin Podiatr Med Surg 1989;6:629–37.
3. Freeman MA, Dean MR, Hanham IW. The etiology and prevention of functional instability of the foot. J Bone Joint Surg Br 1965;47:678–85.
4. Evans DL. Recurrent instability of the ankle-a method of surgical treatment. Proc R Soc Med 1953;46:343–4.
5. Sammarco GJ, DiRaimondo CV. Surgical treatment of lateral ankle instability syndrome. Am J Sports Med 1988;16:501–11.
6. Larsen E. Tendon transfers for lateral ankle and subtalar joint instability. Acta Orthop Scand 1988;59:168–72.
7. Rubin G, Witten M. The subtalar joint and the symptom of turning over the ankle: a new method of evaluation utilizing tomography. Am J Orthop 1962;4:16–9.
8. McCullough CJ. Rotatory stability of the load-bearing ankle. J Bone Joint Surg Br 1985;62:460–4.
9. Sarrafian SK. Anatomy of the foot and ankle. 2nd edition. Philadelphia: JB Lippincott; 1993. p. 163–71, 192–8, 477–521.
10. Colville MR, Marder RA, Boyle JJ, et al. Strain measurement in lateral ankle ligaments. Am J Sports Med 1990;18:196–200.
11. Broström L. Sprained ankles: anatomic lesions in recent sprains. Acta Chir Scand 1964;132:483–95.
12. Lofvenberg R, Karrholm J, Sundelin G, et al. Prolonged reaction time in patients with chronic lateral instability of the ankle. Am J Sports Med 1995;23:414–7.
13. Hyer CF, Lee T, Block AJ, et al. Evaluation of the anterior and middle talocalcaneal facets and the Evans osteotomy. J Foot Ankle Surg 2002;41:389–93.
14. Budny A. Subtalar joint instability: current clinical concepts. Clin Podiatr Med Surg 2004;21:449–60.
15. Heilman A, Braly G, Bishop J, et al. An anatomic study of subtalar instability. Foot Ankle 1990;10:224–8.

16. Weindel S, Schmidt R, Rammelt S, et al. Subtalar instability: a biomechanical cadaver study. Arch Orthop Trauma Surg 2010;130:313–9.
17. Kamada K, Watanabe S, Yamamoto H. Chronic subtalar instability due to insufficiency of the calcaneofibular ligament: a case report. Foot Ankle Int 2002;23:1135–7.
18. Zwipp H, Rammelt S, Grass R. Ligamentous injuries about the ankle and subtalar joints. Clin Podiatr Med Surg 2002;19:195–229.
19. Pisani G. Chronic laxity of the subtalar joint. Orthopedics 1996;19:431–7.
20. Meyer J, Garcia J, Hoffmeyer P, et al. The subtalar sprain: a roentgenographic study. Clin Orthop Relat Res 1986;226:169–73.
21. Hertel J, Denegar C, Monroe M, et al. Talocrural and subtalar joint instability after lateral ankle sprain. Med Sci Sports Exerc 1999;21:1501–8.
22. Chrisman OD, Snook GA. Reconstruction of lateral ligament tears of the ankle. An experimental study and clinical evaluation of seven patients treated by a new modification of the Elmslie procedure. J Bone Joint Surg Am 1969;51:904–12.
23. Lee MS, Hofbauer MH. Evaluation and management of lateral ankle injuries. Clin Podiatr Med Surg 1999;16:659–78.
24. Freeman MA. Instability of the foot after injuries to the lateral ligaments of the ankle. J Bone Joint Surg Br 1965;47:669–77.
25. Schenck RC, Coughlin MJ. Lateral ankle instability and revision surgery alternatives in the athlete. Foot Ankle Clin 2009;14:205–14.
26. Trevino SG, Davis P, Hecht PJ. Management of acute and chronic lateral ligament injuries of the ankle. Orthop Clin North Am 1994;25:1–16.
27. Bosien WR, Staples OS, Russell SW. Residual disability following acute ankle sprains. J Bone Joint Surg Am 1955;37:1237–49.
28. Sammarco VJ. Complications of lateral ankle ligament reconstruction. Clin Orthop Relat Res 2001;391:123–32.
29. DiGiovanni BF, Fraga CJ, Cohen BE, et al. Associated injuries found in chronic lateral ankle instability. Foot Ankle Int 2000;21:809–15.
30. Strauss JE, Forsberg JA, Lippert FG. Chronic lateral ankle instability and associated conditions: a rationale for treatment. Foot Ankle Int 2007;28:1041–4.
31. Kato T. The diagnosis and treatment of instability of the subtalar joint. J Bone Joint Surg Br 1995;77:400–6.
32. Thermann H, Zwipp H, Tscherne H. Treatment algorithm for chronic ankle and subtalar instability. Foot Ankle Int 1997;18:163–9.
33. DiGiovanni CW, Brodsky A. Current concepts: lateral ankle instability. Foot Ankle Int 2006;27:854–66.
34. Frost SC, Amendola A. Is stress radiography necessary in the diagnosis of acute or chronic ankle instability? Clin J Sport Med 1999;9:40–5.
35. Karlsson J, Bergsten T, Lansigner O, et al. Surgical treatment of chronic lateral instability of the ankle joint. Am J Sports Med 1989;17:268–74.
36. Cox JS, Hewes TF. "Normal" talar tilt angle. Clin Orthop Relat Res 1979;140:37–41.
37. Broden B. Roentgen examination of the subtaloid joint in fractures of the calcaneus. Acta Radiol 1949;31:85–91.
38. Keefe DT, Haddad SL. Subtalar instability. Etiology, diagnosis, and management. Foot Ankle Clin 2002;7:577–609.
39. Laurin CA, Ouellet R, St-Jacques R. Talar and subtalar tilt: an experimental investigation. Can J Surg 1968;11:270–9.
40. van Hellemondt FJ, Louwerens JW, Sijbrandij ES, et al. Stress radiography and stress examination of the talocrural and subtalar joint on helical computed tomography. Foot Ankle Int 1997;18:482–8.

41. Sijbrandij ES, van Gils AP, van Hellemondt FJ, et al. Assessing the subtalar joint: the Broden view revisited. Foot Ankle Int 2001;22:329–33.
42. Verhaven EF, Shahbpour M, Handelberg FW, et al. The accuracy of three-dimensional magnetic resonance imaging in the diagnosis of ruptures of the lateral ligaments of the ankle. Am J Sports Med 1991;19:583–7.
43. Mabit C, Boncoeur-Martel MP, Chaudruc JM, et al. Anatomic and MRI study of the subtalar ligamentous support. Surg Radiol Anat 1997;19:111–7.
44. O'Neill PJ, Van Aman SE, Guyton GE. Is MRI adequate to detect lesions in patients with ankle instability? Clin Orthop Relat Res 2010;468:1115–9.
45. Pearce TJ, Buckley RE. Subtalar joint movement: clinical and computed tomography scan correlation. Foot Ankle Int 1999;20:428–32.
46. Beimers L, Tuijthof GJ, Blankevoort L, et al. In-vivo range of motion of the subtalar joint using computed tomography. J Biomech 2008;41:1390–7.
47. Trnka HJ, Ivanic G, Trattnig S. Arthrography of the foot and ankle: ankle and subtalar joint. Foot Ankle Clin 2000;5:49–62.
48. Sugimoto K, Samoto N, Takaoka T, et al. Subtalar arthrography in acute injuries of the calcaneofibular ligament. J Bone Joint Surg Br 1998;80:785–90.
49. Sugimoto K, Takakura Y, Samoto N, et al. Subtalar arthrography in recurrent instability of the ankle. Clin Orthop Relat Res 2002;394:169–76.
50. Ferkel RD, Chams RN. Chronic lateral instability: arthroscopic findings and long-term results. Foot Ankle Int 2007;28:24–31.
51. Hintermann B, Boss A, Schafer D. Arthroscopic findings in patients with chronic ankle instability. Am J Sports Med 2002;30:402–9.
52. Komenda GA, Ferkel RD. Arthroscopic findings associated with the unstable ankle. Foot Ankle Int 1999;20:708–13.
53. DiGiovanni BF, Partal G, Baumhauer JF. Acute ankle injury and chronic lateral instability in the athlete. Clin Sports Med 2004;23:1–19.
54. Webster KA, Gribble PA. Functional rehabilitation interventions for chronic ankle instability: a systematic review. J Sport Rehabil 2010;19:98–114.
55. Hale SA, Hertel J, Olmsted-Kramer LC. The effect of a 4-week comprehensive rehabilitation program on postural control and lower extremity function in individuals with chronic ankle instability. J Orthop Sports Phys Ther 2007;37: 303–11.
56. Keller M, Grossman J, Caron M, et al. Lateral ankle instability and the Broström-Gould procedure. J Foot Ankle Surg 1996;35:513–20.
57. Broström L. Sprained ankles VI. Surgical treatment of "chronic" ligament ruptures. Acta Chir Scand 1966;132:551–65.
58. Gould N, Seligson D, Gassman J. Early and late repair of lateral ligament of the ankle. Foot Ankle 1980;1:84–9.
59. Baumhauer JF, O'Brien T. Surgical considerations in the treatment of ankle instability. J Athl Train 2002;37:458–62.
60. Li X, Killie H, Guerrero P, et al. Anatomic reconstruction for chronic lateral ankle instability in the high demand athlete: functional outcomes after the modified Brotrom repair using suture anchors. Am J Sports Med 2009;37:488–94.
61. Krips R, van Dijk N, Lehtonen H, et al. Sports activity level after surgical treatment for anterolateral ankle instability: a multicenter study. Am J Sports Med 2002;30: 13–9.
62. De Vries JS, Krips R, Sierevelt IN, et al. Interventions for treating chronic ankle instability. Cochrane Database Syst Rev 2006;4:CD004124.
63. Watson-Jones R. Recurrent forward dislocation of the ankle joint. J Bone Joint Surg Br 1952;34:519.

64. Rosenbaum D, Becker HP, Wilke HJ, et al. Tenodeses destroy the kinematic coupling of the ankle joint complex. A three-dimensional in vitro analysis of joint movement. J Bone Joint Surg Br 1998;80:162–8.
65. Colville M, Marder R, Zarins B. Reconstruction of the lateral ankle ligaments. A biomechanical analysis. Am J Sports Med 1992;20:594–600.
66. Hennrikus WL, Mapes RC, Lyons PM, et al. Outcomes of the Chrisman-Snook and modified Broström procedures for chronic lateral ankle instability. A prospective, randomized comparison. Am J Sports Med 1996;24:400–4.
67. Rechtine GR, McCarroll JR, Webster DA. Reconstruction for chronic lateral instability of the ankle: a review of twenty-eight patients. Orthopedics 1982;5:46–50.
68. Riegler HF. Reconstruction for lateral instability of the ankle. J Bone Joint Surg Am 1984;66:336–9.
69. Savastano AA, Lowe EB. Ankle sprains: surgical treatment for recurrent sprains. Am J Sports Med 1980;8:208–11.
70. Snook GA, Chrisman OD, Wilson TC. Long-term results of the Chrisman-Snook operation for reconstruction of the lateral ligaments of the ankle. J Bone Joint Surg Am 1985;67:1–7.
71. Schon L, Clanton T, Baxter D. Reconstruction for subtalar instability: a review. Foot Ankle 1991;11:319–25.

Lateral Ankle Triad: The Triple Injury of Ankle Synovitis, Lateral Ankle Instability, and Peroneal Tendon Tear

Justin Franson, DPM[a,b,*], Bob Baravarian, DPM[c]

KEYWORDS

• Peroneal • Ankle • Instability • Synovitis • Lateral ankle triad

Many articles have been published that discuss various lateral ankle injuries and specific lateral ankle pathology. The purpose of this article is to explore and present a specific combination of findings that the author's multiphysician practice has noticed on a frequently recurring basis. A triple injury of ankle synovitis, ankle instability, and peroneal tendon tear are described herein, termed the Lateral Ankle Triad. While it is common to find each of these specific injuries individually, they are often found in combination. Lateral ankle sprains have been shown to be associated with chronic ankle instability.[1] Peroneal tendon tears are often associated with other disorders such as chronic tenosynovitis, severe ankle sprains, ankle fractures, and chronic ankle instability.[2] Following a discussion of the Lateral Ankle Triad injury complex, a retrospective review of 33 peroneal tendon surgeries is presented and discussed.

DISCUSSION

Twenty-one percent of athletic injuries have been said to be inversion ankle injuries.[3] Lateral ankle injuries are very common, with an estimated 27,000 ankle sprains occurring daily in the United States.[4] Of lateral ankle injuries, a torn anterior talofibular ligament is the most frequent pathologic finding.[4] The majority of lateral ankle sprains successfully heal without sequelae, despite common undertreatment by the general

The author has nothing to disclose.

[a] University Foot & Ankle Institute, 26357 McBean Parkway, Suite 250, Valencia, CA 91355, USA
[b] West Los Angeles VA Medical Center, West Los Angeles, CA 90073, USA
[c] University Foot & Ankle Institute, 212 Wilshire Boulevard, Suite 101, Santa Monica, CA 90403
* University Foot & Ankle Institute, 26357 McBean Parkway, Suite 250, Valencia, CA 91355.
E-mail address: justinjfranson@gmail.com

population and initial treating physicians. Ankle sprains, like broken toes, suffer from a misperception in the general public that there is usually "nothing that can be done for it," so individuals avoid seeking medical evaluation and treatment following an ankle sprain. This could be one reason why there is such a high rate of recurrence and lingering disability following a "routine" ankle sprain. There is minimal initial immobilization, there is rapid return to weight bearing, and there is infrequent rehabilitation and a loss of proprioception.

Although many ankle sprains heal well, approximately 15% to 20% of these patients experience persistent pain or instability.[5] Other sources have related that 40% will continue to report residual disability[6]; this percentage has also been shown to be even much higher.[7,8] One study reported that 73% of ankle sprain patients at a regional primary care facility over a 1-year period had residual symptoms 6 to 18 months following medical evaluation.[7] Another study reported 59% of 380 athletes had residual symptoms and disability that impaired their performance.[8] Many of these patients will not be seen in a foot and ankle physician's office for evaluation until their injury has failed to heal as expected.

The peroneal tendon tear is commonly missed the first time around, as it typically occurs in the presence of an inversion ankle injury. One study reports that only 60% (24 of 40) of peroneal tendon disorders were accurately diagnosed at the first clinical evaluation.[9] These injuries are often carelessly lumped into the diagnosis of "another ankle sprain," which is usually casually treated with some simple PRICE (protection, rest, ice, compression, elevation) advice from the emergency room or urgent care physician, nurse practitioner, or physican's assistant. Despite great evidence that shows that early aggressive treatment with compression and icing can greatly reduce recovery time, ankle sprains are commonly undertreated. A study demonstrated that those who use cryotherapy within 36 hours of injury reached full activity in an average of 13.2 days, compared with an average of 30.4 days for those beginning cryotherapy after 36 hours and 33.3 days for those treated with heat.[10]

What are the common threads among these patients who deal with prolonged pain, swelling, instability, and dysfunction in the lateral ankle? Many will ultimately be found to have chronic ligamentous tears, some with associated peroneal tendon pathology. This condition can range from simple tenosynovitis, to the more involved and recalcitrant tendinosis, and to an assortment of peroneal tendon tears. Peroneal tendon pathology usually is found in the presence of repetitive and prolonged activity, especially following a period of decreased activity.[11] While it is obvious that all recalcitrant ankle sprains will not neatly fit into the Lateral Ankle Triad, it is a common pattern of injury that can help guide in the selection of appropriate imaging modalities, as well as the surgical approach if and when surgery is indicated.

ANATOMY

Anatomy relevant to the Lateral Ankle Triad includes the peroneus longus and brevis with its associated tendon sheath, and the lateral collateral ankle ligaments, including the anterior talofibular, calcaneal fibular, and posterior talofibular ligament.

The peroneal tendons originate from the peroneal muscle, which are innervated by the superficial peroneal nerve and are housed in lateral leg compartment. The peroneus longus tendon runs posterior to the peroneus brevis tendon in the distal leg and at the level of the ankle. The tendons share a synovial sheath beginning about 4 cm above the distal tip of the fibula.[12] The tendons travel along and through the fibrocartilage-lined retromalleolar groove, on the posterior surface of the distal fibula. The shape of this groove can have a bearing on peroneal tendon dislocation and subluxation. The peroneal tendons are secured within the retromalleolar groove by the superficial peroneal retinaculum.

As the peroneal tendons change angle and course around the tip of the lateral malleolus, the common peroneal tendon sheath bifurcates. The peroneus brevis travels a simple and straight path to its insertion at the base of the fifth metatarsal. The peroneus longus has a more complex distal anatomic path: it runs intimate to and just beneath the peroneal tubercle on the lateral wall of the calcaneus on its way to the cuboid notch or groove, where it angles medially to its insertion at the plantar first metatarsal base and medial cuneiform. The os peroneum is a common finding at the lateral cuboid, and is sometimes implicated in the development of a symptomatic peroneus longus tendon.

The peroneus brevis everts and abducts the foot, and plantarflexes the ankle. The peroneus longus also everts the foot, and has a secondary plantarflexion effect on the ankle. It plantarflexes the first ray and stabilizes the medial column during the stance phase of gait. The peroneal tendons are dynamic stabilizers of the lateral ankle ligaments.[12]

The mechanism of acute injury to the peroneal tendons is plantarflexion and inversion of the ankle, with the foot in a weight-bearing position. This stance places the peroneal tendons in a taut position, exposing them to injury.

CLINICAL FINDINGS

Patients who develop the Lateral Ankle Triad will usually present with a history of ankle sprain, complaints of pain, persistent swelling, and a sense of instability in the ankle. Clinical findings include localized edema, which tends to center at the anterolateral ankle joint and the sinus tarsi area, overlying the anterior talofibular ligament. A path of longitudinal edema along the course of the peroneal tendons is a sure sign that the injury is more complex than a typical ankle sprain, and indicates some level of peroneal tendon pathology. Intrasheath edema and tenosynovitis, which often accompanies peroneal tendon tears, will cause this pattern of longitudinal edema.

Palpation tenderness is almost always present directly over the injured ligament(s) and tendon tear. Slow and methodical anterior ankle joint line palpation, combined with minor joint motion and manipulation, can help assess the presence of anterior joint capsule pathology. Palpation of the anterolateral joint with simultaneous inversion stress can help identify the presence of fibrous bands and adhesions, which commonly accompany chronic ankle sprains. Careful evaluation of the ankle joint itself will help direct the possible selection of an arthroscopy in addition to the tendon and ligament repair.

Ankle joint stress maneuvers should be performed in the workup and evaluation of the Lateral Ankle Triad. Inversion stress testing with the ankle joint in a dorsiflexed and plantarflexed position can help evaluate the integrity of the anterior talofibular and calcaneal fibular ligaments. Laxity is usually found in ankle inversion stress, which will also commonly elicit pain. Anterior drawer stress testing evaluates the strength of the anterior talofibular ligament. In the presence of a tear or attenuation of this ligament, increased anterior migration of the ankle joint is felt, and pain is often accompanied with the stress range of motion.

Isolated muscle stress testing of the peroneals is performed bilaterally, with care to note weakness or pain elicited. In the presence of split, longitudinal tears of the peroneal tendons, weakness is not commonly found unless the tear is chronic. Complete ruptures will obviously result in loss of strength in the peroneal tendon complex, but complete tears are much less common than the typical longitudinal pattern.

IMAGING

Routine, 3-view radiographs of the ankle should be obtained in the thorough evalua-tion of suspected Lateral Ankle Triad. Even though the suspicion is for soft tissue pathology, the ankle joint is examined for symmetry, spacing, and alignment; radio-graphs can help rule out avulsion fractures of the distal fibula, osteochondral lesions, exostosis, arthritis and periarticular changes, joint diastasis, angular deformity, bone cysts, lateral process talar fractures, avulsion injury at peroneal retinaculum, and os trigonum pathology. In the presence of distal peroneal tendon symptoms, dorsoplan-tar and lateral oblique radiographs of the foot should also be obtained to rule out avul-sion injury at the fifth metatarsal base or the presence/absence of an os peroneum.

Stress radiography is also recommended, and includes anterior drawer stress and inversion/talar tilt images; these are compared with the asymptomatic contralateral side. Chronic ankle instability is sometimes bilateral, however, though symptoms may be more prominent unilaterally.

Diagnostic ultrasonography has been shown to be an effective imaging modality in the evaluation of the lateral ankle. It can be used to image the lateral collateral ankle ligaments, and has a high specificity and sensitivity in finding peroneal tendon tears.[13] There are some practical advantages to the use of ultrasonography; it can offer imme-diate diagnosis and avoid delays in treatment, it is less expensive than magnetic reso-nance imaging (MRI), it avoids exposure to radiation, and it can be used dynamically.[14] However, ultrasonography does require significant skill by the physician or technician in performing and interpreting the scan to diagnose with confidence.

MRI of the ankle is indicated and recommended in the presence of patients with persistent lateral ankle pain and swelling who have not responded to typical conser-vative treatment. In addition to ruling out osteochondral lesions, MRI is sensitive and specific in the evaluation of the lateral collateral ankle ligaments and the peroneal tendons. It is less reliable in detecting ankle joint synovitis, fibrous bands, and small loose bodies. MRI also does not always offer good visualization of the cuboid tunnel where pathology is likely to exist in distal peroneal tendinitis.[14]

PREDISPOSING FACTORS IN THE LATERAL ANKLE TRIAD

The triple injury of ankle synovitis, ankle instability, and peroneal tendon tears will usually have some common predisposing factors. In most cases, there is a history of lateral ankle sprain, and often there are recurrent sprains. The mechanism of injury that causes peroneal tendon tears has been described as plantarflexion with inver-sion.[15] In the absence of an acute tear, chronic tendon tears can result from repetitive activities in the presence of chronic ankle instability. With this underlying laxity, there is additional excursion available in the ankle joint with normal day-to-day motion, but especially in the presence of strenuous activities and repetitive exercise. Over time, this leads to the development of ankle joint synovitis, and sometimes to the formation of anterolateral joint fibrous bands that are frequently discovered arthroscopically.

Other predisposing and/or contributing factors in the development of the Lateral Ankle Triad include a low-lying peroneal muscle belly, presence of a peroneus quartus muscle, pes cavus foot type, peroneal tendon dislocation or subluxation, abnormal shape and depth of the retrofibular groove, hypertrophic peroneal tubercle, equinus, repetitive activities such as running and dancing, and a sudden onset of aggressive exercise following a period of inactivity.

Equinus is not typically cited as a contributing factor in the cases of chronic ankle ligament and peroneal tendon tears, but its effect should be considered. The mecha-nism of injury to the peroneal tendons is when the foot is weight bearing, and the ankle is plantarflexed and inverted. Patients with significant equinus deformity will function in a constant plantarflexed position of the ankle. Similar to cavus foot type, which places the foot and ankle in an inverted position, equinus can have a strong contributing effect on potential compromise and stress to the lateral ankle by keeping the ankle in a less stable, plantarflexed attitude. The effect of equinus on chronic ankle instability should be examined further, as successful treatment of the lateral ankle requires comprehensive management of the contributing factors. A beautiful peroneal tendon repair in an uncorrected cavovarus foot may be considered unacceptable, just as a simple posterior tibial tendon repair in the presence of a collapsing flatfoot deformity is considered not strong enough to hold up over time.

FACTORS TO CONSIDER

The Lateral Ankle Triad should be considered in all cases of chronic lateral ankle instability, and care should be taken to evaluate all 3 components: integrity of the lateral collateral ligaments, possible presence of intra-articular synovitis, and the level of injury to the peroneal tendons. Acute ankle sprain with peroneal tendon tear that requires surgical repair would have less indication to consider ankle arthroscopy, but strong consideration should be given in cases of chronic ankle instability and chronic peroneal tendon pathology.

MRI will often reveal the presence of a chronically torn anterior talofibular ligament, with pathology in the calcaneal fibular ligament sometimes found as well. Posterior talofibular ligament tears are found less frequently. In an article that analyzed 639 ankle injuries, of 547 patients with ankle sprains that did not cause a fracture, the anterior talofibular ligament was injured 83% of the time (453 of 547). The calcaneal fibular ligament was injured at a rate of 67% (366 of 547), and the posterior talofibular ligament at 34% (187 of 547). Injuries to the ankle joint capsule in this study occurred in 180 cases and to the peroneal tendons in 83 cases.[16]

A study from Germany discussed surgical findings with anterior ankle partial synovectomy. Of the 35 patients studied, 8 were noted to have hyperlaxity of the ankle joint (**Fig. 1**).[17]

One study reported that in the presence of chronic ankle instability, peroneus brevis tendon tears were observed in 25% of the cases, with 77% of patients having tenosynovitis.[18]

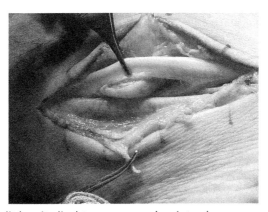

Fig. 1. Common split longitudinal tear, peroneus brevis tendon.

The peroneus brevis tears far more frequently than the peroneus longus. In a retrospective review of peroneal tendon injuries, Dombek and colleagues[9] related that 88% of peroneal tendon tears occurred to the brevis tendon, and only 13% to the peroneus longus (**Fig. 2**).

SURGICAL APPROACH

In terms of surgical correction of the Lateral Ankle Triad, the approach can be somewhat routine and reproducible. Ankle arthroscopy is performed with a standard 2-portal approach to the anterior ankle. In the absence of talar dome lesions, the procedure can typically be performed without a joint distractor. The joint is inspected in a step-wise approach and synovitis and fibrous bands are debrided appropriately (**Fig. 3**).

A longitudinal curvilinear incision is made just posterior to the distal fibula and curved distally along the course of the peroneal tendons. The incision is centered over the peroneal tendon pathology, extending more proximally or distally based on MRI documentation of the location of the tendon tear. Meticulous soft tissue dissection is of ultimate importance in the lateral ankle, as sural neuritis is a far too common postoperative complication following lateral ankle and foot surgery.

Laxity in the peroneal retinaculum can be observed and later tightened and repaired as necessary. The peroneal tendon sheath is exposed and examined. Straw-colored tenosynovitis fluid is often drained on first opening the sheath, a representation of the inflammatory process within the sheath. It is recommended to put the ankle through range of motion and stress testing while visualizing and palpating the peroneal tendon sheath to evaluate for subluxing or dislocating tendons. The peroneal tendon sheath is incised longitudinally above and below the tendon tear to allow for adequate debridement and repair. Achieving adequate exposure is important as attempting repair while tunneling under the proximal or distal extent of the incision can increase the risk of inadvertent sural nerve laceration or entrapment with suture material (**Fig. 4**).

There are commonly accepted principles in the surgical approach to peroneal tendon tears. If less than 50% of the tendon is torn, primary repair, debridement, and tubularization is indicated.[19] For extensive tearing that involves more than 50% of the tendon, tendon grafting or side-to-side anastomosis/tenodesis to the adjacent peroneal tendon is indicated.[19,20] In cases of tendinosis, debridement can be performed, with a consideration for Topaz radiofrequency coblation or platelet-rich plasma.

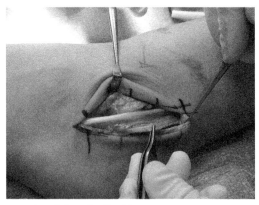

Fig. 2. Chronic peroneus brevis longitudinal tear.

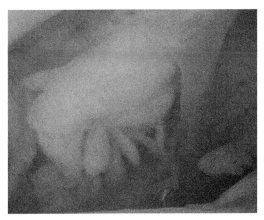

Fig. 3. Ankle synovitis with fibrous band.

Lateral ankle ligament repair can be approached according to the surgeon's preference. The majority of the author's procedures follows the principles outlined by Brostrom[21] and Gould and colleagues,[22] and includes attempts to anatomically restore the anterior talofibular and calcaneal fibular ligaments, reinforced with imbrication of the extensor retinaculum. Bone anchors are sometimes required, and can be directed by MRI findings (which can show avulsion-type ligament tears) or intraoperative findings (**Fig. 5**).

Patients are typically casted for 3 to 4 weeks following surgery for the Lateral Ankle Triad. There has been a recent push to shorten the period of immobilization and to encourage early range of motion, and to initiate physical therapy at 2 to 3 weeks postoperatively.

RETROSPECTIVE ANALYSIS

A retrospective review of peroneal tendon surgery performed by surgeons at the University Foot & Ankle Institute in Southern California was completed for a span of 16 months, extending from September 2008 to December 2009. All peroneal tendon surgeries performed during this time frame were included, with a total of 33 patients

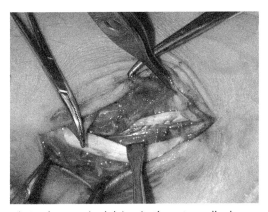

Fig. 4. Peroneus brevis tendon repaired, lying in the retromalleolar groove.

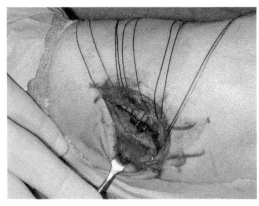

Fig. 5. Modified Brostrom lateral ankle stabilization repair.

and their surgical procedures reviewed. All 33 patients had an MRI performed preoperatively, with 91% showing evidence of peroneal tendinitis, tendinosis, or a peroneal tendon tear. Three cases with peroneal tendon tears observed surgically did not show a tear on the preoperative MRI. Intraoperative findings often show more significant pathology than the MRI.[20]

The average patient age was 45 years, with a range of 14 to 65 years. There were 15 males and 18 females. The average duration of symptoms before surgery was 3.6 years, though 39% (13 of 33) had symptoms for 6 months or less.

The review showed and confirmed that peroneal tendon tears predominantly affect the peroneus brevis tendon. The case review showed that 12% had combined peroneus brevis and longus tendon tears (4 of 33). Eighty-two percent of the cases had an isolated peroneus brevis tear (27 of 33), and solitary peroneus longus tears occurred in only 6% of the study (2 of 33). Including the dual tears found, 94% of cases had a peroneus brevis tendon tear (31 of 33), while 18% had involvement of the peroneus longus tendon (6 of 33) (**Fig. 6**).

The same 33 cases were reviewed in regard of the lateral ankle ligaments. Seventy-three percent of these patients (24 of 33) with a peroneal tendon tear had associated attenuation, chronic thickening, or tears of lateral ankle ligaments, which were surgically repaired concurrently.

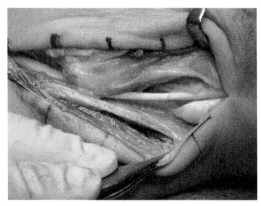

Fig. 6. A neglected peroneus longus rupture with proximal retraction.

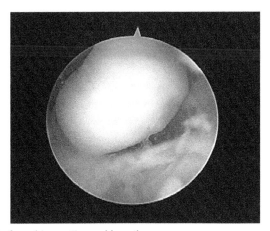

Fig. 7. Loose body found in routine ankle arthroscopy.

Fifty-five percent of the cases included in the review (18 of 33) also underwent an ankle arthroscopy as a combined procedure. Each of the cases that included surgical arthroscopy included anterior ankle synovectomy (18 of 18); none of the cases had a pristine anterior ankle joint, and each of them underwent debridement of the synovitis. Of the 18 arthroscopy procedures reviewed, 33% (6 of 18) had fibrous bands present, which were debrided arthroscopically. Fibrous bands are not typically appreciated on MRI, are usually found at the anterolateral joint gutter, and can cause lateral ankle pain, limitations in joint motion, and an uncomfortable catching sensation of the ankle joint. Especially in athletes, fibrous bands can be a subtle contribution to persistent ankle pain.

Eleven percent of the cases who underwent arthroscopy also noted the presence of loose bodies, which were surgically debrided and excised. As with fibrous bands, MRI does not always pick up the presence of small anterior ankle joint loose bodies (**Fig. 7**).

In cases of lateral ankle pain with an MRI that confirms a peroneal tendon tear or tendinosis with associated ligamentous pathology, the author would assert that strong consideration should be made to include an ankle arthroscopy. It is not always indicated, however. An acute injury, with a fresh peroneal tendon tear, with no anterior or anterolateral joint symptoms would not warrant the inclusion of an ankle arthroscopy. In the analysis, of the 18 cases that included an arthroscopy, the average duration of symptoms before surgical intervention was 5.6 years. The average duration before surgery for all the cases reviewed was 3.6 years. This result shows a trend to consider ankle arthroscopy as an adjunctive procedure to the tendon and ligament repair in the more chronic cases, as these are more likely to have caused damage to the ankle joint itself.

SUMMARY

The Lateral Ankle Triad is a combination of ankle joint synovitis, chronic lateral ankle instability, with a peroneal tendon tear. A follow-up article is already in progress, which will include a 10-year retrospective analysis of the Lateral Ankle Triad procedures performed within the author's multiphysician practice. This analysis will solidify trends and will help direct further treatment, as well as the formation of protocols and clinical and surgical recommendations. The main recommendations to be considered are: obtain MRI in the thorough evaluation of peroneal tendon pathology; assess the lateral collateral ankle ligaments for instability even in the presence of no MRI documentation of ligament tears; consider arthroscopy as an adjunctive procedure to address more subtle changes such as joint synovitis and fibrous bands.

The Lateral Ankle Triad should help clinicians consider this possible combination of injury, which with a careful workup can help uncover more subtle changes that can occur in the presence of chronic ankle instability and peroneal tendon tears.

REFERENCES

1. Hubbard TJ, Kaminski TW, Vander Griend RA, et al. Quantitative assessment of mechanical laxity in the functionally unstable ankle. Med Sci Sports Exerc 2004;36(5):760–6.
2. Clarke HD, Kitaoka HB, Ehman RL. Peroneal tendon injuries. Foot Ankle Int 1998; 19:280–8.
3. Kannus P. Treatment for acute tears of the lateral ligaments of the ankle. J Bone Joint Surg Am 1991;73A:305–12.
4. Mizel MS, Hecht PJ, Marymont JV, et al. Evaluation and treatment of chronic ankle pain. J Bone Joint Surg Am 2004;86:628–32.
5. Bynum JA, Crates JM, Aziz-Jacobo J, et al. Modified Brostrom technique using knotless suture anchors. Tech Foot Ankle 2010;9:29–31.
6. Safran M, Benedetti R, Bartolozzi A, et al. Lateral ankle sprains: a comprehensive review. Part 1: etiology, pathoanatomy, histopathogenesis, and diagnosis. Med Sci Sports Exerc 1999;31:S429–37.
7. Braun BL. Effects of ankle sprain in a general clinic population 6 to 18 months after medical evaluation. Arch Fam Med 1999;8:143–8.
8. Yeung MS, Chan KM, So CH, et al. An epidemiologic survey on ankle sprain. Br J Sports Med 1994;28:112–6.
9. Dombek MF, Lamm BM, Saltrick K, et al. Peroneal tendon tears: a retrospective review. J Foot Ankle Surg 2003;42:250–8.
10. Hocutt JE, Jaffee R, Rylander R, et al. Cryotherapy in ankle sprains. Am J Sports Med 1982;10:316–9.
11. Molloy R, Tisdel C. Failed treatment of peroneal tendon injuries. Foot Ankle Clin 2003;8:115–29, ix.
12. Heckman DS, Reddy S, Pedowitz D, et al. Operative treatment for peroneal tendon disorders. J Bone Joint Surg Am 2008;90:404–18.
13. Grant T, Kelikian A, Jereb S, et al. Ultrasound diagnosis of peroneal tendon tears: a surgical correlation. J Bone Joint Surg Am 2005;87:1788–94.
14. Ritter C. Acute peroneal tendon tears. Tech Foot Ankle Surg 2009;8:106–11.
15. Speer KS, Bassett F. Longitudinal rupture of the peroneal tendons. Am J Sports Med 1993;21:354–7.
16. Fallat L, Grimm DJ, Saracco JA. Sprained ankle syndrome: Prevalence and analysis of 639 acute injuries. J Foot Ankle Surg 1998;37:280–5.
17. Jerosch J, Steinbeck J, Schroder M, et al. Arthroscopic treatment of anterior synovitis of the ankle in athletes. Knee Surg Sports Traumatol Arthrosc 1994; 2(3):176–81.
18. DiGiovanni BF, Fraga CJ, Cohen BE, et al. Associated injuries found in chronic lateral ankle instability. Foot Ankle Int 2000;21:809–15.
19. Krause JO, Brodsky JW. Peroneus brevis tendon tears: pathophysiology, surgical reconstruction, and clinical results. Foot Ankle Int 1998;19:271–9.

20. Redfern D, Myerson M. The management of concomitant tears of the peroneus longus and brevis tendons. Foot Ankle Int 2004;25:695–707.
21. Brostrom L. Sprained ankles: VI. Surgical treatment of "chronic" ligament ruptures. Acta Chir Scand 1966;132:551–65.
22. Gould N, Selingson D, Gassman J. Early and late repair of lateral ligaments of the ankle. Foot Ankle 1980;1:84–9.

Acute and Chronic Achilles Tendon Ruptures in Athletes

Jonathan Thompson, DPM[a,b],*, Bob Baravarian, DPM[c,d]

KEYWORDS

• Achilles tendon rupture • Athletes • Rehabilitation

Achilles tendon injuries are one of the most common injuries in athletes. The Achilles tendon is the largest and strongest tendon in the human body and is composed of the gastrocnemius and the soleus muscles[1] to create a musculotendinous complex (triceps surae) that crosses the knee, ankle, and subtalar joint. The Achilles tendon is subjected to extensive static and dynamic loads and can be subjected to loads 2 to 3 times the body weight with walking and up to 10 times the body weight with certain other athletic activities.[2,3] The Achilles tendon is the most injured tendon of athletes in the lower extremities and has been noted to be the most common tendon to rupture spontaneously.[4]

ANATOMY

The Achilles tendon is in the superficial posterior compartment of the leg and is formed from tendinous continuations of the 2 muscle bellies of the gastrocnemius and soleus muscles, inserting primarily on the central middle portion of the posterior calcaneus as well as providing fibers that extend around the heel to blend in with the plantar fascia.[5] The plantaris tendon (absent in 7%–20% of individuals) is located medial to the Achilles tendon apparatus and inserts medial and anterior to the Achilles complex.[5,6] The Achilles tendon receives its main blood supply to the midportion of the tendon from the paratenon, more proximally from the recurrent branch of the posterior tibial artery and the local small muscular branches and distally from the rete arteriosum calcaneare supplied by the posterior and fibular arteries.[5,7,8] The Achilles tendon is

The author has nothing to disclose.

[a] University Foot and Ankle Institute, Private Practice, 1101 Sepulveda Boulevard, Suite 104, Manhattan Beach, CA, USA

[b] University Foot and Ankle Institute, Private Practice, 2121 Wilshire Boulevard, Suite 101, Santa Monica, CA 90403, USA

[c] University Foot and Ankle Institute, Private Practice, 2121 Wilshire Boulevard, Suite 101, Santa Monica, CA 90403, USA

[d] Santa Monica Orthopedic Hospital, 1250 Sixteenth Street, Santa Monica, CA 90404, USA

* Corresponding author. University Foot and Ankle Institute, Private Practice, 1101 Sepulveda Boulevard, Suite 104, Manhattan Beach, CA.

E-mail address: jonathan.thompson@va.gov

Clin Podiatr Med Surg 28 (2011) 117–135
doi:10.1016/j.cpm.2010.10.002
0891-8422/11/$ – see front matter. Published by Elsevier Inc.

almost entirely composed of type I collagen and approximately rotates 11° to 90° in a medial direction in that the medial fibers proximally come to lie in a posterior position distally.[1] This anatomic construct provides potential energy and mechanical advantage with rotational contraction; however, in doing so, it potentially "strangulates" this portion of the tendon known as the watershed area, making it the most common site of rupture.[9,10] This area of lowest vascularity is approximately 2 to 6 cm proximal to the insertional area.[9–11] Lagergren and Lindholm[10] originally described this zone of reduced vascularity in the midportion of the tendon[1,7,11] and subsequent studies have supported their findings.[7,9,12] Although there remains some dispute regarding the zone of least vascularity,[1,11,13] it is generally expected that the blood flow is diminished with increasing age, with gender (decreased in men), and during certain physical loading conditions.[11,13] Astrom and Westlin[11] evaluated the blood flow of Achilles tendons by comparing 35 patients, most of them competitive runner athletes, with 40 healthy volunteers using Doppler flowmetry and concluded the following: (1) blood flow was evenly distributed throughout the Achilles tendon in both groups, (2) blood flow values progressively declined when tension/contraction increased, (3) values were significantly lower at the distal insertional areas, and (4) symptomatic Achilles tendons had an increase in blood flow to the area. The Achilles tendon lacks a true synovial sheath or lining like other tendons and is surrounded by a peritendinous structure called the paratenon. The paratenon is a multilayered structure that covers the tendon and is composed of an outer layer of which the deep fascia is a portion, the mesotenon, and a very thin and delicate epitenon layer that directly surrounds the tendon.[5] The sural nerve and lesser saphenous vein course in the posterior midline of the leg and need to be accounted for during surgical repair.

INCIDENCE

There is a paucity in the literature with few reported studies documenting the prevalence of Achilles tendon ruptures in the general population and let alone in the athletic population. The incidence of ruptured or spontaneously ruptured Achilles tendons seems to be growing; however, it cannot be determined if this incidence is from a growing population or an increasing percentage of the population. Rates of Achilles tendon rupture have been reported from 2 to 18 ruptures per 100,000.[1,14,15] A large study in Scotland was published in 1999 of a total of 4201 Achilles tendon ruptures between 1980 and 1995, which analyzed data on age- and gender-specific incidence rates, and demonstrated similar rupture rates of 4.7 per 100,000 in 1981 and 6 per 100,000 in 1995.[16] The investigators also determined that the peak incidence in men was from age 30 to 39 years but in women the risk increased after the age of 60 years, and the incidence after the age of 80 years was greater in women than in men.[16] Most studies demonstrated that Achilles tendon ruptures have occurred during sporting-related activities. A study by Postacchini and Puddu[17] showed that in 44% or 12 of 27 cases the rupture occurred during athletic activities. Cetti and colleagues[18] reported that 83% (92/111) of patients in a study injured their tendons during activities. A Scandinavian study of badminton players demonstrated that 58 of 111 patients (52%) with Achilles ruptures were playing badminton at the time of injury.[1,19] A Hungarian study analyzed 749 patients from 1972 to 1985 who were diagnosed and surgically treated for 832 acute tendon ruptures (both upper and lower extremity ruptures).[20] Of the 292 cases, 59% Achilles tendon ruptures occurred during sport-related activities in contrast to 2% of other tendon ruptures.[20] There were no professional athletes included in this study; however, the ruptures occurred most often in participants of recreational soccer (33.5%), track and field (16.2%), and basketball

(13.3%). Furthermore, the investigators also demonstrated that (1) there was a higher prevalence of Achilles tendon ruptures (53.7%) and reruptures (71%) in those with blood group O, (2) most patients commonly ruptured their left Achilles tendon, and (3) most ruptures demonstrated histopathologic alterations on examination.[20] Parekh and colleagues[21] documented 31 cases of Achilles tendon ruptures in the National Football League (NFL) between 1997 and 2002. The average age and time in the league was 29 years (average age of NFL players is 26 years) and 6 years, respectively.[21] About 32% of players (10/31) never played in the NFL again, and those who returned showed a reduction in their performance of more than 50%.[21] There was no study that compared Achilles tendon rupture occurrence rates between professional and recreational athletes. Most studies demonstrated that recreational athletes and furthermore the "weekend warrior" athletes are more prone to ruptures and have increasing rupture rates secondary to a partial sedentary life combined with intermittent activities compared with professional athletes who are consistently exercising. It is postulated that regular exercise allows the tendon diameter to thicken and the tendon to become stronger and, in theory, decreases the chance of rupture compared with inactivity, which results in an atrophied Achilles tendon.[22] Other factors that potentially differentiated the 2 groups of athletes are that the professional athletes are generally younger, are healthier with less associated comorbidities, have potentially lower body mass indexes, and have regular access to physical therapy and a controlled athletic training program.

ETIOLOGY

The exact cause of Achilles tendon ruptures remains unclear, but the condition has been described to be associated with multiple disorders, including, but limited to, inflammatory conditions, autoimmune disorders, collagen abnormalities,[1,23–26] infectious process, exposure to antibiotics (fluoroquinolones),[27,28] systemic or injectable steroid use,[29–32] repetitive microtrauma, tendon variations, decreased blood flow with advanced age,[33,34] abnormal pronation and mechanics, ankle equinus, and Achilles calcification.[35] Some investigators have proposed a possible mechanical theory, whereby injury to the tendon leads to weakening and incomplete regeneration, versus a vascular theory, whereby decreased tendon vascularity secondary to age and/or trauma leading to chronic tendon degeneration.[34,36] It has been debated if a previous history or current symptomatic Achilles tendon increases the risk of Achilles rupture or if most cases are truly spontaneous. Achilles tendon disorders are more prominent in participants of running sports and has been noted to be symptomatic in 7% to 11% of runners,[37] 29% of male runners in one study,[38] and an even higher percentage of runners in other studies. One of the larger studies by Kvist[39] demonstrated that approximately 53% of 455 athletes who developed Achilles tendon disorders were involved in running sports.[40] Because the Achilles tendon is unique compared with other tendons in the body in that it lacks a true synovial sheath it can be a potential for somewhat confusing terminology. Achilles tendon disorders are now grouped together into what is known as Achilles tendinopathy.[41–43] Achilles tendinopathy includes tendinosis and peritendinitis. Tendinosis is differentiated from tendonitis in that there is degeneration of the tendon without inflammation or evidence of intratendinous inflammatory cells.[1,42] This distinction is important not only to understand the pathologic condition but also to dictate the proper and appropriate treatment. Puddu and colleagues[44] in 1976 defined this terminology and classified Achilles tendon disease into 3 categories: (1) pure peritendinitis or inflammation of peritendinous tissue with normal tendon, (2) peritendinitis with tendinosis or inflamed peritendinous tissue and degenerative changes of the tendon and (3) tendinosis or normal peritendinous tissue with degenerative changes of the tendon. The investigators also reported that all so-called spontaneous ruptures (patients without any history of previous pain or swelling to Achilles area) had evidence of degenerative lesions in the tendon tissue and no evidence of peritenon alteration.[44] Astrom and Rausing[45] performed 3 biopsies (one each at the symptomatic and asymptomatic part of Achilles tendon and another at the paratenon) in 163 patients with chronic Achilles tendinopathy among which 75% were athletes. Degeneration or tendinosis was demonstrated in 90% of biopsied specimens from symptomatic parts of the tendon and in only 20% from nonsymptomatic portions, and it was found that the paratenon was mostly normal or revealed slight changes.[45] Partial tendon ruptures were found in 19% of patients and always in the area of tendinosis,[45] which may indicate a predisposition to rupture Achilles tendons that show signs of degeneration even though they may have been asymptomatic.[46] However, Mafulli and colleagues[47] in a study performed bilateral percutaneous muscles biopsies in the triceps surae of 12 asymptomatic athletes within 36 hours of trauma of the affected and normal side and found no significant differences in histochemical analysis, muscle abnormalities, or fiber areas; however, the uninjured side demonstrated slight increase in capillary density.

DIAGNOSIS

The diagnosis of acute Achilles tendon ruptures is usually straightforward and commonly diagnosed with appropriate patient history taking and clinical examination.[1,48–51] Patients present with pain and swelling in the posterior ankle and describe a traumatic event or a feeling of being kicked at the back of the heel.[1] The patients may have heard an audible popping sound[52] and may have difficulty with normal ambulation or walking uphill or climbing stairs.[53–55] On examination there is often calf atrophy when compared with the contralateral leg, loss of Achilles tendon congruity or palpable gap,[51] weakness of ankle joint plantar flexion, and inability to do heel raises.[49] Multiple investigators (Simmonds,[56] Thompson and Doherty,[57] Matles,[58] O'Brien,[59] Copeland[60]) have described clinical tests to diagnose Achilles tendon ruptures. The most commonly used clinical test was originally described by Simmonds[56] and popularized by Thompson and Doherty.[57] Patients are made to lie in a prone position with their feet hanging over the edge of the table, and the examiner squeezes the largest muscle portion of the calf complex to simulate a contraction/shortening of the Achilles tendon complex, which should normally produce a plantar flexion of the foot. An "abnormal" or positive Thompson test result is observed when there is a lack of plantar flexion response. Another reproducible test was described by Matles,[58] which involves having the patient lying prone on the table with the knee flexed at 90° and the examiner evaluating the "resting tension" position of the feet. With an Achilles tendon rupture, the foot shows less plantar flexion and may even be positioned neutrally or slightly dorsiflexed compared with the uninjured leg. Maffulli[50] evaluated the sensitivity, specificity, and predictive values of the calf squeeze test, palpable gap, Matles test, O'Brien needle test, and Copeland sphygmomanometer test of 174 complete Achilles tendon tears. All tests showed a high positive predictive value; however, the calf squeeze (Thompson test) and Matles tests were found to be significantly more sensitive (0.96 and 0.88, respectively) than the other tests.[50] Achilles tendon ruptures have been described to be misdiagnosed approximately a quarter of the time,[53,61] and other potential diagnostic modalities include radiographs, ultrasonography, and magnetic resonance imaging (MRI).

Standard radiography is usually not indicated; however, a lateral ankle view allows the practitioner to rule out a posterior calcaneal avulsion fracture[62] and possible distortion of Kager triangle[63] as well as evaluation of Toygar sign.[1] Ultrasonography and MRI are useful in differentiating between a partial and complete rupture and allow a more detailed evaluation of the tendinous structure with a chronic rupture. Ultrasonography is inexpensive, easy to use, allows dynamic imaging, and is able to measure the residual gap between tendon ends.[49,64] Ultrasonography in an uninjured Achilles tendon demonstrates hypoechogenic bands of parallel fibrillar lines contained between 2 hyperechogenic bands in the longitudinal plane and round or oval shape in the transverse plane.[1,61,64] Ultrasonographic images of a ruptured tendon demonstrate discontinuity of normal fibrillar pattern, gap between torn ends, and an acoustic vacuum.[1,49,64,65] Hartgerink and colleagues[65] evaluated 26 suspected Achilles tendon ruptures with ultrasonography and compared the results of this test with surgical results and demonstrated that ultrasonography was accurate in distinguishing full-thickness tears from partial-thickness tears or tendinopathy with a sensitivity of 100%, a specificity of 83%, an accuracy of 92%, a positive predictive value of 88%, and a negative predictive value of 100%. Some investigators believe that there are some pitfalls with ultrasonography, including false diagnosis of high-grade tear if plantaris tendon remains intact[64] and difficulty in differentiating between all tendinous pathologies including partial ruptures of the Achilles tendon,[66] and MRI should be used in these cases. MRI using sagittal and axial images with T1- and T2-weighted sequences are recommended for the evaluation of Achilles tendon injuries, with normal tendon demonstrating low signal intensity (black) on all images.[1,64] A ruptured tendon shows a signal disruption on T1-weighted images and high signal intensity consistent with hemorrhage/edema with retraction of torn ends with a complete rupture on T2-weighted images.[1,64] MRI allows adequate evaluation of the size of partial and intrasubstance tears, potential gapping of ruptured ends, and the amount of tendon degeneration/scar tissue.[67]

TREATMENT
Conservative

There remains some controversy in the literature regarding whether nonoperative or operative treatment be pursued in the acute rupture of the general population depending on age, time or delayed presentation, activity level, and associated comorbidities.[68] Operative repair has associated risks, including inherent complications from surgery and anesthesia, which have to be accounted for. Studies advocating nonoperative approaches have demonstrated similar results as operative procedures and might be better indicated for high-risk patients.[69,70] Professional and collegiate athletes are generally younger and healthier and have the means for a more appropriate or timely diagnosis. Multiple studies have demonstrated that overall operative repair provides earlier return to sporting activities and less rate of rerupture.[18,71–74] A prospective and randomized study by Cetti and colleagues[18] of 111 patients who were randomly assigned to either an operative or a nonoperative group found that the operative group had a significantly higher rate of resuming sport activities, lesser calf atrophy, more ankle joint range of motion (ROM), and lesser rerupture rates than the conservative group, and is the focus of this article.

Conservative options can be divided into serial casting with gradual decrease in gravity equinus position and splinting devices/boots and early ROM. Multiple casting and rehabilitation protocols are available and are surgeon dependent. An accepted conservative regimen uses either an above-the-knee cast or a below-the-knee cast, with the ankle in plantar flexion (gravity equinus) for approximately 4 weeks.[69] Serial cast changes then begin, gradually reducing equinus for the next 4 to 8 weeks and eventually transitioning to a walking boot with a heel lift while starting ROM exercises and a rehabilitation program. Gradual return to regular tennis shoes with a step-down heel lift is used as well.[23] It is important to implement physical therapy with passive and active ROM exercises. Some investigators argue for early ROM to enhance tendon healing process and to diminish side effects from immobilization. Advocates of early ROM with splint devices argue that this technique provides a speedier recovery and early ambulation.[71]

The Achilles tendon rupture can be severely debilitating and time consuming in the athletic population. The goal of surgical repair is to allow the athlete to return to pre-injury and activity levels with return of normal function, strength, and ROM. A variety of surgical repairs are described in the literature, including open repair, percutaneous repair, and mini-open repair techniques. Open repair can include end-to-end repair with or without graft augmentations and be combined with tendon lengthening, turn-down flaps, or tendon transfers. A retrospective analysis by Ateschrang and colleagues[75] in 104 (20 of them athletes) patients who underwent open augmentation after Silfverskiöld procedure for acute Achilles repair determined that 19 of 20 or 95% versus only 48 of 84 or 57% were able to return to original sport activity.

Operative Repair

End-to-end repair

The patient can be given general, regional, or local anesthesia and is placed in prone position on the operating room table. The affected leg as well as the contralateral leg can be prepped and draped for comparison of proper length/tension of the Achilles tendon. Approximately a 6- to 10-cm incision is placed centrally or made at a more advocated posterior-medial midline of the leg to avoid the sural nerve. Dissection is carried down through subcutaneous tissue and fat with minimal dissection or under-mining until the crural fascia and the overlying tendon can be visualized. The crural fascia and paratenon can then be incised and carefully reflected off the tendon and should be identified to ensure proper anatomic layered closure. The tendon is visual-ized, and once the cleaning or removal of the hematoma formation near rupture ends (**Fig. 1**) is performed, one can attempt to tie or "bundle the horse hair" ends. Unhealthy-appearing tendon ends should be cleaned and debrided before reapprox-imation of tendon. Sometimes the proximal portion of the rupture tendon "retracts" and should lightly be stretched for a short period to promote elongation. Then it must be determined if there is adequate tendon available to reapproximate and repair the rupture ends. Adequate length is evaluated to ensure that a tendon lengthening, turndown or rotational flap, and/or transfer procedure is not indicated. If satisfied, then the end-to-end reapproximation can be carried out.

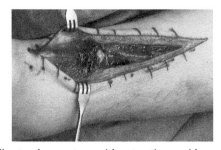

Fig. 1. Complete Achilles tendon rupture with retraction and hematoma formation of the proximal end.

Simple end-to-end repair is most commonly performed via the Bunnel, Kessler, and Krackow techniques.[76] All of these suturing techniques are acceptable for the repair of the Achilles tendon; however, the Krackow method has been shown to be superior in biomechanical and cadaveric studies and has the advantage of allowing 4 threads (and 2 knots) across the rupture site if desired.[77] The size and type of suture available on the market is variable and is usually the surgeon's preference. More recently #2 or 2–0 FiberWire (Arthrex, Naples, FL, USA) has become more popular, and a recent study compared Prolene (Ethicon, a Johnson and Johnson company New Brunswick, NJ, USA), Ticron (Covidien, Mansfield, MA, USA), and FiberWire.[78] The investigators determined that FiberWire has a greater cross-sectional area of similar size and is 10% stronger than Prolene and 25% stronger than Ticron in knotted tensile strength.[78] It should be noted that common to all suturing types the location of failure seems to be located at the knot site regardless of the type of suture used. Some investigators reinforce with simple interrupted sutures across rupture site. The rupture should be repaired with the foot in a position similar to the contralateral side resting in equinus position. The paratenon and crural fascia can be reapproximated as well, and then skin closure via suture or staples is done and dressings are applied.

Augmentation

End-to-end repair with augmentation can be performed with additional autografts, allografts, and synthetic grafts. The most common and easiest autograft to harvest is with the plantaris tendon, which is usually intact after a rupture and easily available through the same surgical wound. The tendon is cut from its insertion on the calcaneus and stretched or "fanned out" and can be placed over the rupture site with absorbable sutures.[79–81] Akgun and colleagues[79] performed 36 acute Achilles tendon end-to-end repair with Krackow technique combined with plantaris augmentation in which 31 of 36 patients participated in sporting activities and returned to preinjury sport activities after a mean of 17 weeks (range 14–20 weeks). In contrast, Aktas and colleagues[82] demonstrated no significant difference in the American Orthopeadic Foot and Ankle Society hind foot clinical outcome scores between the group that underwent single end-to-end repair and the group that underwent end-to-end repair with plantaris tendon. Furthermore, the nonaugmented group demonstrated a slight decrease in local tenderness, scar adhesions, and tendon thickness.[82]

There have been a variety of biologic scaffolds described in the literature and favorable arguments include added strength of repair without sacrificing secondary structures or more dissection to allow early ROM postoperatively.[83–85] Various scaffolds and their cellular makeup, biomechanical strength, and biocompatibility have been described for augmentation in the repair of ruptured Achilles tendons.[86] These scaffolds include, but are not limited to, TissueMend (Stryker, Kalamazoo, MI, USA), Restore (Depuy Orthopaedics, Warsaw, IN, USA), GraftJacket (Wright Medical Technology, Arlington, TN, USA), Conexa (Conexa Reconstructive Tissue Matrix, Tornier, Edina, MN, USA) and Dacron (DuPont, Wilmington, DE, USA) vascular graft. There are limited prospective and randomized trials regarding the use of these grafts in Achilles tendon repairs. TissueMend has been noted to have significantly higher DNA count than most other matrices.[87] A human cadaveric study of 8 matched pairs evaluated simulated Achilles ruptures repaired with end-to-end repair with Krackow technique and 1 limb augmented by human dermal allograft (GraftJacket) and concluded that the augmented limb had significant strength and stiffness.[83] However, there have been no follow-up studies. The graft is usually "wrapped" around the ruptured ends and sutured in place (**Fig. 2**). Every surgeon should be encouraged to

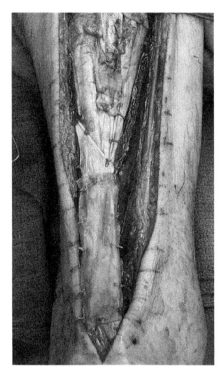

Fig. 2. Sutured onlay graft around ruptured ends.

educate themselves on the differences between these scaffolds, such as the source, tissue type, and inherent properties, to help differentiate between them.

Turndown or rotational flaps

Fascial turn down flaps of the proximal gastrocnemius fascia have also been advocated. The most common being the single strip or Silfverskiöld procedure and the double strip or Lindholm procedure, and these fascial slips are made approximately 3 cm proximal to the rupture site and rotated 180° and flapped down to cover and reinforce rupture site.[88] It should be noted that doing a turndown flap requires a longer proximal skin incision with more dissection that increases the potential for wound healing issues and sural nerve injury. A study by Pajala and colleagues[89] described 66 acute Achilles tendon ruptures in 2 groups, one received end-to-end repair with Krackow locking suture and one group underwent end-to-end repair with augmentation described by Silfverskiöld, and found that it took approximately 25 minutes longer and the incision was 7 cm longer in the augmented repair with no significant advantages regarding ankle score, isolated calf muscle strength, and rerupture rates.

Because the author is dealing with the athletic population, tendon transfers in acute ruptures have been avoided and have been reserved for possible delayed ruptures, chronic ruptures, or reruptures when indicated secondary to the increased dissection, surgical time, and potential morbidity when sacrificing another tendon. In the case that a surgeon feels more comfortable or if indicated, the author recommends using possible plantaris tendon overlay graft or turn down flaps as mentioned earlier. Peroneal tendon transfers for acute Achilles tendon ruptures were described by Perez Teuffer[90] in the 1970s and later popularized by Turco and Spinella[62,91] in 1987. It has been indicated to use these transfers in acute, chronic, and reruptured Achilles tendon injuries. After end-to-end apposition is performed for the acute rupture, then peroneal brevis tendon is detached from the base of the fifth metatarsal brought through to the posterior compartment and tunneled through the distal Achilles tendon in the medial direction and then drawn proximally along the medial Achilles tendon and secured.[62] Turco and Spinella[91] performed a follow-up study in 55 athletes who sustained acute Achilles ruptures in which they found no early evidence of rerupture rate and also that the tendon transfer had minimal loss of strength. Gallant and colleagues[92] concluded that there was only mild objective weakness in eversion strength (14.9% deficit) but no functional or significant loss in eversion strength, plantar flexion strength, ankle instability, or activities of daily living when comparing the peroneal brevis tendon transfer limbs with the normal contralateral side in 8 patients.

Minimal incision techniques

Minimal incisional and percutaneous techniques were introduced and advocated to decrease potential wound complications, scar adhesions, and sural nerve injuries.[93–95] Ma and Griffith[93] first described a percutaneous technique using multiple stab incision of 18 acute Achilles tendon ruptures to minimize postoperative complications and reported no complications of sural nerve injury. The anatomic path of the sural nerve has been well outlined in the literature and is not readdressed in this article, but it should be noted that percutaneous repairs are not completely benign and every surgeon should appreciate this and use caution when placing a proximal and especially proximal lateral incision even with this technique.[96] There have been several modifications of the percutaneous repair described in the literature to decrease potential sural nerve injury by placing percutaneous incisions more in the midline or medial position.[97,98] Martinelli[94] described percutaneous repair on 50 acutely ruptured Achilles tendon. In this study, 30 patients practiced amateur or professional sports and were able to return to preinjury sporting levels after 120 to 150 days.[94] The mini-open technique using the Achillon System (Newdeal, Lyon, France) was introduced to decrease wound complications with smaller incisions.[99–101] Favorable arguments for mini-open technique are allowing for early postoperative ROM and rehabilitation to assist proper tendon healing with the reduction of scar adhesions and allowing athletes an earlier return to sporting activities.[100] Rippstein and Easley[100] used the mini-open technique and Achillon device to repair acutely ruptured Achilles tendons in 89 consecutive patients. Of these patients, 75% participated in sporting activities (5 elite athletes) 1 to 3 or more times per weekend, and all patients returned to sporting activities within 1 year, with an average return to sporting activities at 6 months.[100] The average American Orthopedic Foot and Ankle Society ankle–hind foot score was 98 points.[100] Huffard and colleagues[102] performed a cadaveric study on 10 pairs of matched Achilles tendon specimens comparing the Krackow suturing technique on 1 specimen with the Achillon suturing system on the contralateral limb. In this study the investigators found the latter technique to be biomechanically stronger.

A study by Ceccarelli and colleagues[99] compared acutely ruptured Achilles tendons in 12 paitents who underwent repair via modified Ma and Griffith percutaneous procedure and in 12 who underwent repair using minimally invasive procedure with the Achillon system and found similar results in the time taken to return to work and sports and similar American Orthopedic Foot and Ankle Society Score values.

Rehabilitation of acute repairs

There are a variety of postoperative rehabilitation protocols after acute repair of the Achilles tendon regarding when to initiate ROM, rehabilitation and strengthening, and weight bearing. Mortensen and colleagues[103] prospectively randomized 71 patients who had acute repairs of the Achilles tendon into a group that underwent conventional postoperative management with a cast for 8 weeks and a group that underwent early restrictive ROM with a below-the-knee brace for 6 weeks and concluded that the early ROM group was more satisfied, developed less scar adhesions, had less initial loss of ROM, and returned to sporting activities sooner. The median percentages of strength and heel rise index of the repaired limbs compared with the normal contralateral limbs were similar in both groups.[103] Suchak and colleagues[104] randomized 110 patients into 2 groups of weight bearing and non–weight bearing for 4 weeks after an initial 2 weeks of non–weight-bearing casting. The early weight-bearing group demonstrated improved scores in physical and social functioning with fewer limitations in daily activities at 6 weeks; however, no significant differences were noted at 6 months.[104] Aoki and colleagues[105] allowed early ROM and partial weight bearing with transition to full weight bearing by 16 days in 22 athletes with end-to-end repairs of acute Achilles ruptures. The investigators reported an average period of 13 weeks for returning to the sport.[105] Mandelbaum and colleagues[106] performed the Krackow modified suture technique in 29 athletes who sustained Achilles tendon ruptures and implemented early ROM and rehabilitation programs; 90% of patients demonstrated full ROM at 6 weeks and 92% returned to sport participation by 6 months.

It seems that early ROM most likely allows for earlier return to normal activities of daily living and recreational and sporting activities without a significant increased morbidity or increased rerupture rate regardless of operative technique and is probably the most important aspect that needs to be addressed when dealing with an athletic patient. If a surgeon can provide a solid repair and institute an early ROM and protective weight-bearing protocol, the time missed could be decreased.

CHRONIC, DELAYED, AND RERUPTURE OF ACHILLES TENDONS IN ATHLETES

Chronic or delayed Achilles tendon ruptures in the athletic population are extremely rare. It has been described in the literature that ruptures presenting after 4 to 6 weeks of the injury can be classified as chronic or delayed ruptures.[53,61,107,108] MRI is warranted for more precise evaluation in any patient with a concern of a suspected chronic rupture for better evaluation of the tendinous structure. It is generally accepted that operative repair is recommended for chronic ruptures, delayed ruptures, or reruptures of the Achilles tendon; however, there is no consistent surgical procedure recommendations provided in the literature.[108] The general goal in any ruptured tendon is to attempt end-to-end anastomosis of the ruptured site; however, this attempt becomes more difficult in the ruptures that are presented with delay or in those that are neglected. Accordingly, multiple classification schemes and algorithms have been described to help guide and give surgical recommendations for surgical repair.[53,107–110] There are limited prospective randomized trials to compare these surgical proposals in the general or athletic populations. In delayed ruptures, the tendons usually become a solid mass of scar tissue and it can be difficult to determine healthy or viable tendon and corresponding layers. The surgeon must debride and clean until potentially healthy and functional tendon remains, which obviously results in increase in gapping of the tendon and makes it difficult to oppose the ends. The surgeon must use other potential procedures that include, but are not limited to, lengthening via inverted V-to-Y or tongue-in-groove procedures, turndown rotational flaps, tendon augmentation or bridging, and tendon transfers. Often there requires a combination of the above-mentioned procedures.

Myerson[107] and Kuwada[109] attempted to simplify the operative process and provide recommendations based on this resultant gapping. The classification by Myerson[107] (**Table 1**) recommends the following: type 1 defect that is no more than 1 to 2 cm long can be repaired by an end-to-end anastomosis and a posterior compartment fasciotomy, type 2 defect that ranges from 2 to 5 cm can be repaired via a V-Y lengthening with possible flexor hallucis longus (FHL) tendon transfer, and type 3 defect that is longer than 5 cm and is bridged with FHL tendon transfer with possible V-Y lengthening.

Kuwada[109] classification (**Table 2**) recommends the following: type I lesions are partial tears and can be managed with conservative casting, type II lesions are complete ruptures smaller than 3 cm and can be repaired via end-to-end repair, type III lesions are complete ruptures of 3 to 6 cm and can be repaired with autogenesis turndown flaps and/or synthetic grafts, and type IV lesions are complete ruptures larger than 6 cm and can be repaired with gastrocnemius recession, lengthening, and/or free tendon transfer.

Abraham and Pankovich[111] first described the V-Y advancement for end-to-end repairs of Achilles tendon ruptures in an attempt to allow anastomosis between the 2 ruptured ends. The inverted "V" incision is placed at the musculotendinous junction with the arms approximately 1.5 times the length of the tendon defect and were found to close up to 6-cm gaps in the tendon ends.[111] Parker and Repinecz[112] introduced a tongue-in-groove procedure (**Fig. 3**), which they found was easier to perform, and were able to achieve 50% more length. Single and double turndown flaps can also be used as described earlier for the repair of acutely ruptured Achilles tendon and are not rediscussed.

Tendon transfers have been well described in the literature for acute ruptures, chronic ruptures, and/or reruptures and most commonly use the plantaris,[79] peroneus brevis,[52,62,90,91] flexor digitorum longus (FDL),[43,113] and FHL[61,113,114] tendons. The plantaris tendon is the easiest to harvest; however, most of the time, in chronic ruptures, this tendon has been incorporated into the scarred tendinous mass and is unidentifiable. The peroneus brevis tendon has been described earlier and can be used in similarly for the repair of chronic ruptures. FHL has been advocated over the FDL for Achilles tendon transfers and augmentation because of its anatomic proximity, stronger and longer tendinous structure, and lower-lying muscle belly that can be incorporated into the rupture site for added vascularity and strength.[61,113,115] It is understood that any tendon transfer results in loss of strength, but it is difficult to determine how much of this loss will functionally affect the athlete during sporting activities because there is a lack of published data in the literature as well as difficulty in performing prospective randomized trials with this type of injury and athletic population. Frenette and Jackson[116] determined that there was no disability or activity

Table 1	
Neglected Achilles tendon ruptures	
Size of Defect (cm)	**Recommended Procedure**
1–2	Simple end-to-end anastomosis, can apply tension to "stress relax" myotendinous junction before tying suture for additional length
2–5	V-Y myotendinous lengthening with end-to-end anastomosis, consider flexor hallucis longus (FHL) tendon transfer if warranted
>5	FHL tendon transfer combined with V-Y advancement if needed, turndown flaps, author advocates FHL tendon transfer over flexor digitorum longus or peroneal tendon transfer

Data from Myerson MS. Achilles tendon rupture. Instr Course Lect 1999;48:226, 227; with permission.

Table 2
Kuwada's classification of Achilles ruptures

Type	Recommended Treatment/Procedure
Type I: <50% tear	Cast immobilization for 8 weeks
Type II: defect<3 cm	Simple end-to-end anastomosis
Type III: defect 3–6 cm	End-to-end anastomosis and autogenous or synthetic graft
Type IV: defect>6 cm (includes delayed repairs)	Requires gastrocnemius recession for increased length, end-to-end anastomosis with free tendon graft or synthetic graft

Data from Kuwada GT. Classification of tendo Achillis rupture with consideration of surgical repair techniques. J Foot Surg 1990;29:362.

limitation in 4 athletes who sustained complete laceration of the FHL without repair. The FHL tendon transfer seems to be gaining popularity and has been described and modified by multiple surgeons.[107,114,115] The FHL tendon can be harvested via a single incisional technique or double incisional technique. The single incisional technique uses the same incision with more anterior dissection through posterior fascia that is incised to identify and mobilize the FHL tendon that is cut as distally as possible (**Fig. 4**). The FHL tendon should be easily identified and freed with careful visualization of the neurovascular bundle as the tendon is dissected distally. The double incisional technique requires a secondary incision over the midfoot to identify the FHL near the level of the knot of Henry, which is then incised and retracted through the proximal wound. The single technique has the advantage of not using a secondary incision or dissection and possible neurovascular compromise in the foot incision but provides a potential shorter tendon available for transfer that might require screws and/or anchors for fixation into the calcaneus depending on the surgeon's preferred technique (**Fig. 5**). The 2-incision technique allows for a longer tendon for transfer and augmentation and possibly allows for wrapping around both ruptured ends depending on the technique. An average of additional 3 cm with secondary midfoot incision and harvesting just proximal to the knot of Henry has been described.[116] Furthermore, Wapner and colleagues[115] demonstrated that an additional 10 to 12 cm can be found with transecting the tendon distal to the knot of Henry when compared with a proximal posterior harvesting technique. Once the FHL tendon is harvested, the tendon can be transferred in a variety of ways. The 2-incision approach allows for a longer tendon graft, and the graft can be transferred to the calcaneus in a medial-to-lateral direction through a posterior superior calcaneal drill hole. The graft is then proximally fashioned, and if enough tendon remains, it can be weaved through the proximal and distal

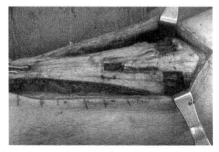

Fig. 3. Open repair with tongue-and-groove lengthening procedure.

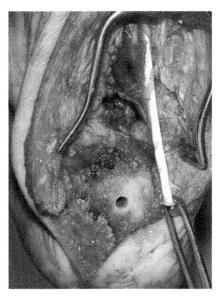

Fig. 4. FHL tendon exposure with single incision approach.

rupture ends of the Achilles tendon.[117] The single incisional approach results in a shorter tendon length and is transferred from a superior- to inferior-directed calcaneal tunnel placed anterior to the Achilles insertional area. The tendon is brought through the osseous tunnel via suture (whip stitch or other suture technique) and out the plantar aspect of the foot and held in tension as an interference screw is placed through the superior hole to secure the tendon in place. Some investigators advocate suturing the FHL muscle belly over the rupture site to provide increased strength and

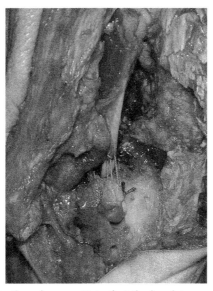

Fig. 5. FHL transferred to the calcaneus. Note that the low-lying muscle belly of FHL can be used to reinforce and provide vascularity to the repaired ruptured tendon.

vascularity. Onlay allograft or synthetic grafts can be wrapped around the tendon once the earlier-mentioned procedure is performed, but this graft adds bulk to the tendon and can make layered closure and wound healing difficult.[118]

Postoperative care and rehabilitation for chronic Achilles tendon ruptures generally require a more conservative approach with longer immobilization and protective casting period. The optimal immobilization and rehabilitation period is still debated.[36] Functional ankle foot orthosis and patellar tendon–bearing braces that limit ankle joint dorsi flexion and allow early ROM and protective weight bearing can be used well in this patient population.

DISCUSSION

Acute and chronic Achilles tendon ruptures in the athletic population are one of the most challenging and time-consuming conditions to deal with for both the athlete as well as the surgeon. These ruptures are becoming more prominent in the medical community, most likely with the increasing number of recreational, amateur, and professional athletes competing in sporting activities. Surgical repair seems to be the standard of care for treatment, especially in this subset of population.

New surgical approaches, including percutaneous and mini-open techniques, are being introduced to potentially diminish perioperative complications, and the advent of early protective ROM and rehabilitation has shown a potential for earlier return to sporting activities for patients with acute Achilles ruptures.

Delayed or chronic ruptures are rare in the athletic population and usually require more extensive surgical approaches with possible tendon lengthening, turndown flaps, tendon augmentation with graft substitutes, and/or tendon transfers. The FHL tendon seems to be more favorable than other tendons available for transfer secondary to its close proximity to the Achilles tendon, in-phase muscle activity, longer and stronger tendinous structure, and low-lying muscle belly for potential incorporation into the repair site for increased strength and vascularity. There remains no clear and identifiable postoperative protocol for rehabilitation and this rehasbilitation regimen remains the surgeon's preference; however, a few studies have determined that early protective ROM has allowed an early return to physical activities. It is hoped that follow-up studies would be performed to define or redefine surgical recommendations and postoperative protocols for the athletic population.

REFERENCES

1. Mafulli N. Current concepts review: rupture of the Achilles tendon. J Bone Joint Surg Am 1999;81(7):1019–36.
2. Soma CA, Mandelbaum BR. Achilles tendon disorders. Clin Sports Med 1994; 13:811–23.
3. Hamilton WG. Surgical anatomy of the foot and ankle. Ciba Clin Symp 1985; 37(3):1–32.
4. Kongsgaard M, Aagaard P, Kjaer M, et al. Structural Achilles tendon properties in athletes subjected to different exercise modes and in Achilles tendon ruptures. J Appl Physiol 2005;99:1965–71.
5. O'Brien M. The anatomy of the Achilles tendon. Foot Ankle Clin 2005;10:225–38.
6. Simpson SL, Hertzog MS, Barja RH. The plantaris tendon graft: an ultrasound study. J Hand Surg 1991;16(4):708–11.
7. Zantop T, Tilmann B, Petersen W. Quantitative assessment of blood vessels of the human Achilles tendon: an immunohistochemical cadaver study. Arch Orthop Trauma Surg 2003;123(9):501–4.

8. Theobald P, Benjamin M, Nokes L, et al. Review of the vascularization of the human Achilles tendon. Injury, Int J Care Injured 2005;36:1267–72.
9. Carr AJ, Norris SH. The blood supply of the calcaneal tendon. J Bone Joint Surg Br 1989;71:100.
10. Lagergren C, Lindholm A. Vascular distribution in the Achilles tendon. An angiographic and micro-angiographic study. Acta Chir Scand 1958–9;116:491–6.
11. Astrom M, Westlin N. Blood flow in chronic Achilles tendinopathy. Clin Orthop Relat Res 1994;308:166–72.
12. Ahmed IM, Lagopoulus M, McConnell P, et al. Blood supply of the Achilles tendon. J Orthop Res 1998;16:591–6.
13. Astrom M, Westlin N. Blood flow in the human Achilles tendon assessed by laser Doppler flowmetry. J Orthop Res 1994;12:246–52.
14. Leppilahati J, Puranen J, Orava S. Incidence of Achilles tendon rupture. Acta Orthop Scand 1996;67:277–9.
15. Moller A, Astros M, Westland N. Increasing incidence of Achilles tendon rupture. Acta Orthop Scand 1996;67:479–81.
16. Waterston S, Squair J, Douglas AS, et al. Changing incidence of Achilles tendon rupture in Scotland. J Bone Joint Surg Br 1994;81:304.
17. Postacchini F, Puddu G. Subcutaneous ruptures of the Achilles tendon. Int Surg 1976;4:145–50.
18. Cetti R, Christensen SE, Ejsted R, et al. Operative versus nonoperative treatment of Achilles tendon rupture. A prospective randomized study and review of the literature. Am J Sports Med 1993;21:791–9.
19. Fahlstrom M, Bjornstig U, Lorentzon R. Acute Achilles tendon ruptures in badminton players. Am J Sports Med 1998;26:467–70.
20. Jozsa L, Kvist M, Balint BJ, et al. The role of recreational sport activity in Achilles tendon rupture. A clinical, pathoanatomical, and sociological study of 292 cases. Am J Sports Med 1989;17(3):338–43.
21. Parekh SG, Wray WH, Brimmo O, et al. Epidemiology and outcomes of Achilles tendon ruptures in the National Football League. Foot Ankle Spec 2009;2(6):283–6.
22. Saltzman CL, Tearse DS. Achilles tendon injuries. J Am Acad Orthop Surg 1998; 6:316–25.
23. Tafuri SA, Daly N. Achilles tendon trauma. In: McGlamry ED, Banks AS, Downey MS, editors. McGlamry's comprehenasive textbook of foot and ankle surgery. 3rd edition. Baltimore (MD): William and Wilkins; 2001. p. 1706–23, chapter 52, part 2.
24. Dent CM, Graham GP. Osteogenesis imperfecta and Achilles tendon rupture. Injury 1991;22:239–40.
25. Rask MA. Achilles tendon rupture owing to rheumatoid disease. JAMA 1978; 239:435.
26. Mahoney PG, James PB, Howell CJ. Spontaneous rupture of the Achilles tendon in a patient with gout. Ann Rheum Dis 1981;490:416.
27. McGarvey WC, Singh D, Trevino S. Partial Achilles tendon ruptures associated with flouroquinolone antibiotics: a case report and literature review. Foot Ankle 1996;17:496–8.
28. Movin T, Gad A, Gunter P, et al. Pathology of the Achilles tendon in association with ciprofloxacin treatment. Foot Ankle 1997;18:297–9.
29. Lee HB. Avulsion and rupture of the tendo calcaneous after injection of hydrocortisone. Br Med J 1957;3:395.
30. Haines JF. Bilateral rupture of the Achilles tendon in patients on steroid therapy. Ann Rheum Dis 1983;42:652–4.

31. Balasubramanium P, Prathrap K. The effect of injection of hydrocortisone into rabbit calcaneal tendons. J Bone Joint Surg Br 1972;54:729–34.

32. Kleinman M, Gross AE. Achilles tendon rupture following steroid injection. A report of three cases. J Bone Joint Surg Am 1983;65:345–7.

33. Strocchi R, DePasquale V, Guizzardi S, et al. Human Achilles tendon: morphological and morphometric variations as a function of age. Foot Ankle 1991;12: 100–4.

34. Kannus P, Natri A. Etiology and pathophysiology of tendon ruptures in sports. Scand J Med Sci Sports 1997;7:107–12.

35. Clement DB, Tauntonn JE, Smart GW. Achilles tendonitis and peritendinitis: etiology and treatment. Am J Sports Med 1984;12:179–84.

36. Deangelis JP, Wilson KM, Cox CL, et al. Achilles tendon rupture in athletes. J Surg Orthop Adv 2009;18(3):115–21.

37. Lysholm J, Wiklander J. Injuries in runners. Am J Sports Med 1987;15:168–71.

38. Kujala UM, Sarna S, Kaprio J. Cumulative incidence of Achilles tendon rupture and tendinopathy in male former athletes. Clin J Sport Med 1994;18:173–201.

39. Kvist M. Achilles tendon overuse injuries [PhD thesis]. University of Turku, Finland; 1991.

40. Kader D, Saxeza A, Movin T, et al. Achilles tendinopathy: some aspects of basic science and clinical management. Br J Sports Med 2002;36:239–49.

41. Mafulli N, Khan KM, Puddu G. Overuse tendon conditions: time to change a confusing terminology. Athroscopy 1998;14:840–3.

42. Jarvinen T, Kannus P, Mafulli N, et al. Achilles tendon disorders: etiology and epidemiology. Foot Ankle Clin 2005;10:255–66.

43. Mann RA, Holmes GB Jr, Seale KS, et al. Chronic rupture of the Achilles tendon: a new technique of repair. J Bone Joint Surg Am 1991;73:214–9.

44. Puddu G, Ippolito E, Postacchini F. A classification of Achilles tendon disease. Am J Sports Med 1976;1(4):145–50.

45. Astrom M, Rausing A. Chronic Achilles tendinopathy: a survey of surgical and histopathological findings. Clin Orthop Relat Res 1995;316:151–64.

46. Fox JM, Blazina ME, Jobe FW, et al. Degeneration and rupture of the Achilles tendon. Clin Orthop 1975;107:221–4.

47. Mafulli N, Testa V, Capasso G. Achilles tendon rupture in athletes: histochemistry of the triceps surae muscle. J Foot Surg 1991;30(6):529–33.

48. Mafulli N, Ajis A. Current concepts review. Management of chronic ruptures of the Achilles tendon. J Bone Joint Surg Am 2008;90:1348–60.

49. Tan G, Sabb B, Kadakia AR. Non-surgical management of Achilles ruptures. Foot Ankle Clin 2009;14(4):675–84.

50. Mafulli N. The clinical diagnosis of subcutaneous tear of the Achilles tendon. A prospective study in 174 patients. Am J Sports Med 1998;26:266–70.

51. Movin T, Ryberg A, McBride DJ, et al. Acute rupture of the Achilles tendon. Foot Ankle Clin 2005;10:331–56.

52. Pintore E, Barra V, Pintore R, et al. Peroneus brevis tendon transfers in neglected tears of the Achilles tendon. J Trauma Injury, Infection, and Critical Care 2001; 50(1):71–8.

53. Padanilam T. Chronic Achilles tendon ruptures. Foot Ankle Clin 2009;14(4): 711–28.

54. Distefano VJ, Nixon JE. Achilles tendon rupture: pathogenesis, diagnosis, and treatment by a modified pullout wire technique. J Trauma 1972;12:671–7.

55. Hartog BD. Insertional Achilles tendinosis: pathogenesis and treatment. Foot Ankle Clin 2009;14(4):639–50.

56. Simmonds FA. The diagnosis of the ruptured Achilles tendon. Practitioner 1957; 179:56–8.
57. Thompson TC, Doherty J. Spontaneous rupture of the tendon of Achilles: a new clinical diagnostic test. J Trauma 1962;2:126–9.
58. Matles AL. Rupture of the tendo Achilles. Another diagnostic sign. Bull Hosp Joint Dis 1975;36:48–51.
59. O'Brien T. The needle test for complete rupture of the Achilles tendon. J Bone Joint Surg AM 1984;66:1099–101.
60. Copeland SA. Rupture of the Achilles tendon: a new clinical test. Ann R Coll Surg Engl 1990;72:270–1.
61. Leslie H, Edwards W. Neglected ruptures of the Achilles tendon. Foot Ankle Clin 2005;10:357–70.
62. Turco VJ, Spinella AJ. Achilles tendon ruptures-peroneus brevis transfer. Foot Ankle 1987;7:253–9.
63. Cetti R, Andersen I. Roentgenopraphic diagnosis of ruptured Achilles tendons. Clin Orthop 1993;286:215–21.
64. Bleakney RR, White LM. Imaging of the Achilles tendon. Foot Ankle Clin 2005; 10:239–54.
65. Hartgerink P, Fessell DP, Jacobson JA, et al. Full- versus partial-thickness Achilles tendon tears: sonographic accuracy and characterization in 26 cases with surgical correlation. Radiology 2001;220(2):401–12.
66. Kayser R, Mahlfeld K, Heyde CE. Partial rupture of the proximal Achilles tendon: a differential diagnostic problem in ultrasound imaging. Br J Sports Med 2005; 39:838–42.
67. Schweitzer ME, Karasick D. MR imaging of disorders of the Achilles tendon. Am J Roentgenol 2000;175:613–25.
68. Leppilahti J, Orava S. Total Achilles tendon rupture. A review. Sports Med 1998; 25:79–100.
69. Nistor L. Surgical and non-surgical treatment of Achilles tendon rupture. J Bone Joint Surg Am 1981;63:394–9.
70. Carden DG, Noble J, Chalmers J, et al. Rupture of the calcaneal tendon. The early and late management. J Bone Joint Surg Br 1987;69(3):416–20.
71. Saleh M, Marshall PD, Senior R, et al. The Sheffield splint for controlled early mobilization after rupture of the calcaneal tendon. A prospective, randomized comparison with plaster treatment. J Bone Joint Surg Br 1992;740(2):206–9.
72. Moller M, Movin T, Granhed H, et al. Acute rupture of tendon Achilles: A prospective randomized study of comparison between surgical and non-surgical treatment. J Bone Joint Surg Br 2001;83:843–8.
73. Weber M, Niemann M, Lanz R, et al. Non-operative treatment of acute rupture of the Achilles tendon: results of a new protocol and comparison with operative treatment. Am J Sports Med 2003;31:685–91.
74. Wong J, Barrass V, Mafulli N. Quantative review of operative and non-operative management of Achilles tendon ruptures. Am J Sports Med 2002;30:565–75.
75. Ateschrang A, Gratzer C, Ochs U, et al. [Open augmented repair according to Silfverskjoid for Achilles tendon rupture: an alternate for athletes?]. Sportverletz Sportschaden 2007;21(2):93–7 [in German].
76. Krackow KA, Thomas SC, Jones LC. A new stitch for ligamentous tendon fixation: brief note. J Bone Joint Surg Am 1986;68:764–6.
77. Watson TW, Jurist KA, Yang KH, et al. The strength of the Achilles tendon repair: an in-vitro study of the biomechanical behavior on human cadaver tendons. Foot Ankle 1995;16:191–5.

78. Scherman F, Haddad R, Scougall F, et al. Cross-sectional area and strength differences of fiberwire, prolene, and ticron sutures. J Hand Surg Am 2010; 35(5):780–4.

79. Akgun U, Erol B, Karahan M. [Primary surgical repair with the Krackow technique combined with plantaris tendon augmentation in the treatment of acute Achilles tendon ruptures]. Acta Orthop Traumatol Turc 2006;40:228–33 [in Turkish].

80. Beskin JL, Sanders RA, Hunter SC, et al. Surgical repair of Achilles tendon ruptures. Am J Sports Med 1987;15:1–8.

81. Rosenzweie S, Azar FM. Open repair of acute Achilles tendon ruptures. Foot Ankle Clin 2009;14(4):699–709.

82. Aktas S, Kocaoglu B, Nalbantoglu U, et al. End-to-end versus augmented repair in the treatment of acute Achilles tendon rupture. J Foot Ankle Surg 2007;46(5): 336–40.

83. Barber FA, McGarry JE, Herbert MA, et al. A biomechanical study of the Achilles tendon repair augmentation using GraftJacket matrix. Foot Ankle Int 2008;29(3): 329–33.

84. Fernandez-Fairen M, Gimeno C. Augmented repair of Achilles tendon ruptures. Am J Sports Med 1997;25(2):177–81.

85. Gilbert TW, Stewart Akers AM, Simmons-Byrd A, et al. Degradation and remodeling of small intestinal submucosa in canine Achilles tendon repair. J Bone Joint Surg Am 2007;89(3):621–30.

86. Stover BS, Zelen CM, Nielson DL. Use of soft tissue matrices as an adjunct to Achilles repair and reconstruction. Clin Podiatr Med Surg 2009;26(4):647–58.

87. Derwin KA, Bkaer AR, Spragg RK, et al. Commercial extracellular matrix scaffolds for rotator cuff tendon repair. Biomechanical, biochemical, and cellular properties. J Bone Joint Surg Am 2006;88:2665–72.

88. Lindholm A. A new method of operation in subcutaneous rupture of Achilles tendon. Acta Chir Scand 1959;117:261–70.

89. Pajala A, Kangas J, Ohtonen P, et al. Augmented compared with non-augmented surgical repair of a fresh total Achilles tendon rupture. A prospective randomized study. J Bone Joint Surg Am 2009;91(5):1092–100.

90. Perez Teuffer A. Traumatic rupture of the Achilles tendon. Reconstruction by transplant and graft using the lateral peroneus brevis. Orthop Clin North Am 1974;5:89–93.

91. Turco V, Spinella AJ. Team physician #2. Peroneus brevis transfers for Achilles tendon rupture in athletes. Orthop Rev 1988;17(8):822–44.

92. Gallant GG, Massie C, Turco VJ. Assessment of eversion and plantar flexion strength after repair of Achilles tendon rupture using peroneus brevis tendon transfer. Am J Orthop 1995;24(3):257–61.

93. Ma G, Griffith T. Percutaneous repair of acute closed ruptured Achilles tendon: a new technique. Clin Orthop Relat Res 1977;128:247–55.

94. Martinelli B. Percutaneous repair of the Achilles tendon in athletes. Bull Hosp Jt Dis 2000;59(3):149–52.

95. Davies M, Solan M. Minimal incision techniques for acute Achilles repair. Foot Ankle Clin 2009;14(4):685–95.

96. Webb JM, Moorjani J, Radford M. Anatomy of the sural nerve and its relation to the Achilles tendon. Foot Ankle Int 2000;21(6):475–7.

97. Webb JM, Bannister GC. Percutaneous repair of the ruptured tendo Achilles. J Bone Joint Surg Br 1999;81(5):877–80.

98. Young J, Sayana K, McClelland D, et al. Percutaneous repair of acute Achilles tendon. Tech Foot Ankle Surg 2006;5(1):9–14.

99. Ceccarelli F, Berti L, Giuriati L, et al. Percutaneous and minimally invasive techniques of Achilles tendon repair. Clin Orthop Relat Res 2007;458:188–93.

100. Rippstein P, Easley M. "Mini-open" repair for acute Achilles tendon ruptures. Tech Foot Ankle Surg 2006;5(1):3–8.

101. Elliott AJ, Kennedy JG, O'Malley M. Minimally invasive Achilles tendon repair using the Achillon repair system. Tech Foot Ankle Surg 2006;5(3):171–4.

102. Huffard B, O'Loughlin PF, Wright T, et al. Achilles tendon repair: Achillon system vs. Krackow suture: an anatomic in vitro biomechanical study. Clin Biomech (Bristol, Avon) 2008;23(9):1158–64.

103. Mortensen N, Skov O, Jensen P. Early motion of the ankle after operative treatment of a rupture of the Achilles tendon: a prospective, randomized clinical and radiographic study. J Bone Joint Surg Am 1999;81(7):983–90.

104. Suchak AA, Bostick G, Beaupré L, et al. The influence of early weight-bearing compared with non-weight-bearing after surgical repair of the achilles tendon. J Bone Joint Surg 2008;90:1876–83.

105. Aoki M, Ogiwara N, Ohta T, et al. Early active motion and weight bearing after cross-stitch Achilles tendon repair. Am J Sports Med 1998;26:794–800.

106. Mandelbaum BR, Myerson MS, Forster R. Achilles tendon rupture: a new method of repair, early range of motion, and functional rehabilitation. Am J Sports Med 1995;23:392–5.

107. Myerson MS. Achilles tendon rupture. Instr Course Lect 1999;48:219–30.

108. Mafulli N, Ajis A, Longo UG, et al. Chronic rupture of tendo-Achillis. Foot Ankle Clin 2007;12:583–96.

109. Kuwada GT. Classification of tendo Achillis rupture with consideration of surgical repair techniques. J Foot Surg 1990;29:361–5.

110. Den Hartog B. Surgical strategies: delayed diagnosis or neglected Achilles tendon ruptures. Foot Ankle Int 2008;29:456–63.

111. Abraham E, Pankovich AM. Neglected rupture of the Achilles tendon. Treatment by V-Y tendinous flap. J Bone Joint Surg Am 1975;57:253–5.

112. Parker RG, Repinecz E. Neglected rupture of the Achilles tendon. Treatment by modified Strayer gastrocnemius resection. J Am Podiatr Med Assoc 1970;69(9):548–55.

113. Lin J. Tendon transfers for Achilles reconstruction. Foot Ankle Clin 2009;14(4):729–44.

114. Hansen ST Jr. Trauma to heel cord. In: Jahss MH, editor, Disorders of the foot and ankle, vol. 3. Philadelphia: WB Saunders; 1991. p. 2355–60.

115. Wapner KL, Pavlock GS, Hecht PJ, et al. Repair of chronic Achilles tendon rupture with flexor hallucis longus tendon transfer. Foot Ankle 1993;14(8):443–9.

116. Frenette JP, Jackson DW. Lacerations of the flexor hallucis longus in the young athlete. J Bone Joint Surg Am 1977;59(5):673–6.

117. Panchbhavi VK. Chronic Achilles tendon repair with flexor hallucis longus tendon harvested using minimally invasive technique. Tech Foot Ankle Surg 2007;6(2):123–9.

118. Schepsis AA, Hugh J, Haas AL. Achilles tendon disorders in athletes. Am J Sports Med 2002;30(2):287–305.

Dance Medicine of the Foot and Ankle: A Review

Bruce Werber, DPM[a,b,*]

KEYWORDS

• Dancer • Foot • Ankle • Injury

The field of dance medicine has grown immensely over the last more than 20 years. Dancers, such as ballet, jazz, modern, tap, or competitive ballroom dancers, are artists and athletes. In dance, the choreographer acts as a sculptor, using the dancer as a medium of expression. This often entails placing the dancer's body in positions that require extraordinary flexibility and movement, which need controlled power and endurance. All forms of dance are highly demanding activities, with a lifetime injury incidence of up to 90%. Most dance types are stressful, particularly on the dancer's forefoot, but certainly, and there is no area of the foot or ankle that is exempt from potential injury.

Who is a typical dancer? In reviewing the literature, both peer-reviewed and trade publications, a profile appears for professional and competitive ballroom dancers.

In a study by Weiss and colleagues,[1] a profile was developed as to the demographics and background of a typical modern dancer. They found that modern dancers are a unique group of artists, performing a diverse repertoire in dance companies of various sizes. The mean age of the dancers was 30.1 ± 7.3 years and they had danced professionally for 8.9 ± 7.2 years. The average body mass index (calculated as the weight in kilograms divided by the height in meters squared) was 23.6 ± 2.4 for men and 20.5 ± 1.7 for women. Women had started taking dance classes earlier (age, 6.5 ± 4.2 years) as compared with men (age, 15.6 ± 6.2 years). Women were more likely to have begun their training in ballet, whereas men more often began with modern classes (55% and 51%, respectively; $P<.0001$). In a survey, the professional modern dancers were found to spend 8.3 ± 6.0 hours in class and 17.2 ± 12.6 hours in rehearsal each week. It was reported that 50% took modern technique class and 67% took ballet technique class. The dancers (N = 84) who specified what modern technique they studied reported between 2 and 4 different techniques. The dancers also participated in a multitude of

[a] InMotion Foot & Ankle Specialists, 10900 North Scottsdale Road, Suite 604, Scottsdale, AZ 85254, USA
[b] Arizona School of Podiatric Medicine, Midwestern University, 19555 North 59th Avenue, Glendale, AZ 85308, USA
* InMotion Foot & Ankle Specialists, 10900 North Scottsdale Road, Suite 604, Scottsdale, AZ 85254.
E-mail address: docwerber@gmail.com

Clin Podiatr Med Surg 28 (2011) 137–154
doi:10.1016/j.cpm.2010.10.005   **podiatric.theclinics.com**
0891-8422/11/$ – see front matter © 2011 Elsevier Inc. All rights reserved.

additional exercise regimens for a total of 8.2 ± 6.6 hours per week, with the most common types being Pilates, yoga, and upper body weight lifting. The dancers wore many different types of footwear, depending on the style of dance being performed. For modern dance alone, dancers wore 12 different types of footwear. Reflecting the diversity of the dancers and companies surveyed, women reported performing for 23.3 ± 14.0 weeks (range, 2–52 weeks) per year, whereas men reported performing 20.4 ± 13.9 weeks (range, 1–40 weeks) per year.

A meta-analysis by Hincapié and colleagues[2] determined that there is a high prevalence and incidence of lower extremity and back injuries, with soft tissue and overuse injuries predominating. For example, lifetime prevalence estimates for injury in professional ballet dancers ranged between 40% and 84%, whereas the prevalence of minor injury in a diverse group of university and professional ballet and modern dancers was 74%. Adolescent dancers account for most ballet injuries.

Among the injuries, 53% occurred in the foot/ankle, 21.6% in the hip, 16.1% in the knee, and 9.4% in the back. There were 1.09 injuries per 1000 athletic exposures, and 0.77 injuries per 1000 hours of dance. Significant differences between injured and noninjured dancers were limited to the history of low-back pain ($P = .017$), right foot pronation ($P = .005$), insufficient right-ankle plantar flexion ($P = .037$), and lower extremity strength ($P = .045$). In a study of Irish dancers by Walls and colleagues,[3] only 3 ankles out of 18 were considered radiologically normal. Achilles tendinopathy, usually insertional, was the most frequent observation (n = 14), followed by plantar fasciitis (n = 7), bone edema (n = 2), and calcaneocuboid joint degeneration (n = 2). There were limited correlations between magnetic resonance imaging (MRI) patterns and clinical scores, indicating that many conditions are subclinical. According to Kadel,[4] the reported injuries occurred in 67% to 95% of ballet dancers and 17% to 24% of modern dancers. Of all dance injuries reported, 34% to 62% are foot and ankle injuries. Female ballet dancers reported more injuries than male ballet and modern dancers, and 23% to 45% foot and ankle injuries in professional musical theater dancers.

No specific demographic data have been developed on competitive ballroom dancing; however, trade information reveals that there is a growing group of 40- to 70-year-old men and women participating in ballroom dancing. The information does not segregate or stratify between competitive ballroom dancing versus noncompetitive dancing. However, the latest trend is an aerobic dance trend called Zumba, a fusion of Latin and international music that creates a dynamic cardio workout. The overall incidence of dance injuries across the spectrum of dance styles varies widely, with a reported annual frequency of 23% to 85% of participants suffering a injury of that percentage; 65% are secondary to overtraining and 35% to trauma.

BIOMECHANICS OF THE FOOT IN DANCE

In any form of dance, great strain is placed on the lower extremity and the foot. A large percentage of injuries to dancers involve the foot and ankle. Understanding the structure, biomechanics, and physics of the lower extremity helps to diagnose and evaluate the mechanics behind these injuries. The lower extremity function is complicated and needs to be studied carefully to understand its laws and principles. For example, relevé can cause sickling and put the foot in an unstable position if there is forefoot instability, such as decreased stiffness of the medial column or a functional or structural hallux limitus or rigidus. If the forefoot is not strong enough, then the leg will externally rotate and the hip joint's muscular support will not be stable during heel raise. In the opposite direction, when a dancer is executing plié, the outcome of an unstable foot is strain on the passive supporting structures, such as the plantar fascia, midtarsal joint capsules, and tarsometatarsal joint complex (Lisfranc joint). This strain leads to faulty bone alignment, increased load when the foot structure is not aligned to dissipate it across a broader surface, and risk of overuse injury.

The en pointe position of maximal plantar flexion through the forefoot, midfoot, and hindfoot requires tremendous flexibility and strength that can only be attained safely through many years of training.

Biomechanically evaluating the function is critical to developing a differential diagnosis and identifying the cause for any type of dancer. The shoe that is required for each type of dance must also be evaluated. There are many companies that fabricate a variety of shoes for each dance specialty. It is only recently that dance shoe manufacturers have started to incorporate biomechanical design features. For example, Capulet has redesigned the ballet pointe shoe to reduce abrasions, reduce impact force, and improve stability as well as by stiffening the shank. Each category of dance must be aesthetically pleasing in addition to being functional for the particular dance style. Competitive ballroom dancing has subcategories for men and women. Many of these dancing shoes are fitted tightly to the foot and leave little room for accomodations to treat biomechanical and structural deformities. Dance shoe evaluation is not only critical to the diagnostic evaluation of a patient's problem but also an integral part of the treatment plan.

Other risk factors that must be considered and related to the dancers foot type and function are dancing barefoot, long training hours, increased flexibility, lifts and throws, increased rotational torque, and insufficient support either mechanically or from shoes.

DANCER EVALUATION AND EXAMINATION

Evaluating dance injuries should be as extensive as any sports injury. The physician must take a careful history including an attempt to understand the mechanism of injury, the patient's preinjury level of activity, history of prior injuries, evaluation of the shoe gear, the type of dance, the frequency and intensity of practice, and the competition or performance schedule, as well as what other activities does the patient participate and what type of shoe gear is used for those activities.

Physical examination includes comparing the unaffected foot with the injured foot, putting each part of the foot through its range of motion, doing active and passive muscle testing and gait analysis, and if possible, evaluating the position or positions that cause the pain. Lastly, having the dance-specific shoe put on while evaluating the fit of the shoe and then doing a dance analysis, if possible, with the dance shoe on, thus recreating the problem.

IMAGING

Diagnostic ultrasonography is a significant tool for this type of patient who typically has soft tissue overuse–type injuries. The tendon and fascial structures are clearly visualized with diagnostic ultrasonography. The metatarsophalangeal (MTP) joint's plantar structures, ganglions, and neuromas can also be clearly visualized using diagnostic ultrasonography.

The use of computed tomography (CT) and MRI has certainly improved the diagnostic specificity of most overuse injuries when compared with plain radiographic evaluation. In a study by Russel and colleagues,[5] the ballet dancers' ankles weight bearing maximum plantar flexion (en pointe) were evaluated to assess whether the pathologic findings of MRI were associated with ankle pain reported by the subjects.

In this study, 9 female ballet dancers (age, 21.0 ± 2.9 years; dance experience, 16.0 ± 4.1 years; en pointe dance experience, 7.0 ± 4.9 years) completed an ankle pain visual analog scale questionnaire and underwent T1- and T2-weighted scans using a 0.25-T open MRI device. The ankle was scanned in 3 positions: supine with full plantar flexion, standing with the ankle in anatomic position, and standing en pointe.

MRI signs of ankle abnormality and anatomic variants were observed. Convergence of the posterior edge of the tibial plafond, posterior talus, and superior calcaneus was noted in 100% of cases. Widened anterior joint congruity and synovitis/joint effusion were present in 71% and 67%, respectively. Anterior tibial and/or talar spurs and Stieda process were each seen in 44%. However, clinical signs did not always correlate with pain reported by the subjects.

Certainly, many other studies have been completed, reporting a multitude of pathologic conditions that have a commonality with the typical dance injuries, and it is beyond the scope of this article to review the CT and MRI literature for foot and ankle injuries.

COMMONLY REPORTED DANCE-RELATED INJURIES AND TREATMENT HIGHLIGHTS

- Fractures varying from incomplete stress fractures to a full comminuted fracture, with no osseous structure exempt from potential injury
- Structural deformities including hallux abducto valgus, hallux limitus, hallux rigidus, and contracted digital deformities. Impingement syndromes (anterior and posterior) of the ankle. Chondral injuries, such as Freiberg disease, and osteochondral avascular necrosis
- Overuse injuries including tendon and fascial injuries, that is, plantar fasciitis, Achilles tendinitis, Achilles enthesopathy, tenosynovitis of the flexors and/or extensors, and shin splints
- Sprains and strains of the ankle and subtalar, midtarsal, tarsometatarsal (Lisfranc joint), and MTP joints.

DISCUSSION OF COMMONLY REPORTED DANCE INJURIES (IN THE ORDER OF FREQUENCY)
Ankle Sprain

Ankle inversion injuries are the most common traumatic injuries in dancers. The lateral ligament complex of the ankle is the most frequently injured structure in the body. Although most simple ankle sprains do not result in long-term disability, a significant number do not completely resolve, leading to residual symptoms that may persist for years. Ankle stability is integral to normal mobilization and to minimizing the risk for ankle sprain. The ability of the dynamic and static stabilizers of the ankle joint to maintain their structural integrity is a major component of the normal gait cycle. Hiller and colleagues[6] attempted to identify intrinsic predictors of lateral ankle sprain and they evaluated 115 adolescent dancers, 94 female and 21 male. They found that in the test group, an increased risk of sprain was predicted by younger age, previous sprain of the contralateral ankle, increased passive inversion range, and the inability to balance on demipointe. Of these predictors, only previous sprain of the contralateral ankle significantly predicted ankle sprain in the validation group. The most commonly reported symptoms, particularly among athletes, include instability, reinjury, and tendinitis. For example, ballet dancers perform in unusual positions, such as en pointe, that place the ankle in extreme plantar flexion, requiring stabilization by surrounding muscles. Dancers' extraordinary performance demands place them at risk for other ankle injuries as well, including inflammation of the Achilles tendon, peroneals, and flexor hallucis longus (FHL) most notably. A literature review by Ritter and Moore[7] reports that numerous studies have investigated ankle sprains and residual complaints, and nearly all studies report that lateral ankle sprains commonly lead to chronic ankle instability. Studies exploring ankle stability have demonstrated that the peroneal muscles play a crucial role in ankle stabilization; electromyographic (EMG) studies confirm that ankle stability is the first to occur during ankle inversion stress. The dancer's need for exceptional ankle stabilization may lead to peroneal overuse and tendinitis. Studies have linked peroneal abnormality to a history of ankle sprain, but there is no dance medicine literature linking peroneal tendinitis to prior ankle sprains. A growing body of literature confirms myriad connections between lateral ankle sprains, residual instability, peroneal muscle increased activity, and tendinitis. Ritter and Moore[7] concluded that ankle sprains lead to instability, particularly en pointe, for which the peroneal muscles attempt to compensate. Peroneal muscle overuse for this static stabilizing function, as well as for dynamic dance movements, then leads to tendonitis.

Symptoms described by dancers when they initially present with an ankle injury are rolled ankle, hearing a "pop" type sound, and swelling and bruising over the lateral ankle, typically occurs after landing with a jump or after a combination of rapid leg movements.

The role of a typical physical examination is to evaluate the lateral collateral ligaments with an anterior drawer test (requires stabilizing the tibia, attempting to bring the talus forward in the mortise, and noting any anterior displacement). Physical examination also includes palpating the lateral collaterals for pain or instability. The examiner should evaluate and attempt to differentiate ankle injury from subtalar joint pain and identify whether the pain is localized at the lateral collaterals or more in the sinus tarsi than the peroneal tendons.

Imaging at this point is extremely important; plain radiography is performed first to rule out osseous pathologic conditions such as stress fracture, acute complete fracture, structural alignment issues, and the presence of Stieda process. Then a diagnostic ultrasonography would be appropriate to image the peroneal tendons and lateral ankle collaterals. Lastly, an MRI can be performed especially in a professional or competitive dancer to isolate the specific area of injury.

Initial therapy for ankle injury is (1) full evaluation, (2) compression using a compression stocking or an equivalent at a pressure of 15 to 20 mm Hg, (3) stabilization using a stiff controlling brace such as AirSport (Aircast) or an equivalent, and (4) contrast temperature therapy using cold application for 10 minutes, followed by heat application for 10 minutes, and then completing the set with a second cold application for 10 minutes. The process of contrast temperature therapy is repeated 4 to 5 times per day for the first 5 days and is then reduced to twice a day until the injury is resolved or imaging studies are completed. A full understanding of the injury is then completed, and a full treatment plan is developed.

Follow-up therapy includes proprioceptive strengthening exercises, possible diagnostic or therapeutic ankle arthroscopy, physical therapy including infrared laser treatment at 800 to 980 nm, ultrasonography, and exercise rehabilitation to return to full strength preinjury level. Additionally, the dancer biomechanics would be assessed and shoe evaluation would be completed to determine if a biomechanical device or modification to the dance shoe is necessary for injury prevention.

Dancers fracture, also known as spiral fracture of the fifth metatarsal base, typically occurs by rolling off pointe or by landing on the lateral aspect of the foot after a jump. Fifth metatarsal fractures are also common with ankle sprains.

The current gold standard for treatment of chronic fracture nonunion in the metaphyseal-diaphyseal region of the fifth metatarsal is intramedullary screw fixation, plating, or tension wire technique. Complications with these procedures, however, are not uncommon. Shock wave therapy can be an effective alternative treatment of fracture nonunions. In a study by Furia and colleagues,[8] 20 of 23 nonunions in the shock wave group and 18 of 20 nonunions in the screw fixation group were healed at 3 months after treatment. One of the 3 nonunions that were not healed by 3 months in the shock wave group was healed by 6 months. There was 1 complication in the shock wave group (posttreatment petechiae) and 11 complications in the screw fixation group (1 case of refracture, 1 cellulitis, and 9 symptomatic hardware). Both open reduction and internal fixation (ORIF) and shock wave therapy are effective treatments of fracture nonunion in the metaphyseal-diaphyseal region of the fifth metatarsal. ORIF is more often associated with complications that frequently result in additional surgery.

Hallux Limitus/Rigidus

A limitation of motion in the first MTP joint can be attributed to several causes including a functional hallux limitus secondary to decreased stiffness of the first ray; with weight bearing, the first ray effectively elevates and the MTP joint is locked. Thus, the hallux cannot dorsiflex on the first metatarsal, forcing the foot to externally rotate and roll off the medial aspect of the hallux; however, in some patients, the hallux interphalangeal joint is forcibly dorsiflexed. Causes of hallux rigidus are also multifactorial; ultimately it can be considered on a continuum with functional hallux limitus. Grading is dependent on the extent of degeneration of the articular surfaces, progressive over time due to the repetitive jamming within the first MTP joint.

Modern, jazz, and ballet dancers complain of the pain in MTP joint earlier than a tap dancer because the shoes and the movements do not require as much motion in the first MTP joint and the shoe sole is much stiffer. Ballet dancers notice the restriction of motion especially in full relevé. Ballet dancers compensate with sickling during demi-pointe, which is not an acceptable alignment and can lead to lateral ankle sprains.

Modern, jazz, and ballroom dancers notice restriction with any dance step or jump that requires push off. The effects of hallux limitus/rigidus are more common among dancers who began dancing at an older age.

Treatment of hallux limitus should begin as early as possible, ensuring excellent function of the peroneus longus, which assists in stabilization of the first ray. Treatment can be performed with proprioceptive exercises, functional foot orthosis, and range of motion exercise of the MTP joint.

If the treatment fails and the limitation of motion continues to develop, then surgical options should be explored, including stabilization of the first ray with arthrodesis of the first metatarsal cuneiform joint and plantar-flexed position of the first metatarsal, possible gastrocnemius recession to achieve lengthening of the Achilles tendon and reduce equinus deformity, or subtalar artheroresis to control rearfoot motion and position during gait and dance. If the limitation of motion has progressed to rigidus and there is osteophytic proliferation around the metatarsal head and base of the proximal phalanx, then cheilectomy or other procedures including joint replacement may need to be considered.

Hallux Abducto Valgus and Turf Toe

Injuries to the MTP joint of the great toe have increased in incidence over the past 30 years following the introduction of artificial playing surfaces and the accompanying use of lighter footwear. Although these injuries are most common in American football players, similar injuries can also occur in other sporting activities including soccer and dance or after trauma to the great toe. The mechanism of injury is typically hyperextension of the MTP joint, but injuries have also been reported secondary to valgus or varus stress or rarely as a result of hyperflexion. The abnormal forces applied to the first MTP joint during injury result in varying degrees of sprain or disruption of the supporting soft tissue structures, leading to the injury commonly referred to as turf toe. The extent of soft tissue disruption is influential in treatment planning and can be used to determine the prognosis.

As with hallux limitus and rigidus, treatment should start early in a dancer's career, addressing the mechanical deficiencies in the foot structure and focusing on improving the stability of the medial column to prevent decreased stiffness of the medial column. When decreased stiffness develops in the medial column, there is an effective elevation of the first ray with weight bearing and this elevation limits motion at the first MTP joint. Over time, this jamming causes degeneration of the cartilaginous surfaces and osteophytic proliferation, moving from available motion and a viable joint space to the end point of severe degenerative arthritis with loss of the joint space within the first MTP joint.

Initially, the dancer needs to focus on reducing posterior muscle tightness (equinus) and maintaining good strength in the peroneal muscle group. Pronatory forces at the subtalar joint are reduced by using a functional foot orthotic, inverting the calcaneal position and loading the lesser metatarsals, and allowing the first ray to function in a more plantar-flexed position. To make a device to fit in a ballet slipper or pointe shoe, it can be fabricated from carbon graphite for minimal thickness and maximal structure and narrow arch area, allowing the heel cup to be wedged inverted (varus, higher medial than lateral) and molded in the forefoot depending on the foot type to hold the forefoot in neutral and allow the first ray to plantar flex as the forefoot loads. Several different modifications can be added to the forefoot placed on an extension from the orthotic to the toes. Using a kinetic wedge as described by Dananberg[9] or reverse the Morton extension, these devices effectively increase the range of motion at the first MTP joint as the forefoot is loaded.

Ultimately, if the progress cannot be slowed sufficiently, then surgical intervention should be considered which may include arthrodesis of the first metatarsal cuneiform joint to plantar flex the first metatarsal to achieve medial column stability with cheilectomy of the osteophytes that have developed around the metatarsal head and base of the proximal phalanx hallux. In an unpublished proof-of-concept (Bruce Werber, DPM, 2009) small group study of 12 patients with hallux limitus, who had a joint space and minimal osteophytic proliferation on radiographs, continued to have joint pain despite the use of appropriate foot orthotics. Their joints were injected with 1.5 mL of autogenous platelet-rich plasma (PRP). After 12 weeks, they reported a significant 80% to 90% reduction in joint pain, which has been effective for 40 weeks on average.

Metatarsalgia

Metatarsalgia is described as forefoot pain that is associated with increased stress/pain in the area of the metatarsal head region. Metatarsalgia is often referred to as a symptom rather than a specific disease. Differential diagnoses of metatarsalgia include interdigital neuroma, MTP synovitis, avascular necrosis, sesamoiditis, and inflammatory arthritis. Female competitive ballroom dancers seem to have a higher incidence of forefoot complaints than other types of dancers. This incidence is attributable to the types of shoes that are typically high heels with very thin soles and extremely tight fit, as well as the motions performed in certain turns and steps, requiring persistent weight focused on the forefoot.

The most common findings and diagnoses in order of frequency as noted in the author's clinic are discussed in the following sections.

Neuritis/nerve entrapment is the most common finding. Dancers are required to perform at the extreme of their physiologic and functional limits. Under such conditions, peripheral nerves are prone to compression. Entrapment neuropathies in dancers can occur at multiple levels. The most common nerve disorders encountered in dancers include interdigital neuromas (second and third interspaces), tarsal tunnel syndrome, anterior tarsal tunnel syndrome, superficial and deep peroneal nerve entrapment, and sural nerve entrapment.

Treatment of these nerve disorders begins with their diagnosis using ultrasonography, MRI, or neurologic testing; in some cases, diagnostic nerve blocks are performed to isolate the cause of pain. Once the abnormality is identified, the treatment protocol is then to address the its mechanics if one exists and to decompress the nerve with physical therapy, change in technique or shoe, or with steroid injection, sclerosing injections of absolute alcohol,[10] or surgical decompression.[11]

Sesamoid injuries of the first metatarsal phalangeal joint in dancers may result in prolonged pain, disability, and career limitation. A thorough understanding of sesamoid function and potential disorders is critical for all dancers, including aerobic, ballroom, and certainly, performance dancers. Sesamoid disorders are common causes of the forefoot pain metatarsalgia. There are significant mechanical stresses and anatomic variations reported and noted regarding the sesamoid complex. Numerous pathologic processes can affect the sesamoid apparatus of the first metatarsal phalangeal joint. These processes include acute fractures, stress fractures, nonunions, osteonecrosis, chondromalacia, and various inflammatory conditions that are grouped as sesamoiditis that is typically caused by synovitis.

Treatment includes activity and weight-bearing restrictions, protective padding, strengthening, functional retraining, and progressive return to dance. Injections of steroid must be used judiciously; bone stimulators have been reported to be successful in the treatment of stress fractures and complete fractures of the sesamoids. This is another area that can be potentially treated with PRP, with minimal risk. The potential loss of hallux plantar-flexion strength due to sesamoidectomy is a major consideration for dancers, and thus, sesamoidectomy should be a procedure of last resort.[12]

Capsulitis and rupture of the plantar plate in lesser metatarsal phalangeal joints potentially lead to the formation of contracture of the proximal interphalangeal joints (hammer toe deformity).

Examination reveals tenderness and palpable fullness of the metatarsal phalangeal joint, painful dorsal drawer sign, adjacent interdigital tenderness, and developing nonrigid hammer toe deformity. Radiography may reveal mild to significant subluxation of the metatarsal phalangeal joint, with the proximal phalangeal base drifting medially or laterally. Diagnostic ultrasonography may reveal rupture of the plantar plate at its attachment to the base of the proximal phalanx, swelling of the flexor tendon, or swelling within the joint itself or a combination of any or all of these findings. Treatment includes intra-articular corticosteroid injection but must be used with caution because the fluid load of the lesser MTP joints is typically less than 1 mL and there is a risk of intrinsic tendon rupture, accelerating capsule tearing, or plantar plate rupture. The use of Budin splint helps reduce pressure and irritation and aligns overlapping digits while encouraging extension of flexible hammer or claw toes during gait. Temporary rocker-sole shoe modification to limit MP joint dorsiflexion helps to off-load the pressure. Restriction and modification of activity is a useful adjunct initially. Surgical options include open arthrotomy with synovectomy, using radio frequency coblation to perform synovectomy and repair plantar plate instability, shortening osteotomy of the metatarsal by performing an oblique osteotomy as described by Weil, and arthrodesis of the proximal interphalangeal joint and flexor transfer. These procedures are successful but must be used with caution in any dancer.[13]

Freiberg disease, or osteonecrosis of the second metatarsal head, is an uncommon cause of forefoot pain that can severely limit a dancer's relevé. Dancers may be predisposed to the condition because of repetitive microtrauma to the ball of the foot during routine dance movements. Freiberg disease is diagnosed by history taking, physical examination, and plain film radiography. Conservative treatment in dancers is disappointing, and surgical options fail to produce uniformly good results.[14] Several alternatives have been reported including an open arthrotomy of the second MTP, a synovectomy using radio frequency coblation under arthroscopic visualization, or injecting the joint with 1 mL of PRP and have protected weight bearing off-loading the forefoot for 2 to 3 weeks, then starting physical therapy and gradual return to activity.[15]

Miscellaneous forefoot complaints that can be concerning and disabling are ingrown toenails with or without infection, subungual bleeding, cracking or breaking of nails, and fungal infections of the skin or nails. Skin injuries are irritating should the dancer develop a blister or corns (hyperkeratosis) on the dorsal aspect of the proximal interphalangeal joints, and included in painful irritations is a viral infection causing a verruca (wart).

Treatment of warts and ingrown nail problems is fairly straightforward and is beyond the scope of this article to review. As far as the development of painful callus or porokeratosis, treatment can be fairly straightforward with periodic debridement, surgical correction of the causative deformity, or as advocated by Balkin,[16] an intradermal injection of liquid silicon (Silikon 1000, Alcon, Fort Worth, TX, USA). Balkin's work has been documented over 40 years using liquid silicon and he has reported significant resolution of painful hyperkeratosis without surgery and solely with injection of liquid silicon intradermally.

Heel Pain, Plantar Fasciitis, Plantar Fasciosis, Heel Spur Syndrome

Heel pain cannot always be assumed to be caused by the pathologic condition in the plantar fascia. It is imperative that all potential causes be investigated and ruled out. Differential diagnosis consists of tarsal tunnel syndrome, entrapment of the medial calcaneal nerve, lumbar radiculopathy, compartment syndrome of the medial and plantar compartments of the foot, rare primary presenting sign of systemic inflammatory disorders, Achilles enthesopathy, stress fracture, bone tumor, and space-occupying lesions.

The cause of heel pain in a dancer is multifactorial; starting from the surface the dancer is working on. For example, whether the floor is sprung or nonsprung; if the floor is hard and unyielding, there will be more force on the foot as the dancer lands and thus increasing strain on the plantar fascia. If the dancer wears heels outside the dance practice and performance arena, then the posterior muscle group can tighten and contribute to increased pronatory forces being created along the plantar fascia.

Diagnosis of heel pain is essential to getting dancers back to their activity. Radiography is essential to evaluate osseous structures and ultrasonography is a tremendous tool to evaluate the plantar fascial thickness. Normal fascia is typically recognized to be approximately 2.5 to 3.5 mm thick at the calcaneal insertion, but as the thickness increases, the fascia becomes scarred and thickened worsening from an inflammatory state to a chronic thickened poorly vascularized state considered to be fasciosis. Lemont and colleagues[17] reviewed histologic findings from 50 cases of heel spur surgery for chronic plantar fasciitis. Findings included myxoid degeneration with fragmentation and degeneration of the plantar fascia and bone marrow vascular ectasia. Histologic findings were presented to support the hypothesis that plantar fasciitis is a degenerative fasciosis without inflammation and not a fasciitis. In the studies by

Almekinders[18] from 1998 through 2002, he demonstrates clearly that there is minimal inflammatory response within the tendon and fascia after direct tissue injury and that there is no inflammatory response in the tissue that has suffered repetitive motion–type injuries. Khan[19] used a rat model to produce acute tendinopathy by exposing the tissues to proinflammatory cytokines. The tissues demonstrated no inflammatory response but did show derangement and degradation of the collagen fibers.

Diagnostic studies for the other differentials include MRI, CT scan, EMG, nerve conduction velocity studies, and possibly, bone scans to fully evaluate the causative factors. The diagnostician must look proximal as well to identify possible causes of heel pain especially in a dancer, for example, lumbar stenosis causing radiculopathy.

Treatment of heel pain varies from modification and change of the types of shoes worn during dancing and nondancing activities to aggressive stretching of the gastrocnemius and soleus and the plantar fascia and intrinsics of the foot. Steroid injections and foot orthotics have been a mainstay in treating plantar fasciitis and fasciosis. New technologies such as radio frequency coblation and injection of PRP show significant promise in combination with traditional therapeutic approaches. Near-infrared diode laser therapy in the frequency range of 800 to 980 nm show significant potential in stimulating the tissue to heal.

When using orthotics for dance shoes, all dance shoes must fit snugly and must be cut narrow and tight to the foot. Pointe shoes are the most difficult to accomodate for any type of biomechanical correction. At times, gluing accommodations directly into the shoe works best or using extremely thin poly prefabricated devices and modifying those shells that typically are 1 to 2 mm in thickness has worked well to stabilize the foot in the pointe shoe. In ballroom, jazz, and tap shoes for men, it is much easier to add thin poly or carbon graphite shells with intrinsic corrections built into the orthosis. It is extremely difficult to modify or accommodate a removable type of orthosis in ballroom shoes for women. In these cases, a shoe repair expert can help to build and modify the inner sole of the shoe, along with the pads and straps to improve foot function.

Achilles Tendinitis, Enthesopathy, and Haglund Deformity

These conditions present with pain in the posterior lower leg and heel. The differentiation between the 3 diagnoses depends on location. Achilles tendinitis or tendinopathy that is found typically 3 to 6 cm from the Achilles tendon insertion presents as a dull ache or discomfort and expands to a nodule within the Achilles tendon, with a feeling of crepitus as the foot is dorsiflexed and plantar flexed. There is swelling and inflammation around the painful area of the tendon. Achilles tendon injuries are typically caused by overtraining to perform relevé and jumps, a case of too much too soon associated with a lack of flexibility of the calf muscles.

The tendon experiences a similar course of events as the plantar fasciosis, with an initiating event occurring to injure the tendon. Initially, an inflammatory reaction occurs, but because of the continued activity or intake of antiinflammatory medications, the normal healing process is interrupted and instead of a healthy tendon a poorly vascularized thickened scar-like tissue is formed. Achilles enthesopathy occurs at the insertion. This condition is typically caused by either repetitive sudden forces at the insertion or chronic equinus with pulling and tearing of the Achilles insertion with reactive bone formation within the tendon insertion. Haglund deformity typically becomes apparent when there is chronic irritation from the shoe on the posterosuperior surface of the calcaneus, resulting in bursa formation and then chronic pain on the posterosuperior aspect of the heel.

Achilles tendon rupture does occur in dancers but is a rare occurrence and must always be in the differential list and ruled out via MRI or diagnostic ultrasonography.

Treatment of Achilles tendinitis and enthesopathy is similar to treating heel pain and is followed by stretching, near-infrared laser therapy, and/or PRP injection if the tendon injury does not respond to the traditional therapy of rest, bracing, and physical therapy. Certainly, using appropriate diagnostic modalities is necessary to confirm the diagnosis; MRI or ultrasonography is an excellent option for visualizing the tendon. If the patient does not respond to conservative modalities, including PRP injection and laser therapy, then an open surgical approach may be necessary to resolve the chronic intractable condition. During surgery for chronic nodule formation and intractable tendinopathy, a posterolateral approach is taken; the tendon is inspected and incised, resecting the poorly organized and formed tissue, radio frequency coblation is performed, and a primary repair is done. This surgical approach is applied for Achilles enthesopathy as well; in addition to repairing the distal tendon, the reactive bone is resected as well, and the author uses knotless anchors to reattach the tendon to the calcaneus.

Ankle Posterior Impingement Syndrome

This syndrome is an impingement at the posterior of the ankle between the talus and tibia. It is also known in the literature as os trigonum syndrome, talar compression syndrome, posterior ankle impingement syndrome, and posterior tibiotalar impingement syndrome.[20–25] The posterior tubercle or elongated posterolateral talar process (Stieda process) of the talus can effectively be pinched between the talus and tibia, causing pain. Hypertrophy or tear of the posteroinferior talofibular ligament (TFL), transverse TFL, tibial slip, or pathologic labrum on the posterior ankle joint can lead to posterior ankle impingement, which can affect the os trigonum or posterior talus of the calcaneus. Shepherd fracture is a synchondrosis of the os trigonum or a fracture of the posterior or trigonal process of the talus.[26]

The dancer describes pain and tenderness at the back of the ankle. Pain is triggered when the ankle is passively plantar flexed to the extreme range of motion. A local anesthetic block injection is given to the affected area, and if passive plantar flexion no longer triggers pain, it is an indication of impingement. This syndrome can also result from abnormality of the os trigonum–talar process, ankle osteochondritis, FHL tenosynovitis, and subtalar joint disease. Pain is elicited by forced plantar flexion and push-off maneuvers.[27] In ballet dancers, forcing a turnout of the foot can predispose to this condition.[27] Hardaker[28] found that in extreme plantar flexion, an os trigonum, a Stieda process, a prominent dorsal process of the calcaneus, or the presence of adhered or loose osteophytes can occupy space within the posterior ankle joint and lead to soft tissue impingement.

Hamilton[29] described a labrum or pseudomeniscus of the posterior lip of the tibia, which can become torn or hypertrophied with ankle sprains and lead to posterior impingement. Excessive plantar flexion at the ankle joint can cause compression of the posterior synovial, capsular, and/or ligamentous tissues against the posterior tibia. With repeated entrapment, the posterior soft tissue structures can undergo inflammatory changes, thickening, and fibrosis, leading to scarring and/or calcification.[30–32]

FHL tendinopathy is a common injury especially in ballet dancers who function frequently en pointe and is included in the differential of posterior impingement syndrome. Repetitive and prolonged plantar flexion leads to tenosynovitis or tendinopathy. Further overuse frequently progresses to frank longitudinal tearing. As in any tendinopathy, there is a thickening of the tendon initially secondary to inflammation, and as the injury goes untreated, the tendon thickens and synovitis develops. As the tendon passes into the flexor sheath in the posterior aspect of the ankle, the thickened tendon essentially gets caught on the edge of the tendon sheath. Inflammation of the FHL tendon generally can occur in one of the following areas: at the fibro-osseous tunnel along the posteromedial ankle, under the base of the first metatarsal where the flexor digitorum longus tendon crosses the FHL tendon (knot of Henry), or where the FHL tendon passes between the great toe sesamoids beneath the metatarsal head.

When the tendon becomes nodular, triggering of the great toe (hallux saltans) can occur and lead to hallux rigidus. Complete tears of the FHL tendon are infrequent, with fewer than 4 cases of acute rupture being reported.

Symptoms described by the dancer include a feeling of the hallux clicking or getting caught, and the dancer will be unable to move into en pointe due to a sense of having no strength and also pain while lowering from demipointe.

Ankle Anterior Impingement Syndrome

This syndrome is an impingement at the anterior portion of the ankle between the talus and tibia. The characteristics of the syndrome are restriction of full plié on one side, pain with deep pliés, swelling may be noted at the anterior ankle joint, and osteophytes may be noted on the anterior aspect of the tibia or the neck of the talus. Bassett and colleagues[33] found and described a separate pathologic fascicle of the anterior TFL in syndesmotic impingement. Following a tear of the anterior TFL, the anterolateral talar dome extrudes anteriorly with dorsiflexion, resulting in impingement. Chronic repetitive microtrauma can lead to bone spur formation (anterior tibiotalar osteophytes), which gradually causes subsequent limitation of movement and pain. The development of anterior ankle impingement in ballet dancers requires hyperdorsiflexion to accomplish the demiplié position, which, in turn, can lead to direct contact and impingement of the anterior lip of the tibia on the talar neck.[34,35] Repetitive impingement secondary to extreme dorsiflexion proliferates exostosis formation at the anterior ankle joint.[28,36]

Conservative treatment of ankle impingement syndromes includes modifying activity, wearing protected bracing or casting, immobilization by rest, physical therapy, heel lifts, dance and regular shoe modifications, antiinflammatory medication, and corticosteroid and PRP injections. If conservative measures fail and the patient continues to experience swelling, tenderness, limitation of motion, and weakness, then surgical management should be considered.

Reach and colleagues[37] investigated the degree to which ultrasonographically guided injections could accurately reach the common foot and ankle injection sites. Using ultrasonographic guidance, a methylene blue–saline mixture was injected into 10 fresh cadaver feet, targeting the FHL sheath as well as the first and second MTP joints, the tibiotalar joint, the Achilles peritendinous space, the posterior tibial tendon sheath, and the subtalar joint. It was reported that the injections for all sites were 100% accurate, whereas that of the subtalar joint was 90% accurate.

Open and arthroscopic techniques have been described for the management of anterior and posterior ankle impingement syndromes. Scranton and McDermott[38] did a comparison of open versus arthroscopic measures for anterior ankle impingement, demonstrating that arthroscopy yielded shorter period of postoperative hospitalization and recovery time.

In a retrospective study, Nihal and colleagues[39] reviewed arthroscopic treatment of the anterior bony and soft tissue impingement of the ankle in elite dancers. Out of the 12 patients, 9 returned to full dance activity at an average of 7 weeks after surgery. It was concluded that arthroscopic debridement is an effective method for the treatment of bony and soft tissue anterior ankle impingement syndrome in dancers and has minimal morbidity.[40–43] The objective for surgical treatment of posterior ankle impingement is excision of the impeding anatomic structure. An open medial approach is recommended if the pathologic condition affects the FHL tendon (eg, tear, tenosynovitis) in addition to posterior bony impingement, whereas a lateral approach would be appropriate if the abnormality is primarily osseous.[19,20,44]

Posterolateral Injuries

Calcaneocuboid joint subluxation and peroneal tendinitis

Cuboid syndrome is defined as a minor disruption or subluxation of the structural integrity of the calcaneocuboid portion of the midtarsal joint. This syndrome is also known as lateral plantar neuritis, cuboid fault syndrome, dropped cuboid, locked cuboid, and subluxed cuboid and is a common cause of lateral foot pain in the dancing population. The chief complaint is that of lateral foot pain and weakness during push off. The pain is described as radiating to the medial plantar aspect of the foot and/or to the anterolateral ankle joint or along the fourth and fifth metatarsals. The patient complaints of an inability to "work through the foot" while moving from a foot flat position to demipointe or a full en pointe position. This syndrome typically occurs acutely when dancers land from jumps or as an overuse syndrome from repetitive pointe work. It is thought that repetitive forces can lead to decreased stability of the midfoot and predispose dancers to cuboid syndrome.[45–47]

Diagnosis of cuboid syndrome is difficult. Radiography, CT scan, and bone scans provide limited information; MRI has a higher diagnostic potential but has limitations. The physician must work through the differential diagnoses including sinus tarsi syndrome, lateral process fracture of the talus, acute tendinitis of the peroneus longus tendon, fracture of the anterior process of the os calcis, fractures (including stress fractures), fracture or dislocation of the os peroneum, and tarsal coalitions (in adolescents).

Treatment is difficult for this syndrome; several investigators suggest reducing the subluxed cuboid by using a manipulative technique, which is defined as a low-amplitude high-velocity mobilization at the end of joint range, to restore proper joint congruency. In addition to or as a primary treatment a cuboid pad can be applied directly under the cuboid and the patients' body weight is used to manipulate the cuboid into a corrected position. A low-Dye taping with a cuboid pad has been suggested to hold the cuboid reduction and stabilize subtalar joint motion. Should these maneuvers be successful, a functional foot orthosis with an intrinsic cuboid raise or an additional pad can be fabricated.

The peroneal muscles make up the lateral compartment of the leg and are innervated by the superficial peroneal nerve. The tendon of peroneus longus courses behind the peroneus brevis tendon at the level of the ankle joint, travels inferior to the peroneal tubercle, and turns sharply in a medial direction at the cuboid bone. The tendon inserts into the lateral aspect of the plantar first metatarsal and medial cuneiform. The peroneus longus plantar flexes the first ray, everts the foot, and assists in plantar flexion of the ankle. A sesamoid bone called the os peroneum may be present within the peroneus longus tendon at about the level of the calcaneocuboid joint. The frequency with which an os peroneum occurs is approximately 20% of the population.

The peroneus brevis inserts onto the base of the fifth metatarsal and everts and plantar flexes the foot.

The peroneal tendons share a common tendon sheath proximal to the distal tip of the fibula. More distally, each tendon is within its own sheath. The common sheath is on the posterolateral aspect of the fibula. When the superior peroneal retinaculum (SPR) is intact, it prevents subluxation of the tendon. The hallmark of disorders of the peroneal tendons is laterally based ankle or foot pain with loss of eversion strength. Tenosynovitis and tendinous disruption (acute or chronic) as well as longitudinal tears of both the longus and brevis also occur. The brevis has been reported to be more susceptible to longitudinal tearing. The os peroneum may be involved with the degenerative process or a singular disorder and can be fractured or fragmented.[48] Brandes and Smith[49] have reported that 82% of patients with primary peroneus longus tendinopathy had a cavovarus hindfoot. Overcrowding from a peroneus quartus muscle also has been reported. The mechanism of injury typically involves an inversion to the dorsiflexed ankle, with concomitant forceful contraction of the peroneals.

Brandes and Smith[49] have described and classified primary peroneus longus tendinopathy into 3 anatomic zones in which the tendon can be injured. Zone A is the level of the SPR. Zone B is the level of the inferior peroneal retinaculum, typically partial ruptures. Zone C is the level of the cuboid notch where complete ruptures are most likely. Sobel and colleagues[50,51] have presented a classification for tears of the peroneus brevis tendon as follows:

- Grade 1, flattened tendon
- Grade 2, partial-thickness split less than 1 cm in length
- Grade 3, full-thickness split less than 2 cm in length
- Grade 4, full-thickness split more than 2 cm in length.

Eckert and Davis[52] have classified SPR abnormality as follows:

- Grade I, SPR elevated from fibula
- Grade II, fibrocartilaginous ridge elevated from fibula with SPR
- Grade III, cortical fragment avulsed with SPR.

The patient typically complaints of laterally based ankle or rearfoot pain increasing with activity and subsiding with rest. There usually is tenderness along the peroneal tendons. To evaluate the peroneal tendon stability, the patient's foot is hung in a relaxed position with the knee at 90° and pressure is applied to the peroneal tendons posterior to the fibula. The patient is then asked to dorsiflex and evert the foot. Pain may be elicited and/or the tendons can be seen subluxing or examiner can feel the subluxation.

Conservative therapy includes modifying activity, modification or changing shoe gear, temporary immobilization, or bracing. Biomechanical therapy with functional foot orthosis adding valgus wedging reduces lateral stress. Consideration should be given to treating with electric stimulation, near-infrared laser therapy, and/or PRP injection with ultrasonographic guidance.

Surgical treatment is best considered under the specific pathology being addressed. With any procedure, it is important to remove abnormal-appearing synovium or tenosynovium. Tenosynovitis may be treated surgically with a simple division of the tendon sheath or radio frequency coblation. Care must be taken to protect the sural nerve. Brandes and Smith[49] advocate adding a lateral closing wedge calcaneal osteotomy (Dwyer type procedure) if the patient has a cavus or varus deformity of the hindfoot. Coughlin recommend tenodesis of the peroneus longus if less than one-third of the tendon remains.[53,54]

SHIN SPLINTS AND DANCERS

Shin splint is a nonspecific term for an overuse syndrome affecting the lower leg. Poorly conditioned and new dancers are especially susceptible to this syndrome. Usually, shin splint pain is found on the inside edge of the lower two-thirds of the tibia. This syndrome is commonly attributed to overuse of the posterior tibialis tendon and/or anterior tibial tendon. Other conditions that can elicit pain on the shin area are stress fractures and compartment syndrome.

Treatment of tibial stress fractures in elite dancers includes rest and activity modification. Miyamoto and colleagues[55] evaluated 1757 dancers; 24 dancers (1.4%) had 31 tibial stress fractures. The mean age at the time of stress fracture was 22.6 years. The mean duration of symptoms was 25.8 months.

Typically, a change in activity and appropriate training along with a posterior muscle group stretching routine are sufficient to resolve shin splint problems. Rarely, as evidenced in Miyamoto and colleagues report, do the dancers require surgical intervention.

FRACTURES AND DANCERS

Fractures in the dance population are common. Radiography, CT, MRI, and bone scan should be used as necessary to arrive at the correct diagnosis after a thorough physical examination. Treatment must address the fracture itself and any surrounding problems such as nutritional/hormonal issues and training/performance techniques and regimens. Compliance issues in dancers are of great concern, and treatment strategies must be developed accordingly. Stress fractures, in particular, can present difficulties for the patient and the physician.

TRAINING CONCERNS AND AGE

The initiation of pointe training for dance students should be determined after careful evaluation. Evaluation of the following criteria is imperative: student's stage of physical development; the quality of trunk, abdominal, and pelvic control (core stability); the biomechanical alignment and strength/stability of the hip, knee, ankle, and foot; and the duration and frequency of dance training. Pointe work should not be considered before the fourth year of training. Students with poor core stability or hypermobility of the feet and ankles require additional strengthening to allow them to safely begin pointe training. Students with insufficient ankle and foot plantar flexion or poor lower extremity alignment should not be allowed to do pointe because it is not worth the risk.[56–58]

SUMMARY

Treatment of dancers can be challenging and rewarding. Dancers often have unusual difficulties related to the dynamic biomechanical forces required by their individual dance form. A thorough understanding of these movements guides the physician to the cause of the injury, particularly in understanding specific overuse injuries. This knowledge, coupled with a meticulous physical examination, is essential for diagnosis and treatment of the dancer, who is both an artist and an athlete. Treatment requires the physician to be creative in some respects to treat the underlying biomechanical issues within the restraints of the particular dance type and shoe gear required.

REFERENCES

1. Weiss DS, Shah S, Burchette RJ. A profile of the demographics and training characteristics of professional modern dancers. J Dance Med Sci 2008;12(2):41–6.
2. Hincapié CA, Morton EJ, Cassidy JD. Musculoskeletal injuries and pain in dancers: a systematic review. Arch Phys Med Rehabil 2008;89(9):1819–29.
3. Walls RJ, Brennan SA, Hodnett P, et al. Overuse ankle injuries in professional Irish dancers. J Foot Ankle Surg 2010;16(1):45–9.

4. Kadel NJ. Foot and ankle injuries in dance. Phys Med Rehabil Clin N Am 2006;17: 813–26.

5. Russell JA, Shave RM, Yoshioka H, et al. Magnetic resonance imaging of the ankle in female ballet dancers en pointe. Acta Radiol 2010;51(6):655–61.

6. Hiller CE, Refshauge KM, Herbert RD, et al. Intrinsic predictors of lateral ankle sprain in adolescent dancers: a prospective cohort study. Clin J Sport Med 2008;18(1):44–8.

7. Ritter S, Moore M. The relationship between lateral ankle sprain and ankle tendinitis in ballet dancers. J Dance Med Sci 2008;12(1):23–31.

8. Furia JP, Juliano PJ, Wade AM, et al. Shock wave therapy compared with intramedullary screw fixation for nonunion of proximal fifth metatarsal metaphyseal-diaphyseal fractures. J Bone Joint Surg Am 2010;92(4):846–54.

9. Dananberg HJ. Gait style as an etiology to chronic postural pain. Part I. Functional hallux limitus. J Am Podiatr Med Assoc 1993;83(8):433–41.

10. Fanucci E, Masala S, Fabiano S, et al. Treatment of intermetatarsal Morton's neuroma with alcohol injection under US guide: 10-month follow-up. Eur Radiol 2004;14(3):514–8.

11. Franson J, Baravarian B. Intermetatarsal compression neuritis. Clin Podiatr Med Surg 2006;23(3):569–78.

12. Cohen BE. Hallux sesamoid disorders [review]. Foot Ankle Clin 2009;14(1): 91–104.

13. Roukis TS. Central metatarsal head-neck osteotomies: indications and operative techniques. Clin Podiatr Med Surg 2005;22(2):197–222.

14. Berkson DA, Cabry R, Shiple B. Freiberg's infraction in an adolescent dancer: condition often mistaken for a stress fracture. Phys Sportsmed 2005; 33(3):42–6.

15. Maresca G, Adriani E, Falez F, et al. Arthroscopic treatment of bilateral Freiberg's infraction. Arthroscopy 1996;12(1):103–8.

16. Balkin SW. Injectable silicone and the foot: a 41-year clinical and histologic history. Dermatol Surg 2005;31(11 Pt 2):1555–9.

17. Lemont H, Ammirati KM, Usen N. Plantar fasciitis: a degenerative process (fasciosis) without inflammation. J Am Podiatr Med Assoc 2003;93(3):234–7.

18. Almekinders LC. Tendinitis and other chronic tendinopathies. J Am Acad Orthop Surg 1998;6(3):157.

19. Kahn MF. Achilles tendinitis and ruptures. Br J Sports Med 1998;32(3):266.

20. Chao W. Os trigonum. Foot Ankle Clin 2004;9(4):787–96.

21. Marotta JJ, Micheli LJ. Os trigonum impingement in dancers. Am J Sports Med 1992;20(5):533–6.

22. Bronner S, Novella T, Becica L. Management of a delayed-union sesamoid fracture in a dancer. J Orthop Sports Phys Ther 2007;37(9):529–40.

23. Julsrud ME. Osteonecrosis of the tibial and fibular sesamoids in an aerobics instructor. J Foot Ankle Surg 1997;36(1):31–5.

24. Quirk R. Common foot and ankle injuries in dance. Orthop Clin North Am 1994; 25(1):123–33.

25. Werter R. Dance floors. A causative factor in dance injuries. J Am Podiatr Med Assoc 1985;75(7):355–8.

26. Shepherd FJ. A hitherto undescribed fracture of the astragalus. J Anat Physiol 1882;17(Pt 1):79–81.

27. Maquirriain J. Posterior ankle impingement syndrome. J Am Acad Orthop Surg 2005;13(6):365–71.

28. Hardaker WT Jr. Foot and ankle injuries in classical ballet dancers. Orthop Clin North Am 1989;20(4):621–7, 16.

29. Hamilton WG. Tendonitis about the ankle joint in classical ballet dancers. Am J Sports Med 1977;5(2):84–8.

30. Hamilton WG, Geppert MJ, Thompson FM. Pain in the posterior aspect of the ankle in dancers: differential diagnosis and operative treatment. J Bone Joint Surg Am 1996;78:1491–500.

31. Meislin RJ, Rose DJ, Parisien JS, et al. Arthroscopic treatment of synovial impingement of the ankle. Am J Sports Med 1993;21:186–9.

32. Van Dijk CN. Anterior and posterior ankle impingement. Foot Ankle Clin 2006; 11(3):663–83.

33. Bassett FH 3rd, Gates HS 3rd, Billys JB, et al. Talar impingement by the anteroinferior tibiofibular ligament. A cause of chronic pain in the ankle after inversion sprain. J Bone Joint Surg Am 1990;72(1):55–9.

34. Hardaker WT Jr, Margello S, Goldner JL. Foot and ankle injuries in theatrical dancers. Foot Ankle Int 1985;6(2):59–69.

35. Kleiger B. Anterior tibiotalar impingement syndromes in dancers. Foot Ankle Int 1982;3(2):69–73.

36. Kim SH, Ha KI. Arthroscopic treatment for impingement of the anterolateral soft tissues of the ankle. J Bone Joint Surg Br 2000;82(7):1019–21.

37. Reach JS, Easley ME, Chuckpaiwong B, et al. Accuracy of ultrasound guided injections in the foot and ankle. Foot Ankle Int 2009;30(3):239–42.

38. Scranton PE Jr, McDermott JE. Anterior tibiotalar spurs: a comparison of open versus arthroscopic debridement. Foot Ankle Int 1992;13(3):125–9.

39. Nihal A, Rose DJ, Trepman E. Arthroscopic treatment of anterior ankle impingement syndrome in dancers. Foot Ankle Int 2005;26(11):908–12.

40. Tol JL, Verhayen CP, van Dijk CN. Arthroscopic treatment of anterior impingement in the ankle. J Bone Joint Surg Br 2001;83(1):9–13.

41. Ogilvie-Harris DJ, Mahomed N, Demaziere A. Anterior impingement of the ankle treated by arthroscopic removal of bony spurs. J Bone Joint Surg Br 1993;75(3): 437–40.

42. Van Dijk CN, Tol JL, Verhayen CC. A prospective study of prognostic factors concerning the outcome of arthroscopic surgery for anterior ankle impingement. Am J Sports Med 1997;25(6):737–45.

43. Coull R, Raffiq T, James LE, et al. Open treatment of anterior impingement of the ankle. J Bone Joint Surg Br 2003;85(4):550–3.

44. Hedrick MR, McBryde AM. Posterior ankle impingement. Foot Ankle Int 1994; 15(1):2–8.

45. Leerar PJ. Differential diagnosis of tarsal coalition versus cuboid syndrome in an adolescent athlete. J Orthop Sports Phys Ther 2001;31(12):702–7.

46. Marshall P, Hamilton WG. Cuboid subluxation in ballet dancers. Am J Sports Med 1992;20(2):169–75.

47. Mooney M, Maffey-Ward L. Cuboid plantar and dorsal subluxations: assessment and treatment. J Orthop Sports Phys Ther 1994;20(4):220–6.

48. Slater HK. Acute peroneal tendon tears. Foot Ankle Clin 2007;12(4):659–74, vii.

49. Brandes CB, Smith RW. Characterization of patients with primary peroneus longus tendinopathy: a review of twenty-two cases. Foot Ankle Int 2000;21(6):462–8.

50. Sobel M, Geppert MJ, Olson EJ, et al. The dynamics of peroneus brevis tendon splits: a proposed mechanism, technique of diagnosis, and classification of injury. Foot Ankle 1992;13(7):413–22.

51. Sobel M, Pavlov H, Geppert MJ, et al. Painful os peroneum syndrome: a spectrum of conditions responsible for plantar lateral foot pain. Foot Ankle Int 1994;15(3): 112–24.
52. Eckert WR, Davis EA Jr. Acute rupture of the peroneal retinaculum. J Bone Joint Surg Am 1976;58(5):670–2.
53. Coughlin MJ. Disorders of tendons. In: Coughlin MJ, Mann RA, editors. Surgery of the foot and ankle. 7th edition. St Louis (MO): Mosby; 1999. p. 786–861.
54. Boya H, Pinar H. Stenosing tenosynovitis of the peroneus brevis tendon associated with hypertrophy of the peroneal tubercle. J Foot Ankle Surg 2010;49(2): 188–90.
55. Miyamoto RG, Dhotar HS, Rose DJ, et al. Surgical treatment of refractory tibial stress fractures in elite dancers: a case series. Am J Sports Med 2009;37(6): 1150–4.
56. Weiss DS, Rist RA, Grossman G. When can I start pointe work? Guidelines for initiating pointe training. J Dance Med Sci 2009;13(3):90–2.
57. Howse AJ. Posterior block of the ankle joint in dancers. Foot Ankle 1982;3(2): 81–4.
58. Peace KAL, Hillier JC, Hulme A, et al. MRI features of posterior ankle impingement syndrome in ballet dancers: a review of 25 cases. Clin Radiol 2004; 59(11):1025–33.

Current Concepts for the Use of Platelet-Rich Plasma in the Foot and Ankle

David J. Soomekh, DPM[a,b,c,*]

KEYWORDS

- Platelet-rich plasma • Plantar fasciitis • Achilles tendonitis
- Tendinopathy • Growth factor

The use of orthobiologics in the treatment of foot and ankle injuries, both in the clinical and surgical venues, is significantly increasing. The clinician and the surgeon continue to seek better ways to accelerate and mediate healing of bone and soft tissue, while incorporating less invasive techniques. The use of autologous platelet-rich plasma (PRP) by foot and ankle specialists over the last few years has emerged in the forefront of biologic tools in this endeavor. Its use has been investigated in the treatment of tendon injuries, chronic wounds, ligamentous injuries, cartilage injuries, muscle injuries, and bone augmentation (intraoperative fusions and fracture repair). PRP has been studied and used over the last 4 decades. Its use had been based on the theory that increased concentrations of autologous platelets, that then yield high concentrations of growth factors and other proteins, will lead to enhanced healing of bone and soft tissue on a cellular level.

PRP is the concentration of platelets derived from the plasma portion of centrifuged or filtered autologous blood. This platelet-rich solution can then be used as an adjunct to healing (as when used in a fresh surgical fusion) or to reinstate healing (as when used in chronic tendon injuries). PRP and related products have different labels throughout the literature, including platelet-rich concentrate, platelet gel, preparation rich in growth factors (PRGF), platelet releasate, and platelet-leukocyte-rich gel (PLRG). When the PRP is acquired, it may or may not be activated by another product. PRP without activation is usually reserved for the treatment of tendon, muscle, and other soft tissue. PRP activated into a gel or fibrin sealant is used clinically and intraoperatively for wound healing and bone augmentation. There have been several

[a] University Foot and Ankle Institute, 2121 Wilshire Boulevard, #101 Santa Monica, CA 90403, USA
[b] Department of Surgery, UCLA Medical Center, 16th Street, CA 90404, USA
[c] Department of Surgery, Cedars Sinai Medical Center, Beverly Boulevard, CA 90048, USA
* University Foot and Ankle Institute, 2121 Wilshire Boulevard, #101 Santa Monica, CA 90403.
E-mail address: drsoomekh@footankleinstitute.com

Clin Podiatr Med Surg 28 (2011) 155–170
doi:10.1016/j.cpm.2010.09.001   **podiatric.theclinics.com**

studies investigating the efficacy of PRP and its applications. It has been widely used in the areas of spine surgery, wound healing, plastic surgery, oral and maxillofacial surgery, orthopedic surgery, and podiatric surgery.[1]

There have been several basic science reviews and studies as well as clinical studies on PRP. Many are both in vitro and in vivo studies. The few controlled clinical studies are based on small numbers of subjects and have many shortcomings. Major factors in the limitation of the studies to date is to the lack of standardization in technique, concentration of platelets, applications of clinical use, volume injected, separation from whole blood, and postinjection care. This article is meant to review the background of PRP and its use for the foot and ankle clinician and surgeon.

BASICS

Platelets are a major player in the clotting cascade. They are colorless, nonnucleated fragments of cells that are derived from megakaryocytes within the bone marrow. They contain cytokines and granules (α, δ, λ) of which α is the most important, containing more than 30 proteins that play a pivotal role in soft-tissue healing and hemostasis.[2] There are several proteins that are generated and secreted by the α granules within minutes of the aggregation of the platelets. Platelet-derived growth factor, insulin-like growth factor, vascular endothelial growth factor, epidermal growth factor, epithelial cell growth factor, osteocalcin, fibrinogen, and fibronectin are some of the secretions from the α granules. These growth factors directly affect their target cells by initiating their growth, morphogenesis, and differentiation. Examples of these target cells are osteoblasts, fibroblasts, endothelial cells, epidermal cells, and mesenchymal stem cells (MSC).[2–4]

The normal 3 phases of wound healing are inflammation, proliferation, and remodeling. At the moment of tissue injury with the inflammatory phase, the platelets are activated. They begin to secrete their proteins (cytokines and growth factors) through the granules. They also produce bioactive factors, such as serotonin, histamine, dopamine, calcium, and adenosine. The serotonin and histamine will act to increase permeability of the capillaries leading to more of these products being delivered to the wound site. Platelets normally do not aggregate together unless there is a stimulant present. Once there is tissue injury, a cellular mix of proteins allows the platelets to initiate clotting and the thrombus process.[5] The platelets are activated by fibronectin, laminins, collagen, von Willebrand factor, and other proteins. Even the platelet's own secretions, such as serotonin and adenosine diphosphate, will trigger platelet aggregation and activation. Once activated, the platelets will begin to form the fibrin clot.[3,6]

The determination of the appropriate concentration of PRP for clinical use is difficult. The normal concentration of platelets in blood ranges from 150,000/μL to 350,000/μL. A level of at least 1,000,000/μL is needed to promote an increase in healing.[7] Most PRP contains a 3- to 5-fold level more than the baseline. However, there have been other studies that have suggested efficacy at 2.0- to 8.5-fold levels.[4]

Current Theory Behind PRP

Essentially PRP is used to increase the concentration of platelets to an injured site. In an acute injury, platelets are normally activated during the inflammatory phase to begin healing. The addition of PRP in the acute injury increases the concentration of platelets at the local tissue over the baseline. Chronic injuries that have failed conservative therapies presumably have ceased the inflammatory phase, and have a paucity of platelets and a decrease in healing potential. PRP in these situations would provide 2 beneficial results. First, the simple act of the application of PRP when used through injection for tendon, ligament, or muscle injuries will stimulate the tissue and restart the inflammatory process, thereby making the chronic injury into a new acute injury; and second, the addition of autologous concentrations of platelets theoretically augments the healing process. This new injury now has a known starting point and can be placed in a controlled postinjection environment (eg, immobilization, bracing, or nonweight bearing). During this time, the use of antiinflammatory medications and therapies are restricted so as not to reverse the desired effect.

Acquiring PRP

To acquire autologous PRP, blood is collected from the cubital vein (**Fig. 1**). The amount of blood acquired is determined by the clinical application (treatment area) and desired concentration. The platelets are then separated from the plasma by means of centrifugation or filtration. Many different systems are available on the market today to obtain the PRP. When using a simple centrifugation process, the blood collected is spun down between 5 and 20 minutes depending on the speed of the centrifuge and the concentration desired. There will be 3 relative layers of product in the tube: plasma layer (platelets), buffy coat layer (white blood cells), and remaining blood products (red blood cells). The platelets are at the top of the tube. There has been debate on the true concentrations obtained through simple centrifugation and the true output of platelet-rich versus platelet-poor product. The platelet-rich plasma is then collected from the tube using a syringe and an 18-gauge needle, being careful not to collect any platelet-poor or red cells.

A similar method of collection uses an automated centrifugation process that separates the platelets from the whole blood and then automatically sends the product to a separate syringe using an infrared microprocessing sensor to differentiate between red blood cells and platelet-rich plasma. This type of system seems to lead to more accuracy and allows for more reproducible concentrations. There is presumably less error with less manual manipulation of the blood product through automated separation. One such devise is the Magellan Autologous Platelet Separator System (Arteriocyte Medical Systems Inc, Cleveland, OH, USA) (**Fig. 2**). With either method, the tube that initially collected the blood must have an anticoagulant. The kits that come with the products usually have tubes already with anticoagulant or come with separate anticoagulant.

The literature seems to be mixed on the idea of activating the platelets before use. Some studies will not mention either way if the PRP was activated; whereas, others

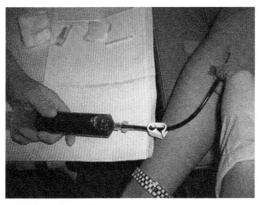

Fig. 1. Acquiring whole blood from the cubital vein.

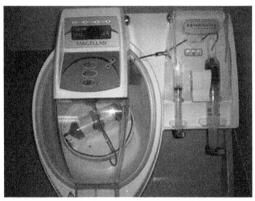

Fig. 2. Preparing PRP with the Magellan Autologous Platelet Separator System (Arteriocyte Medical Systems Inc, Cleveland, OH).

specifically delineate the product used to activate the PRP. A study was presented by de Vos and colleagues[8] on the effects of PRP on Achilles tendinopathy without mentioning activation. In their review article, Foster and colleagues[9] suggest activation with bovine thrombin. Thoms and colleagues[10] mention use of a combination of calcium and thrombin (bovine, human, or recombinant). Fufa and colleagues[11] used type I collagen to activate PRP to create a collagen-PRP gel. The brochure for the Magellan system calls for the activation of PRP by using adenosine diphosphate. The proper way to activate the platelets is determined by the intended use of the PRP.

PRP can be activated into a platelet gel using thrombin and calcium, which creates a product that can both distribute growth factors to stimulate wound healing while constricting blood vessels to reduce bleeding. In addition, the activation will increase the function of the platelets. The gel can improve tissue adhesion as a scaffold and protect from infection with its concentration of leukocytes. It has also been shown to reduce pain postoperatively. The platelet gel material is used mostly for intraoperative situations to promote bone healing and as a wound sealant.[9,12]

With the Magellan system concentrations can easily be determined. A volume of blood is taken and the machine allows the operator to select the volume of PRP desired. For example, if 30 mL of whole blood is collected and the clinician wants to inject 3 mL of PRP, the concentration will be approximately 6-fold more than the baseline; whereas, the same 30 mL will provide a 3-fold concentration more than the baseline if 10 mL of PRP is needed. If 60 mL of whole blood is collected and 3 mL of PRP is required, there will be a 13-fold concentration more than the baseline; whereas, if 10 mL of PRP is needed, only a 5-fold concentration more than the baseline is acquired. This means that as the volume of whole blood collected increases, a higher volume of PRP at a higher concentration is available. Or, when a greater amount of PRP is needed, a lower relative concentration is acquired. In this system, the majority of platelets are recovered in the initial 3 mL of PRP delivered to the 10-mL collected syringe, which means that after the first 3 mL of PRP, the concentrations of PRP are lower because of dilution. Using a smaller volume for applications that only require 10 mL of PRP will allow for an appropriate concentration more than the baseline as discussed earlier in this article. Thus, an area that only needs 10 mL of PRP injected, whether it comes from an initial 60 mL or 30 mL of whole blood collected, will then assure the highest concentrations of PRP.

Clinical Uses

The benefits and safety of PRP have been examined in many animal and human studies. Many of these studies have adequately shown the safety and efficacy of PRP in the clinical and surgical setting.[12–17] The human studies are limited by their inconsistencies, small sample size, and lack of controls.[7] It is difficult to compare studies because of differing concentrations of PRP and postprocedure protocol. There seem to be as many studies that confirm the benefits of PRP as there are studies that are inconclusive. An important distinction that must be made as the use of PRP increases is whether the use of PRP is as beneficial in the acute phases of tissue healing as it may be in chronic pathology.

Foot and ankle applications for PRP can be placed into several categories. These categories include acute and chronic ligamentous injuries, chronic tendinopathy (tendinosis), bone pathology, chronic wounds, and cartilage injury.

Plantar Fasciitis

The use of PRP for plantar fasciitis was investigated in a small study by Barrett and Erredge.[18] They used ultrasound of the fascia before and after treatment and patient pain scale as determination for efficacy. The subjects were weight bearing in a walking boot for 2 days and then in regular shoe gear with limited activity. They were restricted from using antiinflammatories or other modalities. They found that 6 of 9 subjects achieved complete resolution of symptoms after 2 months. One subject had resolution after a second injection. After 1 year, 77.9% of the subjects had no symptoms. They showed that ultrasound measurements of the thickness of the plantar fascia were reduced between preinjection and postinjection. It is unclear how long the patients had their symptoms before treatment.

The author has found promising results using PRP for those patients with chronic, recalcitrant plantar fasciitis. Patients that have failed conservative treatments after 3 to 6 months, including rest, ice, compression, and evaluation (RICE); functional foot orthotics; physical therapy; and cortisone injections, may be candidates for PRP. Diagnosis is confirmed using ultrasound or MRI. A skin marker is used to identify the site of most pain on palpation. An initial anesthetic block is performed at the site. 60 mL of whole blood is drawn using the collection tube supplied with the Magellan system kit. Calcium chloride is used to activate the PRP. Thrombin is not used, to keep the PRP in liquid form for injection. Once the PRP is prepared using the Magellan Autologous Platelet Separator System, using a 10-mL syringe and a 25-gauge needle, patients are injected with 5 mL to 8 mL of PRP from the 60 mL of whole blood collection, yielding a concentration that is a 10 to 6 times more than the baseline, respectively. The author has found that as the concentration increases, the patient's postinjection pain increases. The injection is performed under ultrasound guidance (**Fig. 3**). Several 0.25-mL pulsed injections, while peppering the needle, are placed in the medial plantar fascial band starting at the point of maximum tenderness. In many of the patients, during the injection the fibrosis of the ligament can be appreciated by a crepitus that can be felt and heard as the needle passes in and out of the fascial tissue. After completing the injection, continued peppering of the fascia using the 25-gauge needle is performed to further aggravate the tissue. Patients are restricted from using any antiinflammatories or modalities for up to 3 months using acetaminophen or narcotics for pain as needed. The author has found better results with a postinjection protocol of a walking boot and crutches with no weight bearing for 3 to 5 days, and then walking in the boot for 2 to 3 weeks. Activity begins gradually around the third or fourth week in an athletic shoe and functional foot orthotic,

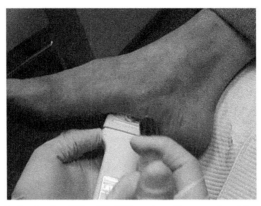

Fig. 3. Treatment of plantar fasciitis with PRP under ultrasound guidance.

increasing over a 4-week period. Some patients have benefited from a second injection when the first yielded only some relief in symptoms given about 6 weeks afterwards. Those patients that have no change in their symptoms after the first injection rarely benefit from a follow-up injection.

Achilles Tendinopathy and Rupture Repair

Recent studies have shown that PRP can positively affect gene expression and matrix synthesis in tendon and tendon cells.[9] It is important, however, to distinguish acute tendon injury from chronic cases when discussing and studying PRP and its use for tendon pathology. The use of PRP specifically for the treatment of Achilles pathology has been investigated. Tendon injury leads to a cascade of degenerating events leading to eventual rupture. These events include hypovascularity, repetitive microtrauma, and the addition of fibrous tissue that can then lead to degeneration and weakness of the tendon. PRP is thought to reverse the effects of tendinopathy by stimulating revascularization and improving healing at the microscopic level.[19] Alfredson and Lorentzon categorize Achilles tendon pathology into paratendinitis, paratendinitis with tendinosis, and pure tendinosis.[19] In paratendinitis, there are adhesions formed between the paratenon and the tendon. Paratendinitis with tendinosis involves degenerative changes within the substance of the tendon as well as inflammation in the paratenon. In cases of pure tendinosis there is a palpable nodule that often presents. It is hypothesized that the introduction of PRP into the pathologic tendon will aid in the repair and remodeling of the tendon by tenocytes.

Lyras and colleagues[20] studied the effect of PRP on angiogenesis during tendon healing. The study was performed on the Achilles tendon of rats against a control group injected with saline. They found a significant increase in angiogenesis in the PRP group compared with the control group during the first 2 weeks of the healing process (ie, the inflammatory and proliferative phases), and the number of the newly formed vessels in the PRP group was significantly reduced at 4 weeks compared with the controls, suggesting the healing process was shortened. They observed that the orientation of collagen fibers in the PRP group was better organized. They concluded that PRP seems to enhance neovascularization, which may accelerate the healing process and promote scar tissue of better histologic quality.

Gaweda and colleagues[21] performed a prospective study on 15 subjects with Achilles tendonitis. Subjects were followed for 18 months. They found improvement in pain scores and ultrasound imaging. The American Orthopaedic Foot and Ankle

Society scores improved from a medial of 55 points to 96 points, and the achilles tendon score improved from 24 points to 96 points. They concluded PRP to be a viable treatment alternative for Achilles tendonitis.

A recent study by de Vos and colleagues[8] was performed on subjects with tendinopathy. Their study was stratified, block randomized, double blind, and placebo controlled. They included subjects age 18 to 70 years old. Diagnosis was made clinically with findings of a painful and thickened tendon in relation to activity and on palpation with symptoms lasting greater than 2 months. The subject base included 27 in the PRP group and 27 in the control group. They used 54 mL of whole blood to derive the PRP that was mixed with sodium bicarbonate to match the pH of tendon tissue. A undisclosed amount of PRP was injected into 5 sites along the injured tendon under ultrasound guidance. subjects were only allowed to walk short distances indoors in the first 48 hours. In days 3 to 7, subjects were allowed to take walks up to 30 minutes. After 1 week an exercise routine was started with 1 week of stretching and a 12-week daily eccentric exercise program with heel drops off a step. No weight-bearing sports activities were allowed for 4 weeks, and then a gradual return was instructed. They were only to use acetaminophen during the follow-up period. Their results were based on subject questionnaires that quantify pain and activity level. The results showed an improvement in 24 weeks by 21.7 points in the PRP group and 20.5 points in the placebo group. They concluded that there was no significant difference between the groups.[8] This study is limited by several factors. They did not identify any characteristics of the anatomy of the tendon preinjection and postinjection, neither clinically nor with imaging techniques. Their sample size was small. They could not quantify the concentrations of PRP that were used in each subject.

PRP in the form of a fibrin gel (when combined with thrombin) can also be used as a tendon scaffold. It can be used as a bridge and augmentation within the rupture defect, or it can be wrapped around the tendon repair. In most cases, it will be combined with Bone marrow aspirate (BMA) for further enhancement of the PRP matrix. The introduction of PRP in the repair of Achilles rupture has also been evaluated in the rat model.[19,22,23] In one study, surgically transected tendons treated with PRP showed a 42% increase in their force to failure, a 61% increase in ultimate stress, and a 90% increase in energy after 2 weeks compared with control.[22] In another study, those tendons treated with PRP had a 30% increase in strength and stiffness after 1 week.[24] Sánchez and colleagues[25] investigated the augmentation of Achilles tendon rupture repair with PRP in athletes (6 in both the PRP group and control group). They used 2 PRP preparations on the primary repair of the Achilles as compared with controls. A total of 4 mL of PRP was mixed with $CaCl_2$ and after 30 minutes a fibrin scaffold was produced and incorporated into the repair site between the tendon ends. The remaining PRP was again mixed with $CaCl_2$ but immediately sprayed onto the wound site before closure. Subjects were followed for 1 year by ultrasound imaging and physical examination. They found that as compared with the control, the PRP group was able to return to mild running with earlier range of motion and without wound complication.

Sarrafian and colleagues[26] performed a study to compare a cross-linked acellular porcine dermal patch (APD) against a platelet-rich plasma fibrin matrix (PRPFM) for repair of acute Achilles tendon rupture in a sheep model. The 2 surgically transected tendon ends were re-approximated in groups 1 and 2; whereas, a gap was left between the tendon ends in group 3. APD was used to reinforce the repair in group 2, and autologous PRPFM was used to fill the gap, which was also reinforced with APD, in group 3. Tensile strength testing showed a statistically significant difference in elongation between the operated limb and the unoperated contralateral limb in groups 1 and 3, but not in group 2. In group 1, all surgical separation sites were identifiable and healing occurred via increasing tendon thickness. In group 2, healing occurred with new tendon fibers across the separation, without increasing tendon thickness in 2 out of 6 animals. Group 3 showed complete bridging of the gap, with no change in tendon thickness in 2 out of 6 animals. In groups 2 and 3, peripheral integration of the APD to tendon fibers was observed. They concluded that the use of APD, alone or with PRPFM, to augment Achilles tendon repair in a sheep model is a viable and strong repair.

The author has used PRP for the treatment of chronic Achilles tendinopathy and rupture repair in many cases (**Fig. 4**). The treatment protocol is similar to that of plantar fasciitis. Patients are chosen based on the chronicity of their symptoms and the quality of the tendon. Those patients that have failed conservative therapies after 3 to 6 months are good candidates. In addition to pain, decreased activity, and loss of function, most patients present with nodular thickening within the substance of the tendon. Some may even have multiple fibrotic nodules. Patients that have an associated retrocalcaneal exostosis have also been treated with PRP with varying results. Diagnosis is confirmed with ultrasound or MRI. A local anesthetic block is placed well above the site of injection. The PRP is then prepared at the desired concentration from the whole blood collection and activated by calcium citrate. Between 6 and 10 mL of PRP is injected within the substance of the tendon beginning at the site of pathology (pain and any bulbous mass). The medial or lateral aspect of the tendon is approached with patients in a prone position under ultrasound guidance. Several pulsed (peppered) doses of approximately 0.25 mL at a time are injected using a 25-gauge needle, fenestrating the tendon. Patients are then placed in a walking boot on crutches and nonweight-bearing for up to 1 week, and then allowed to bear weight in the boot for the next 1 to 3 weeks. They are then transferred into an athletic shoe with a slow increase in weight-bearing activity over a 4-week period. The author has seen a significant reduction in pain, decrease in the size of fibrous nodules within the tendon, and a sooner return to regular and sporting activity after PRP. Most patients have been able to return to increased exercise and activity within 2 months of the injection. Again, some patients have benefited by a second injection approximately 6 weeks after the first.

Cartilage Injury

Many studies have been performed examining the role of PRP in aiding the repair of cartilage in early osteoarthritis (OA). In vitro studies have shown that PRP has the

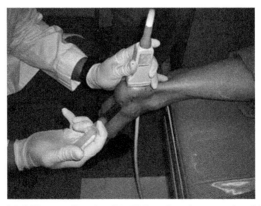

Fig. 4. Treatment of Achilles tendinosis with PRP under ultrasound guidance.

potential of increasing proteoglycan and collagen synthesis in chondrocytes.[27] Sun and colleagues[28] evaluated the effect of PRP on cartilage defects in a rabbit model. They looked at the cartilage specimens after 4 and 12 weeks, macroscopically, with computed tomography, and histologically and found a significant increase in newly formed cartilage and bone as compared with the untreated group. They concluded that PRP improves osteochondral healing in the rabbit model. In vivo studies have also been promising.[29,30] Sánchez and colleagues[31] reported results on a retrospective study for human subjects with OA of the knee. They compared PRP injections and hyaluronan injections with 3 injections over 3 weeks. By week 5, the pain scale success reached only 10.0% for the hyaluronan group and 33.4% for the PRP group. Kon and colleagues[32] studied 115 osteoarthritic knees with PRP injections. They found improvements in pain scale at 6 months follow-up. Cugat and colleagues[33] investigated PRGF on athletes with chondral defects with positive results. As discussed earlier, mesenchymal stem cells can differentiate into chondrocytes and cartilage. Mishra and colleagues[34] studied the effect of MSC treated with PRP on cartilage regeneration in vitro. They found that a 10% PRP treatment increased cellular proliferation of chondrogenic differentiation more than 10-fold versus control. Investigation by Wu and colleagues[35] suggested promising results by using PRP as a chondrocyte carrier to fill acute cartilage lesions in the knee. A scaffold made with PRP and thrombin was used to transfer chondrocytes to the lesion.

The author has not found recent studies that show the effect of PRP on OA of the foot and ankle. Theoretically, however, there is evidence that suggests improvement in pain and cartilage regeneration that could prove effective in the treatment of OA in the foot and ankle. At present, foot and ankle surgeons perform microfractures into cartilage lesions (osteochondral drilling) to initiate fibrocartilage repair. The marrow cells that are presented into the joint after microfracture are similar to those from BMA, MCS, and PRP. It would seem logical that the introduction of such cell products by percutaneous injection or surgical transfer would in fact increase cartilage regeneration and repair.

Bone Augmentation

PRP can be used in the augmentation of bone or bone grafting. Concentrating platelets will increase the level of growth factors that could stimulate a prematurely terminated bone healing process.[36,37] Initially, PRP was used for graft augmentation in oral and maxillofacial surgery by Marx and colleagues[17] finding significant improvements in fusion rates and bone density in the mandible. It has been used as a percutaneous injection for fresh fractures to facilitate healing of nonunions, to augment fresh arthrodesis procedures with and without bone graft, for surgery using autologous or allogenic bone graft, and to fill bone defects. The effect of PRP on bone healing has been studied in great detail both in vitro[38–41] and in vivo.[36,37,42] It is thought that the increase in platelets and their growth factors will stimulate and enhance levels of osteoprotegerin, osteopontin, osteoblast differentiation of myoblasts and osteoblastic cells, and osteoclastlike cells.[39,41,43,44]

BMA has been studied and used for several years and shown to enhance the healing of bone.[45] There are 2 types of stem cells that originate in the bone marrow: hematopoietic and mesenchymal. It is the hematopoietic stem cells (HSC) that are pluripotent stem cells and give rise to all blood types. HSCs are fond in large numbers in the bone marrow and play a role in hard-tissue formation and differentiate into platelets. Mesenchymal stem cells are multipotent stem cells and are found in human tissues, including synovial tissue, bone marrow, and adipose tissues. They differentiate into cartilage, bone, muscle, and adipose tissue.[46] Studies have shown MSCs to regenerate articular cartilage in animal models and in bone for human models.[47–51] Investigators have shown that PRP and its growth factors and cytokines enhance MSC proliferation.[52,53] Theoretically, combining BMA and PRP together can create an environment where platelets and stem cells can act together to even further enhance bone healing than when used alone. The efficacy of PRP and BMA in the augmentation of bone and bone-graft healing is divided. There are many studies that show promise; whereas, others show little difference versus control or traditional products.

Gandhi and colleagues[15] used PRP in nonunion fractures of the foot and ankle that were present for 4 months or more. Their findings suggest a decreased level of growth factors around nonunion fracture sites as compared with fresh fracture sites. The addition of PRP in this area could then increase nonunion healing potential through increases in growth factors. They found a 60-day mean resolution of the nonunions after the addition of PRP.[19]

High-risk elective foot and ankle surgical subjects were studied by Bibbo and colleagues.[54] The risk factors included previous poor osseous healing, osteomyelitis, tobacco use, diabetic neuropathy, malnutrition, immunosuppression, and alcohol abuse. Their results showed that 116 fusion sites (94%), using either autogenous or allogenic graft, went on to fusion in a mean of 41 days. They concluded that PRP may aid in union rates for high-risk patients.

Bielecki and colleagues[55] used what they called platelet-leukocyte-rich gel percutaneously in delayed and nonunions of the humerus, femur, tibia, radius, and clavicle. They followed 32 subjects using radiograph and absorptiometry examinations. Results showed a total union in 9.3 weeks for all those delayed union cases treated with PLRG. In the nonunion group, union was seen in 13 of the cases with an average of 10.3 weeks with PLRG. They found that delayed and nonunions that were more than 11 months had the least favorable results. They concluded that percutaneous injection of PLRG into nonunion and delayed union fractures may be sufficient to facilitate union and can replace more invasive bone marrow injections.

Coetzee and colleagues[56] studied the benefits of PRP in the union of the syndesmosis with use of total ankle arthroplasty. The retrospective study compared 66 subjects with the addition of PRP and 114 without augmentation. The control group had a fusion rate of 61% at 8 weeks and 85% at 6 months. The PRP group had a fusion rate of 76% at 8 weeks and 97% at 6 months. They also found and increase in the fusion rate of those subjects treated with PRP that had a history of tobacco use.[55] Similar results were reported by Barrow and Pomeroy[57] who found an 85% union rate at 8 weeks and 100% at 6 months in their prospective study.

The author has been using PRP in conjunction with BMA to facilitate midfoot and hindfoot surgical fusions. Patients are chosen as candidates for augmentation of fusion with PRP based on the patient history and risk factors. Those patients that have a history of tobacco use, alcohol abuse, previous nonunions, diabetic neuropathy, and osteoporosis are good candidates. PRP has been used in conjunction with BMA in cases with or without the need for bone autograft or allograft. The author will harvest the BMA from the calcaneus or the proximal tibial metaphysis. The technique for acquiring the percutaneous BMA from these areas is documented by Schweinberger and Roukis.[58] The whole blood acquired for the PRP and BMA are combined together and prepared in the centrifuge. The final PRP and BMA mixture can be applied as a liquid or a gel. The gel is formed by adding thrombin to the final mixture. Exposure of PRP to thrombin will induce platelet degranulation, increasing the concentration of growth factors. The use of bovine thrombin can lead to the development of antibodies to the clotting factors V, XI, and autologous thrombin, which can lead to multisystem failure.[59] Techniques can now use the same blood sample used to make PRP to generate autologous thrombin from prothrombin. This generation can be achieved by adding calcium chloride during the processing of the PRP, forming a dense fibrin matrix that traps the platelets resulting in a small amount of thrombin, minimizing activation that leads to a slow release of growth factors over 7 days.[9] The fibrin mass that is created is a gelatinous scaffold that is a malleable product that can be introduced between bones to be fused when used with or without a bone graft and introduced into bone defects (**Fig. 5**). The liquid form can be used to coat a bone graft. The author has seen significant promising results with an increase in bone healing rates with less pain and earlier radiographic evidence of fusion using a combination of PRP and BMA.

Wound Healing

Many foot and ankle surgeons are faced with diabetic, iatrogenic, decubitus, and venous chronic wounds. A plethora of biologic materials have been produced and investigated to aid in the closure of chronic wounds. PRP seems to also have the properties to augment wound healing. During the inflammatory phase of wound healing, an environment rich in cellular proteins form an initial clot. This clot is composed of collagen, platelets, thrombin, and fibronectin. In addition to aiding in hemostasis these products lead to the release of growth factors and cytokines that will stimulate the cascade that ends in a healed wound. PRP full of these growth factors could potentially significantly aid in the closure of chronic wounds. PRP is usually used in conjunction with bone marrow aspirate when applied to wounds.

Several in vitro and in vivo studies have shown PRP can increase the potential of wound-healing cell products. Smith and Roukis[4] reviewed several studies investigating PRP used on chronic wounds (diabetic and nondiabetic) of the lower extremities. The majority of these studies found that wounds treated with PRP healed significantly sooner than their control groups. In most of the studies, the control groups were eventually treated with PRP with closure achieved because of its effectiveness. Some studies have shown the ability of PRP to combat wound infection.[60–62] Bielecki and colleagues[60] found that PRP gel inhibited the growth of *Escherichia coli* and *S aureus*.

Lacci and Dardik[63] performed a literature review between July of 2008 and March of 2009 to evaluate the number of studies and their outcomes with the use of PRP on

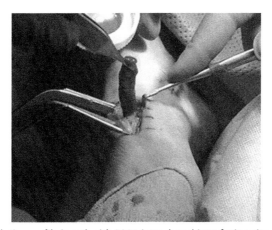

Fig. 5. PRP formulation as fibrin gel with BMA introduced into fusion site at first metatarsal cuneiform joint.

chronic wounds. They found PRP to be effective in several case-control studies and noncontrolled clinical trials. They only found 1 prospective, randomized, controlled clinical trial on PRP in the treatment of diabetic foot ulcers by Driver and colleagues[64] with significant results. Lacci and Dardik[63] concluded that there is promise for the use of PRP in chronic wounds of varying etiology and diabetic foot ulceration.

Cervelli and colleagues[65] performed a study on 30 chronic lower-extremity wounds. They used the theory that MSC is present in adipose tissue, which can accelerate the effects of PRP by using PRP and autologous fat grafts. Their results showed an improvement from minor to moderate in 100% of subjects after 3 weeks, healing in less than 6 weeks in 47% of subjects, and complete wound healing in 57% of subjects within 3 months. They concluded that there is the ability of the combination of PRP and autologous adipose graft to regenerate tissue and epithelialization with wound closure, with a significant healing-time reduction. They found it to be well accepted by subjects with a relative reduction in cost. This group also studied the role of PRP used as an autologous scaffold for cellular growth, in combination with hyaluronic acid as a temporary dermal substitute for chronic wounds with exposed tendon, and found that PRP aided healing of acute and chronic open wounds of the foot and ankle.[66]

A recent study by Frykberg and colleagues[67] evaluated the use of PRP gel in the initial wound-healing trajectories of chronic, nonhealing wounds of various etiologies and in different care settings. They followed 65 nonhealing wounds (mean duration 47.8 weeks, range 3.0 to 260.0) at 8 long-term acute care hospitals and 3 outpatient foot or wound clinics and applied PRP gel on their wounds. The majority of subjects had low albumin, hematocrit, or hemoglobin levels. The most common wounds were pressure ulcers, venous ulcers, and diabetic foot ulcers. Following a mean of 2.8 weeks with 3.2 applications, reductions in wound volume area, undermining, and sinus tract/tunneling were observed. For all wound etiologies, 97% of wounds improved. Their results suggest the application of this PRP gel can reverse nonhealing trends in chronic wounds.

Most patients with chronic lower extremity wounds are good candidates for the use of PRP with BMA. The PRP is prepared with a 60 mL blood draw. The platelet-poor portion is set aside to spray over the inner dressings. The BMA is acquired and prepared with the PRP and thrombin is added to create the gel. While the gel is forming, extensive debridement of the ulcerating is performed to healthy bleeding tissue. The gel is formed into the shape of the wound and placed directly to the wound site. The dressings are applied with a standard wet-to-dry dressing for the first few days, to allow the patch to fully breakdown and begin the healing process. After the first few days (4–6), the dressing should be changed. Mineral oil can also be used to aid in the dressing.

DISCUSSION

Clearly the importance of platelets, their α granules, and their release of growth factors on bone and tissue repair cannot be overstated. The literature is full of studies suggesting the potential for the augmentation of bone, soft tissue, and wound healing with PRP. In vitro and in vivo animal studies have shown PRP to have a positive effect on tissue repair on the cellular level. The safety and risk profile for PRP proves to have low morbidity and associated complications.[19] It has a low chance of rejection because it is produced from the patients' own blood. PRP is easy to acquire and apply because it can be produced in the clinical or operative setting at the time it is needed. It is also less expensive than other orthobiologics and modes of tissue augmentation.

The research and use of PRP also has potential limitations. There is a lack of uniformity on several levels. Many different concentrations of PRP are used, although some simply cannot quantify the concentrations used. There is no optimal dose presented for the potential application and uses of PRP. The literature is not standardized on the acquisition, the method of preparation, or the addition of supplements to activate PRP.

There are several studies investigating PRP; however, many are poorly designed and few involve the foot and ankle. Further human, large, consistent, and well-performed prospective studies of PRP and its use in the foot and ankle are critical to better understand and apply its potential and benefits of use. Future studies that investigate the benefits of using PRP in acute versus chronic cases would also be beneficial. It will be important that future studies be able to suggest consistent concentrations of PRP, appropriate dosing, improved technique, and the best postinjection protocol.

SUMMARY

PRP presents promise for the treatment of many foot and ankle pathologies, including tendinopathy (Achilles, peroneal, posterior tibial, flexor hallucis longus, anterior tibial), ligamentous injury (plantar fasciitis, lateral ankle), augmentation of bone intraoperatively with primary fusions, fresh fractures, nonunions, tendon rupture repairs, cartilage injury (ankle, subtalar, metatarsal cartilage lesions), sesamoiditis, and chronic wounds. The author has even seen promising results in a small sample of patients treated for sesamoiditis and chronic lateral ankle pain.

The author has been using PRP over the last 2 years. The results have been increasingly promising with regard to decreased pain, increased activity, improved function, faster recovery, and increased strength. The use of PRP in the clinical setting may be advantageous for its ease of use, relative availability, low side effects, and tolerability, as compared with more invasive techniques. Although the theory behind the use and effectiveness of PRP and some positive clinical evidence have shown promise, it is evident that additional well-designed prospective studies on PRP and its use in foot and ankle pathology are needed to measure its true effectiveness.

REFERENCES

1. Mehta S, Watson JT. Platelet rich concentrate: basic science and current clinical applications. J Orthop Trauma 2008;22(6):432–8.
2. Harrison P, Cramer EM. Platelet alpha-granules. Blood Rev 1993;7(1):52–62.
3. Broughton G 2nd, Janis JE, Attinger CE. Wound healing: an overview. Plast Reconstr Surg 2006;117(Suppl 7):1e-S–32e-S.
4. Smith SE, Roukis TS. Bone and wound healing augmentation with platelet-rich plasma. Clin Podiatr Med Surg 2009;26(4):559–88.
5. Plow E, Abrams C. The molecular basis for platelet function. 4th Edition. Philadelphia: Elsevier, Churchill, Livingstone; 2005.
6. Witte MB, Barbul A. General principles of wound healing. Surg Clin North Am 1997;77(3):509–28.
7. Marx RE. Platelet-rich plasma (PRP): what is PRP and what is not PRP? Implant Dent 2001;10(4):225–8.
8. de Vos RJ, Weir A, van Schie HT, et al. Platelet-rich plasma injection for chronic Achilles tendinopathy: a randomized controlled trial. JAMA 2010;303(2):144–9.
9. Foster TE, Puskas BL, Mandelbaum BR, et al. Platelet-rich plasma: from basic science to clinical applications. Am J Sports Med 2009;37(11):2259–72.
10. Thoms RJ, Marwin SE. The role of fibrin sealants in orthopaedic surgery. J Am Acad Orthop Surg 2009;17(12):727–36.

11. Fufa D, Shealy B, Jacobson M, et al. Activation of platelet-rich plasma using soluble type I collagen. J Oral Maxillofac Surg 2008;66(4):684–90.
12. Bhanot S, Alex JC. Current applications of platelet gels in facial plastic surgery. Facial Plast Surg 2002;18(1):27–33.
13. Camargo PM, Lekovic V, Weinlaender M, et al. Platelet-rich plasma and bovine porous bone mineral combined with guided tissue regeneration in the treatment of intrabony defects in humans. J Periodontal Res 2002;37(4):300–6.
14. Eppley BL, Pietrzak WS, Blanton M. Platelet-rich plasma: a review of biology and applications in plastic surgery. Plast Reconstr Surg 2006;118(6):147e–59e.
15. Gandhi A, Bibbo C, Pinzur M, et al. The role of platelet-rich plasma in foot and ankle surgery. Foot Ankle Clin 2005;10(4):621–37, viii.
16. Kassolis JD, Rosen PS, Reynolds MA. Alveolar ridge and sinus augmentation utilizing platelet-rich plasma in combination with freeze-dried bone allograft: case series. J Periodontol 2000;71(10):1654–61.
17. Marx RE, Carlson ER, Eichstaedt RM, et al. Platelet-rich plasma: Growth factor enhancement for bone grafts. Oral Surg Oral Med Oral Pathol Oral Radiol Endod 1998;85(6):638–46.
18. Barrett S, Erredge S. Growth factors for chronic plantar fasciitis. Podiatry Today 2004;17(11):37–42.
19. Alfredson H, Lorentzon R. Chronic Achilles tendinosis: recommendations for treatment and prevention. Sports Med 2000;29(2):135–46.
20. Lyras DN, Kazakos K, Verettas D, et al. The influence of platelet-rich plasma on angiogenesis during the early phase of tendon healing. Foot Ankle Int 2009;30(11):1101–6.
21. Gaweda K, Tarczynska M, Krzyzanowski W. Treatment of Achilles tendinopathy with platelet-rich plasma. Int J Sports Med 2010;31(8):577–83.
22. Virchenko O, Aspenberg P. How can one platelet injection after tendon injury lead to a stronger tendon after 4 weeks? Interplay between early regeneration and mechanical stimulation. Acta Orthop 2006;77(5):806–12.
23. Virchenko O, Grenegard M, Aspenberg P. Independent and additive stimulation of tendon repair by thrombin and platelets. Acta Orthop 2006;77(6):960–6.
24. Aspenberg P, Virchenko O. Platelet concentrate injection improves Achilles tendon repair in rats. Acta Orthop Scand 2004;75(1):93–9.
25. Sanchez M, Anitua E, Azofra J, et al. Comparison of surgically repaired Achilles tendon tears using platelet-rich fibrin matrices. Am J Sports Med 2007;35(2):245–51.
26. Sarrafian TL, Wang H, Hackett ES, et al. Comparison of Achilles tendon repair techniques in a sheep model using a cross-linked acellular porcine dermal patch and platelet-rich plasma fibrin matrix for augmentation. J Foot Ankle Surg 2010;49(2):128–34.
27. Akeda K, An HS, Okuma M, et al. Platelet-rich plasma stimulates porcine articular chondrocyte proliferation and matrix biosynthesis. Osteoarthr Cartil 2006;14(12):1272–80.
28. Sun Y, Feng Y, Zhang CQ, et al. The regenerative effect of platelet-rich plasma on healing in large osteochondral defects. Int Orthop 2010;34(4):589–97.
29. Nakagawa K, Sasho T, Arai M, et al. Effects of autologous platelet-rich plasma on the metabolism of human articular chondrocytes. Osteoarthr Cartil 2007;15(Suppl 2):B134.
30. Saito M, Takahashi K, Arai Y, et al. The preventative effect of platelet-rich plasma and biodegradable gelatin hydrogel microspheres on experimental osteoarthritis in the rabbit knee. Osteoarthr Cartil 2007;15(Suppl 3):C232.

31. Sanchez M, Anitua E, Azofra J, et al. Intra-articular injection of an autologous preparation rich in growth factors for the treatment of knee OA: a retrospective cohort study. Clin Exp Rheumatol 2008;26(5):910–3.

32. Kon E, Buda R, Filardo G, et al. Platelet-rich plasma: intra-articular knee injections produced favorable results on degenerative cartilage lesions. Knee Surg Sports Traumatol Arthrosc 2010;18(4):472–9.

33. Cugat R, Carrillo JM, Serra I, et al. Articular cartilage defects reconstruction by plasma rich in growth factors. Bologna (Italy): Timeo Editore; 2006.

34. Mishra A, Tummala P, King A, et al. Buffered platelet-rich plasma enhances mesenchymal stem cell proliferation and chondrogenic differentiation. Tissue Eng Part C Methods 2009;15(3):431–5.

35. Wu W, Zhang J, Dong Q, et al. Platelet-rich plasma - A promising cell carrier for micro-invasive articular cartilage repair. Med Hypotheses 2009;72(4):455–7.

36. Dallari D, Fini M, Stagni C, et al. In vivo study on the healing of bone defects treated with bone marrow stromal cells, platelet-rich plasma, and freeze-dried bone allografts, alone and in combination. J Orthop Res 2006;24(5):877–88.

37. Gandhi A, Doumas C, O'Connor JP, et al. The effects of local platelet rich plasma delivery on diabetic fracture healing. Bone 2006;38(4):540–6.

38. Granzi F, Ivanoski S, Cei S, et al. The in vitro effect of different PRP concentrations on osteoblasts and fibroblasts. Clin Oral Implants Res 2006;17:212–9.

39. Kanno T, Takahashi T, Tsujisawa T, et al. Platelet-rich plasma enhances human osteoblast-like cell proliferation and differentiation. J Oral Maxillofac Surg 2005;63(3):362–9.

40. Ogino Y, Ayukawa Y, Kukita T, et al. The contribution of platelet-derived growth factor, transforming growth factor-beta1, and insulin-like growth factor-I in platelet-rich plasma to the proliferation of osteoblast-like cells. Oral Surg Oral Med Oral Pathol Oral Radiol Endod 2006;101(6):724–9.

41. Tomoyasu A, Higashio K, Kanomata K, et al. Platelet-rich plasma stimulates osteoblastic differentiation in the presence of BMPs. Biochem Biophys Res Commun 2007;361(1):62–7.

42. Weibrich G, Hansen T, Kleis W, et al. Effect of platelet concentration in platelet-rich plasma on peri-implant bone regeneration. Bone 2004;34(4):665–71.

43. Bolander ME. Regulation of fracture repair by growth factors. Proc Soc Exp Biol Med 1992;200(2):165–70.

44. Gruber R, Karreth F, Fischer MB, et al. Platelet-released supernatants stimulate formation of osteoclast-like cells through a prostaglandin/RANKL-dependent mechanism. Bone 2002;30(5):726–32.

45. Yamaguchi Y, Kubo T, Murakami T, et al. Bone marrow cells differentiate into wound myofibroblasts and accelerate the healing of wounds with exposed bones when combined with an occlusive dressing. Br J Dermatol 2005;152(4):616–22.

46. Szilvassy SJ. The biology of hematopoietic stem cells. Arch Med Res 2003;34(6):446–60.

47. Barry FP. Mesenchymal stem cell therapy in joint disease. Novartis Found Symp 2003;249:86–96 [discussion: 96–102, 104–70, 141–239].

48. Caplin A. Mesenchymal stem cells. J Orthop Res 1991;9:641–50.

49. Carter DR, Beaupre GS, Giori NJ, et al. Mechanobiology of skeletal regeneration. Clin Orthop Relat Res 1998;(355 Suppl):S41–55.

50. Murphy JM, Fink DJ, Hunziker EB, et al. Stem cell therapy in a caprine model of osteoarthritis. Arthritis Rheum 2003;48(12):3464–74.

51. Wakitani S, Goto T, Pineda SJ, et al. Mesenchymal cell-based repair of large, full-thickness defects of articular cartilage. J Bone Joint Surg Am 1994;76(4):579–92.

52. Kocaoemer A, Kern S, Kluter H, et al. Human AB serum and thrombin-activated platelet-rich plasma are suitable alternatives to fetal calf serum for the expansion of mesenchymal stem cells from adipose tissue. Stem Cells 2007;25(5):1270–8.

53. Vogel JP, Szalay K, Geiger F, et al. Platelet-rich plasma improves expansion of human mesenchymal stem cells and retains differentiation capacity and in vivo bone formation in calcium phosphate ceramics. Platelets 2006;17(7):462–9.

54. Bibbo C, Bono CM, Lin SS. Union rates using autologous platelet concentrate alone and with bone graft in high-risk foot and ankle surgery patients. J Surg Orthop Adv 2005;14(1):17–22.

55. Bielecki T, Gazdzik TS, Szczepanski T. Benefit of percutaneous injection of autologous platelet-leukocyte-rich gel in patients with delayed union and nonunion. Eur Surg Res 2008;40(3):289–96.

56. Coetzee JC, Pomeroy GC, Watts JD, et al. The use of autologous concentrated growth factors to promote syndesmosis fusion in the Agility total ankle replacement. A preliminary study. Foot Ankle Int 2005;26(10):840–6.

57. Barrow C, Pomeroy G. Enhancement of syndesmotic fusion rates in total ankle arthroplasty with teh use of autologous platelet concentrate. Foot Ankle Int 2006;26: 458–61.

58. Schweinberger MH, Roukis TS. Percutaneous autologous bone marrow harvest from the calcaneus and proximal tibia: surgical technique. J Foot Ankle Surg 2007;46(5):411–4.

59. Anitua E, Andia I, Ardanza B, et al. Autologous platelets as a source of proteins for healing and tissue regeneration. Thromb Haemost 2004;91(1):4–15.

60. Bielecki TM, Gazdzik TS, Arendt J, et al. Antibacterial effect of autologous platelet gel enriched with growth factors and other active substances: an in vitro study. J Bone Joint Surg Br 2007;89(3):417–20.

61. El-Sharkawy H, Kantarci A, Deady J, et al. Platelet-rich plasma: growth factors and pro- and anti-inflammatory properties. J Periodontol 2007;78(4):661–9.

62. Everts PA, Overdevest EP, Jakimowicz JJ, et al. The use of autologous platelet-leukocyte gels to enhance the healing process in surgery, a review. Surg Endosc 2007;21(11):2063–8.

63. Lacci KM, Dardik A. Platelet-rich plasma: support for its use in wound healing. Yale J Biol Med 2010;83(1):1–9.

64. Driver VR, Hanft J, Fylling CP, et al. Autologel Diabetic Foot Ulcer Study G. A prospective, randomized, controlled trial of autologous platelet-rich plasma gel for the treatment of diabetic foot ulcers. Ostomy Wound Manage 2006;52(6): 68–70, 72, 74 passim.

65. Cervelli V, De Angelis B, Lucarini L, et al. Tissue regeneration in loss of substance on the lower limbs through use of platelet-rich plasma, stem cells from adipose tissue, and hyaluronic acid. Adv Skin Wound Care 2010;23(6):262–72.

66. Cervelli V, Lucarini L, Spallone D, et al. Use of platelet rich plasma and hyaluronic acid on exposed tendons of the foot and ankle. J Wound Care 2010;19(5):186 188–90.

67. Frykberg RG, Driver VR, Carman D, et al. Chronic wounds treated with a physiologically relevant concentration of platelet-rich plasma gel: a prospective case series. Ostomy Wound Manage 2010;56(6):36–44.

Pathology-Designed Custom Molded Foot Orthoses

Kevin B. Rosenbloom, CPed

KEYWORDS

- Foot orthoses • Custom orthoses • Orthotic devices
- Pathology-designed orthoses • Orthosis design

Treating patients with custom foot orthoses for common pathologies is a rewarding experience when the proper steps are taken during foot casting and custom-orthosis prescription writing. This article describes successful methods for orthoses casting and prescription writing for custom-molded orthoses for Achilles tendonitis, pes planus, hallux limitus, plantar fasciitis/heel spurs, lateral ankle instability, metatarsalgia, and pes cavus. In addition, a summary of orthotic laboratory instructions for each pathology-designed orthosis is provided, which should be considered by orthotic laboratories.

ACHILLES TENDONITIS

When treating Achilles tendonitis with custom-molded foot orthotics, the most important function of the orthosis is to relieve tension on the Achilles tendon by plantar-flexing the foot and then reducing any internal or external rotation of the Achilles tendon by supporting the heel with corrective posting and custom contour inferior of the midtarsal joints.[1] Plantar flexion of the foot can be achieved with a simple heel lift in a shoe or by wearing shoes with elevated heels such as running shoes or clogs. It is important for patients to forgo wearing flat shoes and soft surfaces where the heel has a tendency to sink below the grade of the forefoot; walking barefoot should also be avoided.

In a foot with normal mechanics, controlling eversion or inversion of the calcaneus is critical for prevention of rotational torsion of the Achilles. A deep heel cup with extrinsic varus or valgus posting will control any subtalar eversion or inversion while ambulating (**Figs. 1** and **2**). The full contact orthosis shell is important for full functionality of the rearfoot posting and controlling midtarsal joint articulation. Proper casting is also critical. While suspension casting with plaster or a similar material, one must load the midtarsal joints to a pronated position while keeping the subtalar joint neutral.[2,3] It is very important that the laboratory replicate the casted position with the positive model using minimal medial arch fill and no plaster build-up on the medial aspect of the

Kevin Orthotics, Foot In Motion, 3232 23rd Street, Santa Monica, CA 90405, USA
E-mail address: kevin@kevinorthotics.com

Clin Podiatr Med Surg 28 (2011) 171–187
doi:10.1016/j.cpm.2010.11.001 **podiatric.theclinics.com**

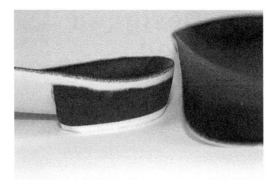

Fig. 1. Achilles tendonitis pathology-designed orthosis, medial posterior view of 16-mm heel cup, extrinsic post with 3-mm heel lift. Anterior view of custom molded polypropylene shell with vinyl top cover terminating proximal to the metatarsal heads.

heel. A high-quality polypropylene shell material that is semirigid and selected according to the patient's weight for 5% to 10% give and rebound should be employed for optimal results in comfort and control.[4] A slim vinyl top cover keeps the custom-molded orthosis shell intimate with foot contour. The custom orthosis should terminate proximal to the metatarsal heads to position the forefoot below the elevation of the heel throughout the gait cycle (**Fig. 3**). Custom orthoses designed for Achilles tendonitis should be worn by the patient full-time after the break-in period and should then be worn for the life of the patient to prevent recurrence. For orthotic laboratory instructions, see **Box 1**.

PES PLANUS

Pes planus can be a difficult yet rewarding pathology to treat with orthoses. Fighting gravity, mechanical inefficiencies, and accommodating bony prominences in the foot is challenging for the foot and ankle specialist. Careful casting is critical for pes planus foot architecture. A foam impression may prove sufficient if the goal is merely to support and accommodate the present foot structure. However, custom orthosis correction is usually desirable in order to prevent degenerative mechanics and inefficient gait. Suspension casting is preferred.[3]

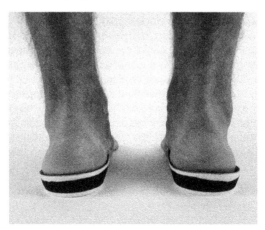

Fig. 2. Achilles tendonitis pathology-designed orthosis, posterior view, with 4° extrinsic rearfoot posting and 3-mm heel lift.

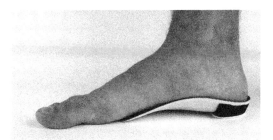

Fig. 3. Achilles tendonitis pathology-designed orthosis, medial view, terminating proximal to the metatarsal heads. Polypropylene custom-molded shell, 4° extrinsic rearfoot posting, 3-mm heel lift.

To position the foot for correct casting, a full understanding of the weight-bearing position is needed to determine how much deformity is present during ambulation. A subtalar neutral position with a fully pronated midtarsal joint captures a corrected foot position that is tolerable.[3] Bony prominences require button-out accommodations, especially the navicular and talus head. Button-out accommodations should be slightly greater than their respective size to allow for some orthosis shear and movement. The orthotic laboratory should be familiar with proper placement and sizing of button-out accommodations; however, the laboratory may require prominences to be marked accordingly on the negative cast. A forefoot varus wedge inferior to the metatarsal heads posted to the degree of forefoot varus is an effective method to prevent mid- and rear-foot compensation for the forefoot varus deformity. Attention to proper shoe gear that allows enough room for the forefoot wedge is required. Medial flange and lateral clip, coupled with proper shoe gear, minimizes foot eversion, abduction, and lateral sliding off the orthosis. Vinyl top covers over a shell constructed of polypropylene will control and support the foot with comfort. Shell reinforcement is usually necessary in the form of an ethyl vinyl acetate (EVA) arch fill to provide long-lasting support. A very deep heel cup and extrinsic posting to correct subtalar eversion creates a solid foundation for the pes planus foot (**Figs. 4–6**). Pes planus designed

---

Box 1
Achilles tendonitis: custom foot orthosis laboratory instructions

Orthotic Type: Semirigid functional

Cast Balancing: Forefoot perpendicular to rearfoot

Plaster Cast Fill: Minimal

Shell Material: Polypropylene per weight

Heel Cup Depth: 16 mm (deep)

Shell Width: Standard (medial edge bisecting the sesamoids, lateral edge bisecting the fifth metatarsal head)

Rearfoot Posting: Extrinsic crepe posted to correct reducible varus or valgus heel position with 3-mm heel lift bilateral

Extension: None

Top Cover: Vinyl

Bottom Cover: None

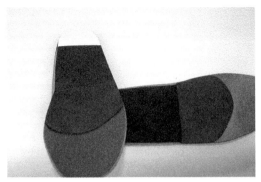

Fig. 4. Pes planus designed orthosis, inferior view, forefoot varus posting inferior of the metatarsal heads.

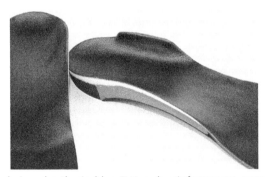

Fig. 5. Pes planus designed orthosis, blue EVA arch reinforcement, varus rearfoot posting, medial flange, lateral clip to prevent lateral slipping.

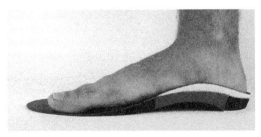

Fig. 6. Foot with pes planus designed orthosis, forefoot varus wedge under the metatarsal heads, blue EVA arch reinforcement, medial flanged polypropylene custom-molded shell, varus extrinsic heel post and deep heel cup.

orthoses should be broken in accordingly and should be worn for the lifetime of the patient. For orthotic laboratory instructions, see **Box 2**.

HALLUX LIMITUS

Treatment of functional hallux limitus with custom-molded foot orthoses is rewarding, and positive mechanical results are present nearly immediately when orthosis prescriptions are written correctly and when the orthotic is correctly dispensed. The primary function of the orthosis is to increase range of motion of the first metatarsal phalangeal joint by preventing jamming moments of the first metatarsal phalangeal joint. Underlying mechanical pathology of overpronating midtarsal and subtalar joints is often present with functional hallux limitus. The goal of orthotic treatment is to correct hind- and mid-foot mechanics while enhancing dorsiflexion of the hallux with forefoot modifications.[5,6] Suspension casting while the subtalar joint is neutral and the midtarsal joint is fully pronated is crucial. Standard laboratory modification of the positive model is preferred: 3 mm of allowance for medial arch pronation and fat pad expansion. A custom-molded polypropylene shell is desirable for semirigid control along with rearfoot posting to correct calcaneus eversion or inversion. An extension that incorporates a functional modification to promote dorsiflexion of the hallux is critical to achieve desirable first metatarsal phalangeal joint range of motion. A dynamic wedge that elevates the second through fifth metatarsal heads at least 1.5 to 3 mm relative to the first metatarsal head allows the first metatarsal to plantar-flex, thus enhancing hallux dorsiflexion. A 1.5- to 3-mm elevation under the hallux further promotes hallux dorsiflexion (**Fig. 7**). This modification is essentially a balancing of the first metatarsal head and elevation of the distal hallux (**Figs. 8** and **9**). Vinyl top covers allow intimate control of the mid- and rearfoot and allow the dynamic wedge to function without the extra bulk of padding in the forefoot. Orthoses for hallux limitus require a break-in period, and should be worn for the lifetime of the patient to ensure proper mechanics and prevent degenerating stress on the first metatarsal phalangeal joint. For orthotic laboratory instructions, see **Box 3**.

Box 2
Pes planus: custom foot orthosis laboratory instructions

Orthotic Type: Semirigid functional

Cast Balancing: Forefoot perpendicular to rearfoot

Plaster Cast Fill: Standard

Shell Material: Polypropylene per weight

Shell Arch Fill: EVA

Heel Cup Depth: 20 mm (very deep)

Shell Width: Wide (medial edge medial to tibial sesamoid, lateral edge lateral to fifth metatarsal head) with medial flange and button out accommodations for bony prominences

Rearfoot Posting: Extrinsic crepe posted to reduce varus heel position

Forefoot Posting: Extrinsic crepe wedge to stabilize and accommodate forefoot varus position

Extension: 3-mm cushion to toes

Top Cover and Padding: Vinyl top cover and moderate padding

Bottom Cover: Suede or similar

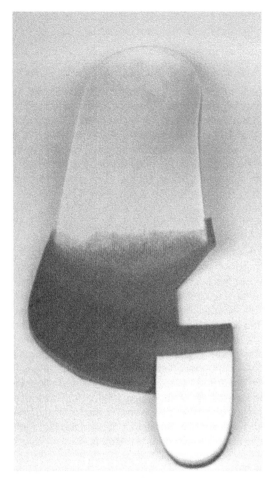

Fig. 7. Hallux limitus designed orthosis, without top cover, revealing dynamic wedge extension.

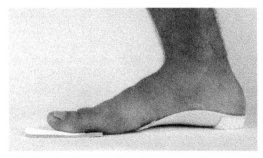

Fig. 8. Hallux limitus designed orthosis, without top cover, showing dynamic wedge extension assisting dorsiflexion of the hallux.

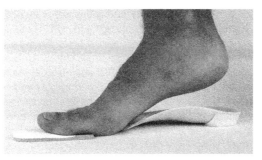

Fig. 9. Hallux limitus designed orthosis, without top cover, showing dynamic wedge extension assisting dorsiflexion of the hallux.

HALLUX RIGIDUS

Hallux rigidus can be a challenging pathology to treat, given the compliance of shoe gear that is required by the patient. The goal of custom-molded foot orthoses is to restrict all motion and moments in the first metatarsal phalangeal joint by creating a splinting type of modification across the joint on the plantar aspect to withstand and transfer dorsiflexion moments to the orthosis shell or shoe gear. These types of splints or modifications are commonly called Morton extensions.[7] Proper suspension casting is critical for distribution of pressure and overall comfort. Neutral subtalar joint positioning and fully pronated midtarsal joint positioning is ideal during suspension casting. A polypropylene shell with rigid Morton extension is the best method to prevent movements in the pathologic joint (**Fig. 11**). This orthosis modification is an extension of the orthosis shell made from polypropylene, which extends from the heel distal to the first metatarsal phalangeal joint. Complications of fitting shoe gear with fully rigid devices are often present with rigid Morton extensions. Conversations with the patient to educate him or her on shoe-gear selection and expectations are paramount for successful outcomes with modifications of rigid Morton extensions. Because of the limited shoe-gear selection and fitting issues with rigid Morton

---

Box 3
Hallux limitus: custom foot orthosis laboratory instructions

Orthotic Type: Semirigid functional

Cast Balancing: Forefoot perpendicular to rearfoot

Plaster Cast Fill: Standard

Shell Material: Polypropylene per weight

Shell Arch Fill: None

Heel Cup Depth: 10 mm (standard)

Shell Width: Standard (medial edge bisecting the sesamoids, lateral edge bisecting the fifth metatarsal head)

Rearfoot Posting: Extrinsic crepe posted to correct reducible varus or valgus heel position

Extension: Dynamic wedge extension (to promote hallux dorsiflexion) to toes

Top Cover: Vinyl

Bottom Cover: Suede or similar

extensions, very often semiflexible Morton extensions are prescribed to provide some relief to the rigid first metatarsal phalangeal joint (**Fig. 10**). These semiflexible extensions absorb some dorsiflexion moments of the first metatarsal phalangeal joint, and satisfactory results are achieved in mild to moderate cases. The semiflexible extension should be crafted from a firm cushioning material such as EVA or crepe and extend from the distal shell, proximal to the metatarsal heads, extending distally past the first metatarsal phalangeal joint. Laterally, the rigid or semiflexible Morton extension should terminate at the first interspace. With a rigid or semiflexible Morton extension, a 1.5- to 3-mm cushioned top cover is desirable for comfort and acceptance of the topographic features of the Morton extension. Patients with hallux rigidus should use a proper break-in period to become accustomed to their custom-molded orthoses, and the orthoses should be worn for the lifetime of the patient. For orthotic laboratory instructions, see **Box 4**.

PLANTAR FASCIITIS AND HEEL SPURS

Treating plantar fasciitis and heel spurs with custom-molded foot orthoses is effective when accomplished through a modification used to offload the inflamed tissue and a mechanical correction to reduce tension on the plantar fascia.[8] During suspension casting, it is critical to load the mid-tarsal joint to maximum pronation while keeping the subtalar joint neutral. It is also critical to take note of the swelling in the affected heel(s) and palpate for extra tissue mass on the plantar surface of the heel. If

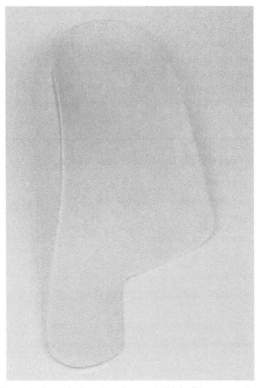

Fig. 10. Hallux rigidus pathology designed orthoses, rigid shell incorporating Morton extension.

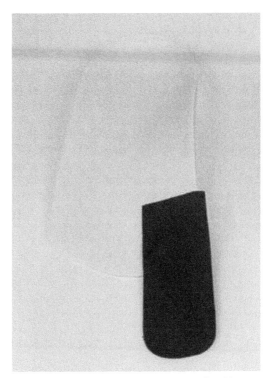

Fig. 11. Hallux rigidus pathology designed orthoses, crepe flexible Morton extension.

inflammation or asymmetric plantar mass is present at any location along the plantar surface of the heel, it is critical to write on the orthotic prescription that extra heel tissue expansion or accommodation is required for the pathologic heel. Modifications of the heel cup should accommodate for the inflamed area and for the spurring of the

---

Box 4
Hallux rigidus: custom foot orthosis laboratory instructions

Orthotic Type: Rigid functional

Cast Balancing: Forefoot perpendicular to rearfoot

Plaster Cast Fill: Minimum

Shell Material: Polypropylene per weight

Shell Arch Fill: None

Heel Cup Depth: 10 mm (standard)

Shell Width: Standard (medial edge bisecting the sesamoids, lateral edge bisecting the fifth metatarsal head)

Rearfoot Posting: Extrinsic crepe posted to correct reducible varus or valgus heel position

Extension: Morton extension, rigid or semiflexible

Top Cover: Cushioned

Bottom Cover: Suede or similar

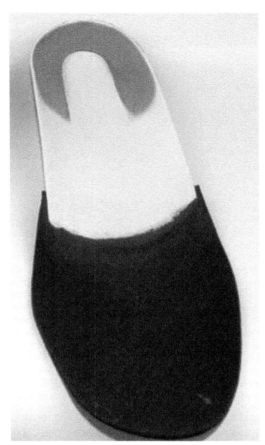

Fig. 12. Heel spur pathology designed orthosis, uncovered custom-molded orthosis with horseshoe pad.

calcaneus by offloading that area with a horseshoe-shaped pad (**Fig. 12**). The horseshoe-shaped pad should consist of a material that is firm yet cushioning. If spurs are not present, a heel cushion is recommended to provide extra comfort and heel elevation (**Fig. 13**). Three-millimeter cushion top covers provide sufficient cushion and comfort. An extrinsic post that corrects subtalar eversion or inversion by posting to the reducible position is also desirable to reduce rotational tension on the plantar fascia and underlying biomechanical pathology. A 3-mm heel lift bilateral, regardless of unilateral spurring and heel pain, helps reduce overall length of the plantar fascia. Deep heel cups help control calcaneus eversion and inversion; in addition they help contain excessive fat-pad expansion during weight bearing. Patients should follow a structured break-in period and continue to wear functional orthoses during rigorous activities for the duration of their lifetime to prevent reoccurrence. For orthotic laboratory instructions, see **Box 5**.

LATERAL ANKLE INSTABILITY

Treating lateral ankle instability with custom-molded orthoses is a challenge; one must fight a tendency toward lateral rolling and ankle sprains while making a comfortable, tolerable device.[9–11] First and foremost, a cast that positions the subtalar joint in

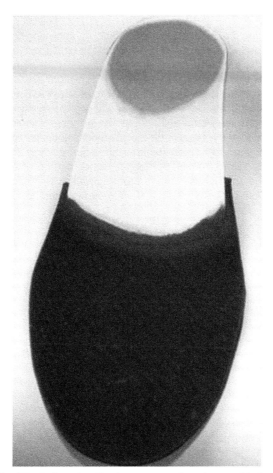

Fig. 13. Plantar fasciitis designed orthosis, uncovered custom-molded orthosis with heel cushion.

Box 5
Plantar fasciitis and heel spurs: custom foot orthosis specifications

Orthotic Type: Semirigid functional

Cast Balancing: Forefoot perpendicular to rearfoot

Plaster Cast Fill: Standard

Shell Material: Polypropylene per weight

Shell Arch Fill: None

Heel Cup Depth: 16 mm (deep)

Shell Width: Standard (medial edge bisecting the sesamoids, lateral edge bisecting the fifth metatarsal head)

Rearfoot Posting: Extrinsic crepe posted to correct reducible varus or valgus heel position

Extension: Thin cushion to toes

Top Cover and Padding: Cushion to toes with horseshoe pad or heel cushion

Bottom Cover: Suede or similar with 3 mm heel lift bilateral neutral while pronating the midtarsal joints is critical for achieving comfort and control. Then, standard fat pad expansion of 3 mm around the heel and 3-mm lowering of the arch are advisable in the cast. When patients present with high-arch, non-weight bearing that flattens to a pes planus position during weight bearing, maximum arch fill in the cast is desirable to lower the medial arch so as to prevent medial ground reaction force while wearing the orthosis. Any medial ground reaction force should be avoided. Modifications for lateral ankle instability orthoses should have an oblique valgus post that reduces the tension on the posterior talofibular ligament and calcaneofibular ligament (**Fig. 14**). Three degrees of valgus posting is ideal for patients whose calcaneus is aligned under the leg. A higher degree of correction may be needed for pes cavus foot types in the rearfoot as well as valgus posting in the forefoot. A cuboid pad should be added for the reduction of anterior talofibular ligament tension (**Fig. 15**). A cushioned extension to the toes is desirable for comfort. Lateral ankle instability designed orthoses should be worn by the patient for their lifetime and especially during intense activity. For orthotic laboratory instructions, see **Box 6**.

METATARSALGIA

Treating metatarsalgia with custom-molded foot orthoses is rewarding in most cases because the patient will experience a "wow" moment. Upon dispensing carefully crafted devices that offload pressure from the metatarsal heads during the propulsion phases of gait, significant relief is often experienced.

First and foremost, a suspension cast that positions the subtalar joint in neutral while pronating the midtarsal joints is critical for achieving a contour of the arch that is in a functional position for propulsion as a rigid lever.[2] Minimal lowering of the arch in the cast is desirable to ensure close contact of the orthosis and arch during gait. Close contact of the arch will allow pressure to transfer from the metatarsal heads to the proximal osseous structures. The extension of the orthosis should offload the affected metatarsal heads when the patient describes pain in the precise location of 1 or 2 metatarsal heads. If general pain in the ball of the foot is the chief compliant and the patient has a Morton foot, a foot cookie modification in the extension is helpful in transferring propulsion moments to the first and fifth metatarsal heads while offloading the second, third, and forth metatarsal heads (**Fig. 16**). A metatarsal pad that is sized appropriately for the foot is also helpful for more severe cases that require more metatarsal shaft elevation, to attempt to offload the affected metatarsal

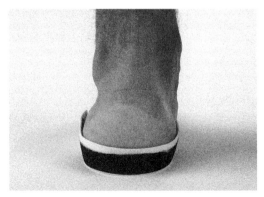

Fig. 14. Lateral ankle instability pathology designed custom-molded orthosis, extrinsic valgus posting, lateral clip (left foot posterior view).

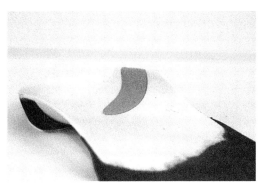

Fig. 15. Lateral ankle instability pathology designed orthosis, uncovered, blue cuboid pad, lateral clip, extrinsic oblique rearfoot post.

head.[12,13] A small pad no larger than 3 mm in thickness is usually satisfactory. Mechanically the rearfoot should not be overlooked. Internal rotation of the metatarsal heads in the pronating foot can often cause an improper tracking of the lesser metatarsal phalangeal joints. This improper joint articulation can cause metatarsalgia, and attention to correct even the slightest pronation movement should be attempted with varus posting of the rearfoot. A 1.5-mm cushion top cover will allow full functionality of balance pads and foot cookie and metatarsal pad modifications, while providing comfort and cushioning. The designed orthosis should be worn by the patient for his or her lifetime to prevent recurring symptoms. For orthotic laboratory instructions, see **Box 7**.

PES CAVUS

The pes cavus foot is a demanding foot type to treat with custom-molded foot orthoses. Several mechanical pathologies proximal to the foot result from rigid foot architecture. Identifying the specific structure of the cavus foot can be a challenge. Plantar-flexed first rays are most common, causing the rearfoot to invert, resulting

---

Box 6
Lateral ankle instability: custom foot orthosis laboratory instructions

Orthotic Type: Semirigid functional

Cast Balancing: Forefoot perpendicular to rearfoot

Plaster Cast Fill: Standard

Shell Material: Polypropylene per weight

Shell Arch Fill: None

Heel Cup Depth: 10 mm

Shell Width: Wide (medial edge medial to tibial sesamoid, lateral edge lateral to fifth metatarsal head) with lateral clip

Rearfoot Posting: Extrinsic crepe oblique valgus post

Extension: 3 mm cushion to toes

Top Cover and Padding: Vinyl, cuboid pad

Bottom Cover: Suede or similar

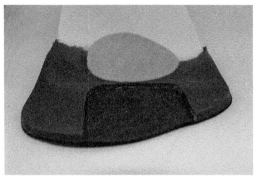

Fig. 16. Metatarsalgia pathology designed orthosis, uncovered, with foot cookie modification and metatarsal pad.

in a foot that is unstable and at risk. To treat these foot types, a suspended cast is not as crucial due to the inflexibility of the foot. Foam box impression casting usually works as well as suspension slipper casting.[3,14] A loaded midtarsal joint that is fully pronated, and a neutral subtalar joint are preferred during casting and impression taking. If it presents, a plantar flexed first ray should be captured during the impression technique. The positive cast modification at the laboratory should contain minimal to no medial arch lowering, and standard fat pad expansion in the heel. A forefoot to rearfoot balancing is desired in the positive cast.

The orthosis should have a rearfoot extrinsic post at neutral to valgus degree, depending on the angle of calcaneal varus. Forefoot balancing is also important to elevate the lesser metatarsal heads, allowing the first metatarsal head to drop. The trick of balancing the cavus foot with orthoses is to clinically observe the reduction of calcaneus varus obtainable and the severity of the plantar flexed first ray. Balancing by coupling moderate rearfoot post in the range of 2° to 4° valgus with a forefoot post of 2° to 4° valgus is usually effective. This balancing should also be coupled with a first metatarsal head balancing if there is a true plantar flexed first-ray deformity (**Fig. 17**). Not all cavus foot types have plantar flexed first rays; some have a forefoot

---

Box 7
Metatarsalgia: custom foot orthosis laboratory instructions

Orthotic Type: Semirigid functional

Cast Balancing: Forefoot perpendicular to rearfoot

Plaster Cast Fill: Minimal fill in medial arch

Shell Material: Polypropylene per weight

Shell Arch Fill: None

Heel Cup Depth: 10 mm

Shell Width: Standard (medial edge bisecting the sesamoids, lateral edge bisecting the fifth metatarsal head)

Extension: Foot cookie modification (balance second, third, and forth metatarsal heads)

Top Cover and Padding: Cushion top cover and metatarsal pads under affected metatarsals

Bottom Cover: Suede or similar

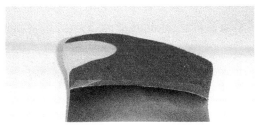

Fig. 17. Pes cavus pathology designed orthosis, Coleman modification (valgus forefoot wedge with first metatarsal head cut-out filled in) (inferior view).

perpendicular to the rearfoot or even a forefoot varus.[15] For the latter foot architectures, a cushioned, full-contact semirigid orthosis should be employed. Cavus foot patients should take care in breaking in orthoses and wear them for their lifetime in order to ensure a mechanically stable gait. For orthotic laboratory instructions, see **Box 8**.

ORTHOTIC BREAK-IN

With all custom-molded foot orthoses, a break-in schedule should be followed by the patient before wearing full time. Patient instructions with a preferred break-in schedule is as follows (but should be adjusted to consider patient age and health, and orthosis history; **Box 9**).

PATIENT EDUCATION AND FOLLOW-UP

It is important to educate patients in accommodating custom foot orthoses with properly fitting shoe gear for functionality and comfort. Custom-molded foot orthoses should never be forced into shoes, and they should sit flat and level within the shoe. Custom-molded foot orthoses should be checked annually for posting, top cover,

---

Box 8
Pes cavus: custom foot orthosis laboratory instructions

Orthotic Type: Semirigid functional

Cast Balancing: Forefoot perpendicular to rearfoot

Plaster Cast Fill: Minimal to none

Shell Material: Polypropylene per weight

Shell Arch Fill: None

Heel Cup Depth: 10 mm

Shell Width: Standard (medial edge bisecting the sesamoids, lateral edge bisecting the fifth metatarsal head)

Rearfoot Posting: Extrinsic crepe valgus posting

Extension: Coleman modification (valgus forefoot wedge posted to specific degree and first metatarsal head cut out with cushion fill-in)

Top Cover: Vinyl

Bottom Cover: None

Box 9
Custom foot orthotic break-in period instructions (provide to patient when dispensing orthoses)

It usually takes 10 days to become accustomed to your orthotics
Follow the daily schedule for proper break-in:

First day: Wear no longer than 1 hour

Second day: Wear no longer than 2 hours

Third day: DO NOT wear orthotics; take a break

Fourth day: Wear no longer than 3 hours

Fifth day: Wear no longer than 5 hours

Sixth day: DO NOT wear orthotics; take a break

Seventh day: Wear no longer than 7 hours

Eighth day: Wear no longer than 9 hours

Ninth day: DO NOT wear orthotics; take a break

Tenth day: Wear up to 10 hours

Eleventh day: Wear all day long!

Do not wear orthotics for athletic activity during break-in period. Wait until after the 10th day before doing any intense activity like running or playing sports.
If you experience any joint pain while wearing your orthotics, stop wearing your orthotics and contact the office.
Your orthotics are custom made for you and your needs. They may require you to follow alternative instructions from your doctor.

---

and shell breakdown. Orthoses should be replaced or repaired if posting or shells have lost their shape or if the top cover has become worn.

SUMMARY

These methods for foot casting and custom-orthosis prescription writing will provide positive outcomes for their intended pathology. Establishing a relationship with an orthotic laboratory that provides quality custom orthoses and quality service through communication will allow patients to receive the highest quality care and best possible outcome.

REFERENCES

1. Donoghue OA, Harrison AJ, Laxton P, et al. Orthotic control of rear foot and lower limb motion during running in participants with chronic Achilles tendon injury. Sports Biomech 2008;7(2):194–205.
2. Lee WE. Podiatric biomechanics: a historical appraisal and discussion of the root model as a clinical system of approach in the present context of theoretical uncertainty. Clin Podiatr Med Surg 2001;18(4):555–684.
3. Losito JM. Impression casting techniques. In: Valmassy RL, editor. Clinical biomechanics of the lower extremities. St Louis (MO): Mosby; 1996. p. 279–94.
4. Olson WR. Orthotic materials. In: Valmassy RL, editor. Clinical biomechanics of the lower extremities. St Louis (MO): Mosby; 1996. p. 307–26.

5. Scherer PR, Sanders J, Eldredge D, et al. Effect of functional foot orthoses on first metatarsophalangeal joint dorsiflexion in stance and gait. J Am Podiatr Med Assoc 2006;96(6):474.

6. Hetherington VJ, Johnson RE, Albritton JS. Necessary dorsiflexion of the first metatarsophalangeal joint during gait. J Foot Surg 1990;29:218.

7. Jones JL. Prescription writing for functional and accommodative foot orthoses. In: Valmassy RL, editor. Clinical biomechanics of the lower extremities. St Louis (MO): Mosby; 1996. p. 295–306.

8. Cheung JT, Zhang M, An KN, et al. Effect of Achilles tendon loading on plantar fascia tension in the standing foot. Clin Biomech (Bristol, Avon) 2006;21(2): 194–203.

9. Hertel J. Functional anatomy, pathomechanics, and pathophysiology of lateral ankle instability. J Athl Train 2002;37:364.

10. Orteza LC, Vogelbach WD, Denegar CR. The effect of molded and unmolded orthotics on balance and pain while jogging following inversion ankle sprain. J Athl Train 1992;27:80.

11. Richie DH. Effects of foot orthoses on patients with chronic ankle instability. J Am Podiatr Med Assoc 2007;97:19–30.

12. Chang AH, Abu-Faraj ZU, Harris GF, et al. Multistep measurement of plantar pressure alterations using metatarsal pads. Foot Ankle Int 1994;15:654–60.

13. Hsi WL, Kang JH, Lee X. Optimum position of metatarsal pad in metatarsalgia for pressure relief. Am J Phys Med Rehabil 2005;84:514–20.

14. Marzano R. Fabricating shoe modifications. In: Janisse D, editor. Introduction to pedorthics. Columbia (MD): Pedorthic Footwear Association; 1998. p. 226–31.

15. Burns J, Crosbie J, Hunt A, et al. The effect of pes cavus on foot pain and plantar pressure. Clin Biomech 2005;20(9):877–82.

Physical Therapy and Rehabilitation of the Foot and Ankle in the Athlete

Suzanne T. Hawson, PT, MPT, OCS

KEYWORDS

• Foot • Ankle • Injuries • Athletes • Physical therapy

Injuries to the foot and ankle in athletes are well documented in research. An epidemiologic study by Garrick and Requa[1] found that 25% of 12,681 injuries seen in a multispecialty sports medicine clinic occurred at the foot and the ankle. A study by Dane and colleagues[2] found that the foot and the ankle were the most frequently injured body regions in basketball, volleyball, soccer, and running, and that injury rates are associated with sport. In 1997, Bronner and Brownstein[3] documented that the majority of dance injuries in a Broadway ballet show involved the foot and the ankle, and in 2008 Gamboa and colleagues[4] found that 53% of injuries in ballet dancers occurred in the foot and ankle.

Recreational and elite athletes alike sustain foot and ankle injuries that can hamper their ability to return to sport. If self-treatment does not resolve their condition, most athletes will seek professional consultation from a physician, podiatrist, chiropractor, or other sports medicine professional. Conservative management of injuries and rehabilitation from surgical repair frequently involves physical therapy. Athletic injuries involving musculoskeletal issues benefit significantly with physical therapy to optimize return to function and sports participation. Physical therapists specialize in the evaluation and treatment of movement dysfunction that result from injury. Their expertise should be employed to maximize outcomes after foot and ankle injuries have been sustained in athletes.

A brief survey was completed by calling podiatry offices in California listed in http://footweb.net to estimate the percentage of patients, with sports medicine conditions of the foot and ankle that are referred to physical therapy. Of the 76 podiatrists that were contacted, 52 reported that they treated sports medicine related injuries. Of those 52 respondents, the reported average number of sports medicine patients referred to physical therapy was 37.93%, with a median of 20%. The results of this brief survey

The author has nothing to disclose.

Physical Therapy Department, University Foot and Ankle Institute, 26357 McBean Parkway, Suite 250, Valencia, CA 91355, USA

E-mail address: suzanne@footankleinstitute.com

can only be applied to the population that was contacted during the survey. It is beyond the scope of this article to determine whether this is statistically significant and whether the results would apply to a larger population. According to the Physical Therapy Board of California,

> Physical therapists in California are required to have a diagnosis from a licensed health care professional who is authorized by his/her license to diagnose (ie, physicians, dentists, podiatrists, chiropractors, etc.) Although a physical therapist may perform an evaluation without a diagnosis, one is required before the physical therapist providing any physical therapy treatment.[5]

Because podiatrists and physicians are primary health care providers in sports medicine, they can recommend physical therapy as part of treatment. Some of the challenges that affect the inclusion of physical therapy in injury management are awareness and access. Archer and colleagues[6] found that physicians and physical therapists differ in opinion regarding initiation and timing of physical therapy after traumatic lower extremity injury. The difference may result from lack of awareness of physical therapy interventions that can benefit athletes during the early stages of injury. With the advent of obtaining information through the Internet and increasing costs of health care, athletes may choose self-treatment instead of receiving professional physical therapy care. Physicians and podiatrists who have increased awareness of the skills and services that physical therapists offer can educate their patients about the benefits of physical therapy and encourage them to seek services.

According to the American Physical Therapy Association's (APTA) Guide to Physical Therapist Practice, physical therapists:

> (1) Diagnose and manage movement dysfunction and enhance physical and functional abilities, (2) Restore, maintain, and promote not only optimal physical function but optimal wellness and fitness and optimal quality of life as it relates to movement and health, (3) Prevent the onset, symptoms and progression of impairments, functional limitations, and disabilities that may result from disease, disorders, conditions or injuries.[7]

Physical therapists have the education, tools, capabilities, and expertise that would greatly benefit injured athletes to optimize outcomes. Through their skills and competence, physical therapists prescribe functional rehabilitation programs for athletes that Title and Katchis[8] have said is the best means to rapidly return the player to competing and to prolong athletic careers. Functional limitation is defined as the "inability to perform the actions, tasks and activities that constitute the usual activities for a given individual,"[7] and disability is defined as "the inability or restricted ability to perform actions, tasks and activities related to required self-care, home management, work, community and leisure roles in the individual's sociocultural context and physical environment."[7] For the athlete, an example of a functional limitation is not being able to run, and the resulting disability is the inability to participate in sports such as soccer or competing in a running race.

Physical therapists that have additional training in functional biomechanical evaluation, or who have attended residency program and completed advanced studies to specialize in sports medicine and orthopedics are likely to offer the best care for athletes. The American Board of Physical Therapy Specialties (ABPTS) offers certification for physical therapists to develop a "greater depth of knowledge and skills related to a particular area of practice."[9] Physical therapists with specialties in orthopedics and sports have formal recognition of having more knowledge, experience, and skills.[9] Physicians, podiatrists, and other health care personnel are encouraged to develop good relationships with physical therapists with whom they refer patients, and to familiarize themselves with specialist to maximize patient outcome and satisfaction when treating foot and ankle related conditions in athletes.

COMPREHENSIVE EVALUATION OF INJURED ATHLETES

Physical therapy is indicated for athletes who present with impairments and functional limitations that may be severe enough to be considered a disability, which for athletes would be the inability to participate in sports. Management of injured athletes involves an extensive examination process whereby subjective history taking is coupled with tests and measures to determine impairments and functional limitations with which each athlete presents. This dynamic process between the athlete and the physical therapist allows for the collection of information regarding mechanism of injury, previous level of function, current level of function, and symptoms. The information is pertinent for differential diagnosis and formulation of a treatment plan.

It is important for physical therapists to determine the mechanism of injury to guide treatment plans. Athletic injuries to the foot and ankle can result either from overuse or trauma. Regardless of the mechanism of injury, there is almost always resulting muscle and joint dysfunction that could potentially affect proper functioning of the injured body part. The mechanism of injury for traumatic injuries is fairly easy to determine. It is usually triggered by a specific incident, and the onset of signs and symptoms are usually immediate following an incident, such as an acute ankle sprain. On the other hand, the mechanism of injury for overuse syndromes in the foot and ankle is usually more difficult to determine. For instance, typical questions for runners would include details about their training program, type of footwear, to what extent their shoes are worn out, running style and technique, preferred running terrain, and others. It has been found that training volume or mileage and the occurrence of previous injuries are the most consistent risk factors for overuse injuries in runners.[10,11] There can be multiple factors that have contributed to an athlete's condition, which physical therapists have to decipher through history taking and, later, through tests and measures.

It is also during this stage of the examination process that the athlete can relate his or her expected outcomes and goals. Each athlete presents with different expectations regarding length of rehabilitation, anticipated return to sport, and performance. For example, competitive athletes' concerns may include the negative stresses of missing workouts, games, or events, and an unrealistic expectation of returning to their activity almost immediately. For professional athletes, injuries to the foot and ankle may present a variety of issues such as loss of pay and at worst, the end of a career. Oztekin and colleagues[12] completed a retrospective descriptive study of time lost for professional soccer players with foot and ankle injuries, and found that the most common diagnosis is ankle sprain and the most common hindfoot injury is from Achilles tendinopathy. The investigators conclude that time lost to play dramatically increases through the presence of severe foot and ankle injuries, and results in players being out of professional competition for about 2 months.[12] These considerations for professional athletes may affect the athlete's expectations during the rehabilitative process, thus influencing outcomes and satisfaction levels.

The establishment of rapport between the athlete and the physical therapist also starts here. The bond between the athlete and the physical therapist can greatly influence outcomes. Roberts and Bucksey[13] have determined that physical therapists spend an increased amount of time during history taking and reciprocating to patient concerns by giving advice, discussing psychosocial factors, and explaining treatment options. Physical therapy appointments can last from 30 minutes to an hour, with follow-up sessions that can range from once a week to 3 times per week. If there is a good relationship between the athlete and the physical therapist, then time can be used productively for learning and support. Increasing effective communication and active listening in addition to providing social support and encouragement can help athletes in their recovery.[14] Chevan and Haskvitz[15] found that physical therapists exercise more when compared with the United States adult population and other health diagnosing professional such as physicians, nurses, and physician assistants. Physical therapists who are athletes themselves can contribute to the bond and mutual understanding of issues that may concern the athlete.

TESTS AND MEASURES

During the initial encounter of athletes with foot and ankle injuries, objective tests and measures are completed to determine impairment. Impairment is defined as "alterations in anatomic, physiologic or psychological structures or function."[7] Tests and measures can include observation of foot type, gross deformities, noting pathologic changes in skin and appearance; measurement of swelling, range of motion, strength deficits, leg length symmetry, assessment of arthrokinematics, gait evaluation, balance, sensory changes, nerve tension relationships, balance issues, movement dysfunctions, and an overall biomechanical evaluation. Gathering all this information is sometimes not feasible during the initial visit because of time constraints, or can sometimes be limited by the athlete's presentation. For example, a running gait evaluation could not be completed for an athlete who has recently had Achilles tendon rupture repair and remains with non–weight-bearing restrictions. This part of the evaluation process would have to be completed at a later time, when appropriate (**Fig. 1**).

Foot type is considered during the biomechanical evaluation to determine if it is a contributor to injury or if it needs to be addressed during treatment for successful rehabilitation. The foot, ankle, knee, hip, and trunk are examined in a non–weight-bearing position and in a weight-bearing position, both statically and dynamically. Trained physical therapists can reliably use visual appraisal methods to classify gross foot type abnormalities with good reliability.[16] There is evidence[17,18] that foot type can lead to certain musculoskeletal conditions in athletes. Ryan and colleagues[19] have shown that abnormal or excessive pronation of the foot is a risk factor for developing

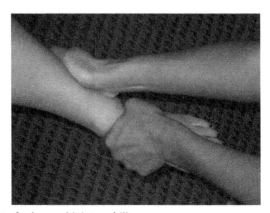

Fig. 1. Assessment of talocrural joint mobility.

medial tibial stress syndrome. Achilles mid-portion tendinopathy is associated with increased pronation at the subtalar joint. High arched runners have a greater incidence of ankle injuries, bony injuries, and lateral injuries whereas low-arched runners exhibit more knee injuries, soft tissue injuries, and medial injuries; these relationships should be considered when planning treatment.[20] Burns and colleagues[21] found that a supinated foot type was more likely to sustain an overuse injury in triathletes not wearing foot orthoses. Regardless of the foot type, the physical therapist determines how the foot type affects the biomechanics of the lower extremities and how that relates to a particular athlete's needs.

Evaluation of footwear is also completed. Athletes present with different types of footwear depending on their sport. Cleats, ballet shoes, running shoes, and the like are assessed for appropriate fit and to rule out contributing factors to injury. For instance, athletic shoe companies such as Asics, Brooks, New Balance, and others have attempted to accommodate foot type in their running shoe selections. The shoes are marketed based on 3 basic foot types: supinated, neutral, or pronated. A recent study by Cheung and Ng[22] indicates that with increased running mileage, plantar force in medial foot structures is higher and that recreational runners with more than 6° of foot pronation should consider motion control shoes. However, there is evidence[23] that running footwear prescription should not be based on foot type, but instead should be based on mechanics.[24] In addition, physical therapists can assess footwear for defects that may have caused the athlete's condition. A defective running shoe has been documented[25] as a contributor to development of plantar fasciitis in a competitive triathlete.

The development of movement dysfunction along the entire kinetic chain is also assessed. Physical therapists assess other areas that may have resulted or contributed to the foot and ankle condition, especially for athletes who present with chronic conditions. Immobilization after injury or surgical repair in the foot and ankle has effects on the knee, hip and trunk as the body will likely adapt with compensatory mechanisms to maintain functional mobility. What may have started as a compensation for the foot and ankle injury can eventually contribute to the athlete's condition. For instance, it has been determined[26] that alignment of the lower extremity up to the pelvic girdle can be altered, due to forces acting on the foot. Therefore, for excessive pronators, issues such as weakness in the hip abductors and external rotators as well as patellofemoral and tibiofemoral joint issues will also be addressed by the physical therapist for appropriate treatment.[27]

Clinical judgments based on this gathered information allow the physical therapist to establish a plan of care that includes the prognosis and treatment interventions for the athlete. Compliance to a rehabilitation program is viewed as important for successful recovery from injury.[28] Establishment of short-term and long-term goals and agreement between the athlete and the physical therapist for the defined treatment plan are necessary for successful rehabilitation. Goal setting in injury rehabilitation has a positive effect on athlete compliance and adherence to rehabilitation.[29] During the early phases of rehabilitation, athletes may be anxious to return to activity as soon as possible. Laying out realistic short-term goals for athletes during each phase of recovery establishes attainable and tangible goals to keep athletes compliant and motivated in their recovery. Unrealistic expectations between the athlete and the physical therapist must be addressed as the establishment of rapport continues to develop during this important phase of evaluation and leads to compliance in treatment. The athlete must feel as if his or her concerns will be addressed in the treatment plan, and the physical therapist must also be able to justify his or her judgments based on clinical reasoning.

REHABILITATION: PROGRESSION FROM INJURY TO RETURN TO SPORT

The multifaceted nature of foot and ankle conditions in athletes is best addressed when physical therapy is appropriately tailored to the condition. Physical therapy interventions used in foot and ankle rehabilitation can include the use of electrotherapeutic modalities, physical agents, manual therapy, orthotic fabrication, assistive device prescription such as bracing, application of therapeutic exercises, and neuromuscular reeducation. Selection, timing, and proper application of appropriate treatment interventions are based on tissue properties as one goes through the healing process.

The initial phase of healing is the inflammatory phase. This phase is initiated by injury or by surgery, and the goal of this phase is to prepare the area of injury for repair. The application of RICE (rest, ice, compression, and elevation) is commonly used to regulate the inflammatory process. Too little inflammation would retard healing and too much inflammation poses a risk of excess scarring.[30] During this phase, physical therapists can apply techniques to help control inflammation, such as the use of cryotherapy and intermittent compression devices, and apply other modalities such as electrical stimulation to help quell pain.[31]

The inflammatory phase is followed by the fibroplastic or proliferative phase, which is when fibroblasts work to repair damaged tissues. Collagen is assembled and the margin of the wound closes as scar tissue forms. Because the tensile strength of the scar is weak during this phase, physical therapy activities are limited to controlled motions to avoid breaking down the scar tissue.[30] However, there is concern for formation of joint contractures during this phase if too much scar tissue is laid down. Physical therapists use their clinical judgment to determine the appropriate amount of force to prevent excessive scar tissue formation and avoid breaking down healthy scar tissue. Manual therapy techniques such as joint mobilizations using oscillations or sustained glides can be applied during this phase,[32] as well as gentle range of motion exercises to help minimize this risk. Isometric strengthening exercises are appropriate, and range of motion exercises can be progressed as long as they do not interrupt the healing process.[31] If the scar is overly stressed, secondary inflammation can occur and disrupt healing.

The remodeling phase, which can last for more than 1 year from injury, follows the fibroplastic phase. It is during the remodeling phase that the wound continues to heal and the scar matures. The orientation of the collagen fibers determines the strength and the function of the healing tissue.[30] Exercises for flexibility and strengthening as well as manual techniques to affect muscles, tendons, and joints are used during this phase to effectively remodel the scar tissue to serve its appropriate function (**Fig. 2**). Progression of activity is based on Wolf's Law, which states that both bone and soft tissue will remodel or realign based on physical demands placed on them.[31]

Physical agents such as heat and cold applications are used to help alleviate pain and improve circulation, and can facilitate or suppress muscle function with the aim of returning to function.[33] These techniques can be in the forms of fluidotherapy, cryotherapy, ultrasound, and laser, to name a few. Low-level laser has been shown to improve symptoms of Achilles tendinopathy when coupled with eccentric exercises as compared with eccentric exercises completed alone (**Fig. 3**).[34–36] Electrical stimulation can improve motor recruitment or strengthen healthy muscle weakened by disuse atrophy, and muscle contractions can help minimize swelling.[33] The application of a direct current to chemicals by way of iontophoresis has been shown to help relieve symptoms of plantar fasciitis when used with acetic acid.[37,38]

Manual therapy techniques are applied to joints, ligaments, tendons, muscles, and skin to affect a physical change in the structure. For example, the purpose of friction

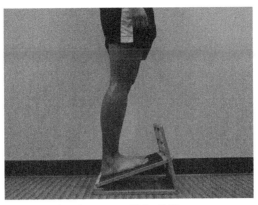

Fig. 2. An incline board is used to improve calf flexibility.

massage is to reduce local muscle spasms and loosen adherent fibrous tissues, and can also be used to incite the inflammatory process in chronic conditions such as Achilles tendinitis.[31] Joint mobilization can alter connective tissue remodeling through oscillations, sustained glides, thrust maneuvers, and capsular stretching.[32] Manual therapy has been shown to help relieve heel pain,[39] and a combination of manual physical therapy and exercise is superior to electrophysical agents and exercise alone in managing plantar heel pain.[40]

In addition, no other health professional best understands the application of therapeutic exercises for return to function than physical therapists do. Progression of exercises in athletes recovering from foot and ankle injuries, whether postsurgical or not,

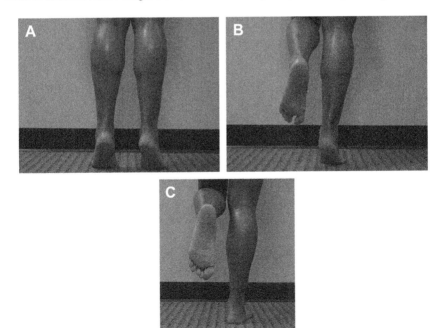

Fig. 3. (*A–C*) Procedure for eccentric strengthening of the gastroc-soleus complex for right lower extremity Achilles tendinitis.

relies on the theory of tissue strain and application of appropriate stress to improve tissue function. The inherent tensile strength of tissues dictates the intensity of exercise applied to those tissues. Care is taken with initiation of therapeutic exercises and movement stresses that the healing tissue can handle. Khan and Scott[41] discuss the theory of mechanotherapy, which is described as therapeutic exercise prescribed to promote the repair and remodeling of injured tissue. It is through the practical application of this theory that physical therapists are able to prescribe appropriate exercises. The delicate balance between tissue loading and the amount of stress that tissues can handle is always considered during prescription of exercises. The initiation of weight-bearing exercises for foot and ankle injuries has to take into consideration the appropriateness of adding this additional stress on healing tissues.

Progression during this phase includes exercises in weight bearing to load the foot and the ankle. Functional tolerance to weight-bearing activities are addressed, and completion of gait analysis is indicated if it has not been previously completed, such as in postsurgical cases that may have had weight-bearing restrictions. In addition to completing exercises to tissues directly affected by the specific foot and ankle injury, physical therapists can also prescribe appropriate cross-training activities that can help the athlete either maintain or regain aerobic health.

A common foot and ankle injury treated in physical therapy is a lateral ankle sprain, which is also a common recurrent injury that leads to chronic ankle sprains and instability. Physical therapy is indicated for prevention of recurrence of injury after the initial injury, because it has been found that previous injuries to the ankle are strong predictors of recurrence.[42] Studies also indicate the persistence of dysfunction and limitations with sporting activities after an ankle sprain. Gerber and colleagues[43] found that in a young athletic population at the United States Military Academy, 95% of cadets who sustained ankle injuries returned to sports activities within 6 weeks. However, during a 6-month follow-up, 40% of those injured athletes reported residual symptoms especially in syndesmosis sprains. In 2002, Denegar and Miller[44] published an article suggesting that a treatment approach to preventing chronic ankle instability requires protection for healing tissues during the inflammatory process, with proper application of stress and lower extremity biomechanics needing to be addressed to restore normal joint function. For complete rehabilitation to occur, preventing recurrence of injury is always addressed by educating athletes about graded return to activity and use of assistive devices when appropriate. Prescription of activities to address balance and proprioceptive awareness, and issues with postural control and compensations along the kinetic chain may be overlooked when athletes focus on treating only the foot and ankle injury. Balance problems occur after acute ankle sprains because of proprioception deficits, and the reflexive aspect of proprioception is more severely affected than voluntary proprioception.[45] In addition, an exercise program to improve kinesthetic awareness is needed for individuals with multiple ankle sprains (**Fig. 4**).[46] Chronic ankle instability can alter supraspinal motor control mechanisms, and should be treated as a global injury instead of just locally at the site.[47] Compensations may emerge in the athlete's biomechanics as a response to lack of mobility or function in multiple joints. Exercises that integrate foot and hip function and activities that address the kinetic chain are appropriate when treating running injuries.[48]

Impairments in proprioception affect coordination, and it is essential that athletes regain timing and sequencing to prevent recurrence of injury. Exercises, muscle reeducation, and coordination drills that address the multiplanar activities in the foot and ankle are specifically addressed. Twisting, turning, and cutting are all part of sports, and these activities present lateral and rotational stresses to the foot, ankle, knee,

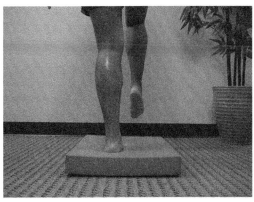

Fig. 4. Unilateral stance on a soft surface integrates the foot and hip to address kinesthetic awareness.

hip, and trunk. These higher-level activities are completed in physical therapy when tissues have enough tensile strength and flexibility to withstand these rotational stresses. Use of bracing initially is helpful, but eventually the activity should be completed without bracing. Giza and colleagues[49] found that injuries in soccer are caused by tackles involving lateral or medial forces that create corresponding eversion or inversion rotation of the foot or ankle on the weight-bearing limb. Withstanding these same rotational forces need to be addressed in order for soccer players to return to sport successfully. Bracing and taping can minimize deviations in single leg balance and jumping performance than when not braced or taped at all.[50] Bracing also contributes to rotational stiffness at the ankle[51] and can be helpful in modified return to sporting activities whereby athletes can work on sagittal plane activities, yet still avoid activities in the transverse and coronal planes.

Regaining speed and intensity of movement are necessary for optimal return to function for all athletes. Plyometric exercises produce fast repetitive movements that require a muscle to be loaded and then contracted quickly to improve elasticity, for muscle hypertrophy, and for the tendon to tolerate higher tensions and improve sport performance.[52] Plyometric exercises in combination with weight training are essential for strength performance.[53] Finally, sport-specific training for optimal return

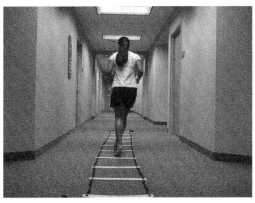

Fig. 5. An agility ladder is used to improve an athlete's timing, coordination, and sequencing.

to activity is worked into the athlete's rehabilitation program. For instance, a basketball player benefits from plyometric exercises designed for the foot and ankle to improve jumping ability. A gymnast would benefit from plyometrics to improve explosiveness during his or her routines (**Fig. 5**).

Assessment of the athlete occurs throughout the rehabilitation process to ensure that impairments and functional limitations are addressed thoroughly. Differences within individuals and factors such as time, compliance, and other preexisting conditions can all affect outcomes of a rehabilitation program. Without a comprehensive physical therapy approach to treating foot and ankle injuries, athletes are at risk for recurrence of injury or not being able to return to sporting activities at all. For many athletes, continuing in their sport is a fundamental part of their lifestyle, and the preservation of this lifestyle is essential for maintaining their quality of life.

SUMMARY

The role of physical therapy in the rehabilitation of foot and ankle injuries is documented in research. Physical therapists have the knowledge and expertise from which athletes can benefit greatly in returning to function after a foot and ankle injury. In the American College of Foot and Ankle Surgeons practice guidelines[54] for the treatment of heel pain, physical therapy is not specifically mentioned as a treatment option even though ice and stretching are recommended. It is noted in research[55] that exercises learned only from a brochure without being monitored by a physical therapist resulted in fewer improvements in impairments, and were done correctly only half the time when compared with a group that was supervised by physical therapists. When completing their rehabilitation, athletes who have the access to physical therapists who have a good understanding of their specific sport or are athletes themselves have an advantage. Even with the recognition of the benefits of physical therapy, some medical schools and residency programs in orthopedic surgery do not educate residents on how physical therapy is useful to their patients.[56] Although it is not necessary that medical schools or podiatry schools contain curricula on the specifics of physical therapy, it is important for physicians, podiatrists, and other health care providers to consider the benefits of physical therapy for all athletic injuries and to familiarize themselves with physical therapists who can best help with the management of sports injuries in their patients.

REFERENCES

1. Garrick JG, Requa RK. The epidemiology of foot and ankle injuries in sports [abstract]. Clin Podiatr Med Surg 1989;6(3):629–37. Available at: PubMed. Accessed May 18, 2010.
2. Dane S, Can S, Gursoy R, et al. Sport injuries: relations to sex, sport, injured body region [abstract]. Percept Mot Skills 2004;98(2):519–24. Available at: ProQuest Nursing & Allied Health Source. Accessed May 30, 2010.
3. Bronner S, Brownstein B. Profile of dance injuries in a Broadway show: a discussion of issues in dance medicine epidemiology. J Orthop Sports Phys Ther 1997; 26(2):87–94.
4. Gamboa JM, Roberts LA, Maring J, et al. Injury patterns in elite preprofessional ballet dancers and the utility of screening program to identify risk characteristics. J Orthop Sports Phys Ther 2008;38(3):126–36.
5. California Physical Therapy Board Website. Updated June 14, 2010. Available at: http://www.ptbc.ca.gov/consumers/consumer_info_faq.shtml#obtain, http://www.ptbc.ca.gov/consumers/. Accessed June 14, 2010.

6. Archer KR, MacKenzie EJ, Castillo RC, et al. Orthopedic surgeons and physical therapists differ in assessment of need for physical therapy after traumatic lower-extremity injury. Phys Ther 2009;89(12):1337–49.
7. Guide to physical therapist practice, 2nd edition. Phys Ther 2001;81(1):30–55.
8. Title CI, Katchis SD. Traumatic foot and ankle injuries in the athlete [abstract]. Orthop Clin North Am 2002;33(3):587–98. Available at: PubMed. Accessed May 16, 2010.
9. American Physical Therapy Association Website. Updated June 14, 2010. Available at: http://apta.org. Accessed June 14, 2010.
10. Wen DY. Risk factors for overuse injuries in runners [abstract]. Curr Sports Med Rep 2007;6(5):307–13. Available at: PubMed (PMID: 17883966). Accessed May 29, 2010.
11. Korpelainen R, Orava S, Karpakka J, et al. Risk factors for recurrent stress fractures in athletes [abstract]. Am J Sports Med 2001;29(3):304–10. Available at: PubMed. Accessed June 6, 2010.
12. Oztekin HH, Boya H, Ozcan O, et al. Foot and ankle injuries and time lost from play in professional soccer players [abstract]. Foot (Edinb) 2009;19(1):22–8. Available at: PubMed. Accessed June 5, 2010.
13. Roberts L, Bucksey SJ. Communicating with patients: what happens in practice? Phys Ther 2007;87(7):586–94.
14. Christakou A, Lavallee D. Rehabilitation from sports injuries: from theory to practice [abstract]. Perspect Public Health 2009;129(3):120–6. Available at: PubMed. Accessed June 5, 2010.
15. Chevan J, Haskvitz EM. Do as I do: exercise habits of physical therapists, physical therapist assistants, and student physical therapists. Phys Ther 2010;90:726–34.
16. Dahle LK, Mueller MJ, Delitto A, et al. Visual assessment of foot type and relationship of foot type to lower extremity injury. J Orthop Sports Phys Ther 1991;14(2):70–4.
17. Moen MH, Tol JL, Weir A, et al. Medial tibial stress syndrome: a critical review [abstract]. Sports Med 2009;39(7):523–46. Available at: PubMed. Accessed June 6, 2010.
18. Tweed JL, Campbell JA, Avil SJ. Biomechanical risk factors in the development of medial tibial stress syndrome in distance runners. J Am Podiatr Med Assoc 2008; 98(6):436–44.
19. Ryan M, Grau S, Krauss I, et al. Kinematic analysis of runners with Achilles mid-portion tendinopathy [abstract]. Foot Ankle Int 2009;30(12):1190–5. Available at: PubMed. Accessed May 17, 2010.
20. Williams DS 3rd, McClay IS, Hammill J. Arch structure and injury patterns in runners [abstract]. Clin Biomech 2001;16(4):341–7. Available at: PubMed. Accessed June 5, 2010.
21. Burns J, Keenan AM, Redmond A. Foot type and overuse injury in triathletes. J Am Podiatr Med Assoc 2005;95(3):235–41.
22. Cheung RT, Ng GY. Influence of different footwear on force on landing during running. Phys Ther 2008;88:620–8.
23. Richards CE, Magin PJ, Callister R. Is your prescription of distance running shoes evidence-based? [abstract]. Br J Sports Med 2009;43(3):159–62 [serial online]. Available at: CINAHL, Ipswich, MA. Accessed May 30, 2010.
24. Butler RJ, Davis IS, Hamill J. Interaction of arch type and footwear on running mechanics [abstract]. Am J Sports Med 2006;34(12):1998–2005. Available at: CINAHL, Ipswich, MA. Accessed May 30, 2010.
25. Wilk BR, Fisher KL, Gutierrez W. Defective running shoes as a contributing factor in plantar fasciitis in a triathlete. J Orthop Sports Phys Ther 2000;30(1):21–8.

26. Khamis S, Yizhar Z. Effect of feet hyperpronation on pelvic alignment in a standing position [abstract]. Gait Posture 2007;25(1):127–34. Available at: PubMed. Accessed June 6, 2010.

27. Snyder KR, Earl JE, O'Connor KM, et al. Resistance training is accompanied by increases in hip strength and changes in lower extremity biomechanics when running [abstract]. Clin Biomech 2009;24(1):26–34. Available at: PubMed. Accessed June 6, 2010.

28. Niven A. Rehabilitation adherence in sport injury: sports physiotherapists' perception [abstract]. J Sport Rehabil 2007;16(2):93–110. Available at: PubMed. Accessed June 5, 2010.

29. Evans L, Hardy L. Injury rehabilitation: a goal-setting intervention study. Res Q Exerc Sport 2002;73(3):310–9. Available at: ProQuest Health and Medical Complete. (Document ID: 183109231). Accessed June 6, 2010.

30. Hardy MA. The biology of scar formation. Phys Ther 1989;69:1014–24.

31. Prentice WE. Therapeutic modalities for allied health professionals. United States: McGraw-Hill; 1998.

32. Threlkeld AJ. The effects of manual therapy on connective tissue. Phys Ther 1992;72:893–902.

33. Hayes KW. Manual for physical agents, 5th edition. New Jersey (NJ): Prentice Hall, Inc; 2000.

34. Stergioulas A, Stergioula M, Aarskog R, et al. Effects of low-level laser therapy and eccentric exercises in the treatment of recreational athletes with chronic Achilles tendinopathy [abstract]. Am J Sports Med 2008;36(5):881–7. Available at: PubMed. Accessed May 18, 2010.

35. Tumilty S, Munn J, Abbott JH, et al. Laser therapy in the treatment of Achilles tendinopathy: a pilot study [abstract]. Photomed Laser Surg 2008;26(1):25–30. Available at: PubMed. Accessed May 18, 2010.

36. Oliviera FS, Pinfildi CE, Parizoto NA, et al. Effect of low level laser therapy (830 nm) with different therapy regimens on the process of tissue repair in partial lesion calcaneous tendon [abstract]. Lasers Surg Med 2009;41(4):271–6. Available at: PubMed. Accessed May 18, 2010.

37. Osborne HR, Allison GT. Treatment of plantar fasciitis by low dye taping and iontophoresis: short term results of a double blinded, randomized, placebo controlled clinical trial of dexamethasone and acetic acid. Br J Sports Med 2006;40(6):545–9. Available at: PubMed. Accessed May 18, 2010.

38. Japour CJ, Vohra R, Vohra PK, et al. Management of heel pain syndrome with acetic acid iontophoresis. J Am Podiatr Med Assoc 1999;89(5):251–7. Available at: PubMed. Accessed June 6, 2010.

39. Young BA, Strunce J, Walker MJ, et al. A combined treatment approach emphasizing impairment-based manual physical therapy for plantar heel pain: a case series. J Orthop Sports Phys Ther 2004;34(11):725–33.

40. Cleland JA, Abbott JH, Kidd MO, et al. Manual physical therapy and exercise versus electrophysical agents and exercise in the management of plantar heel pain: a multicenter randomized clinical trial. J Orthop Sports Phys Ther 2009; 39(8):573–85.

41. Khan KM, Scott A. Mechanotherapy: how physical therapists' prescription of exercise promotes tissue repair. Br J Sports Med 2009;43:247–51.

42. Malliaropoulos N, Ntessalen M, Papacostas E, et al. Reinjury after acute lateral ankle sprains in elite track and field athletes [abstract]. Am J Sports Med 2009; 37(9):1755. Available at: ProQuest Health and Medical Complete. (Document ID: 1858575491). Accessed May 31, 2010.

43. Gerber JP, Williams GN, Scoville CR, et al. Persistent disability associated with ankle sprains: a prospective examination of an athletic population [abstract]. Foot Ankle Int 1998;19(10):653–60. Available at: PubMed. Accessed May 18, 2010.
44. Denegar CR, Miller SJ III. Can chronic ankle instability be prevented? Rethinking management of lateral ankle sprains. J Athl Train 2002;37(4):430–5. Available at: ProQuest Health and Medical Complete. Accessed June 5, 2010.
45. Akbari M, Karimi H, Farahini H, et al. Balance problems after unilateral lateral ankle sprains. J Rehabil Res Dev 2006;43(7):819–24. Available at: ProQuest Health and Medical Complete. (Document ID: 1254164401). Accessed May 31, 2010.
46. Garn SN, Newton RA. Kinesthetic awareness in subjects with multiple ankle sprains. Phys Ther 1988;68:1667–71.
47. Hass C, Bishop M, Doidge D, et al. Chronic ankle instability alters central organization of movement. Am J Sports Med 2010;38(4):829. Available at: ProQuest Health and Medical Complete. (Document ID: 2006895871). Accessed May 31, 2010.
48. Geraci MC Jr, Brown W. Evidence-based treatment of hip and pelvic injuries in runners [abstract]. Phys Med Rehabil Clin N Am 2005;16(3):711–47. Available at: PubMed. Accessed June 6, 2010.
49. Giza E, Fuller C, Junge A, et al. Mechanisms of foot and ankle injuries in soccer [abstract]. Am J Sports Med 2003;31(4):550–4. Available at: ProQuest Health and Medical Complete. (Document ID: 376719001). Accessed May 31, 2010.
50. Ozer D, Senbursa G, Baltaci G, et al. The effect of neuromuscular stability, performance, multi-joint coordination and proprioception of barefoot, taping or preventative bracing [abstract]. Foot (Edinb) 2009;19(4):205–10. Available at: PubMed. Accessed May 16, 2010.
51. Zinder S, Granata K, Shultz S, et al. Ankle bracing and the neuromuscular factors influencing joint stiffness. J Athl Train 2009;44(4):363–9. Available at: ProQuest Health and Medical Complete. (Document ID: 1815486791). Accessed May 31, 2010.
52. LaStayo PC, Woolf JM, Lewek MD, et al. Eccentric muscle contractions: their contributions to injury, prevention, rehabilitation, and sport. J Orthop Sports Phys Ther 2003;33(10):557–71.
53. Saez-Saez De Villareal E, Requena B, Newton RU. Does plyometric training improve strength performance? A meta-analysis [abstract]. J Sci Med Sport 2010;13(5):513–22. Available at: PubMed. Accessed May 16, 2010.
54. Schroeder BM. American College of Foot and Ankle Surgeons: diagnosis and treatment of heel pain. Am Fam Physician 2002;65(8):1686–8. Available at: ProQuest Health and Medical Complete. (Document ID: 116970016). Accessed May 31, 2010.
55. Friedrich M, Cermak T, Maderbacher P. The effect of brochure use versus therapist teaching on patients performing therapeutic exercise and on changes in impairment status. Phys Ther 1996;76:1082–8.
56. Urbscheit N, Sanchez LB. Survey of orthopedic residents' exposure to physical therapy during residency. J Orthop Sports Phys Ther 1986;7(6):335–8.

Current Concepts and Techniques in Foot and Ankle Surgery

Primary Subtalar Joint Arthrodesis with Internal and External Fixation for the Repair of a Diabetic Comminuted Calcaneal Fracture

Zacharia Facaros, DPM[a], Crystal L. Ramanujam, DPM[b], Thomas Zgonis, DPM[c,d,*]

KEYWORDS

- Calcaneus • Fracture • Internal fixation • External fixation
- Diabetes • Subtalar joint fusion

Calcaneal fractures are debilitating injuries because of the anatomy distortion and severely limited and painful joint motion. An annual incidence has been reported in 11.5 out of 100,000 persons per year; most are sustained from falls of 2 m or higher and are seen more commonly in men.[1] Fractures of the tarsal bones are infrequent but calcaneal involvement is the most frequently traumatized bone in this area.[2] The fracture is typically a result of direct trauma, such as a fall from a height, or possibly motor vehicle accidents, stress-related injuries, or Charcot neuroarthropathy.[3] These injuries often require reconstructive surgery and thus a significant recovery period with potential long-term disability.

Contemporary strategies for proper restoration of anatomy and function following a calcaneal fracture involve a combination of internal and external fixation. Surgical intervention should aim to restore the height, length, width, and axis of the calcaneus,

[a] Reconstructive Foot and Ankle Surgery, Division of Podiatric Medicine and Surgery, Department of Orthopaedic Surgery, University of Texas Health Science Center at San Antonio, San Antonio, TX, USA
[b] Division of Podiatric Medicine and Surgery, Department of Orthopaedic Surgery, University of Texas Health Science Center at San Antonio, San Antonio, TX, USA
[c] Division of Podiatric Medicine and Surgery, Department of Orthopaedic Surgery, University of Texas Health Science Center at San Antonio, San Antonio, TX, USA
[d] Research and Reconstructive Foot and Ankle Fellowships, University of Texas Health Science Center at San Antonio, San Antonio, TX, USA
* Corresponding author. Division of Podiatric Medicine and Surgery, Department of Orthopaedic Surgery, University of Texas Health Science Center at San Antonio, San Antonio, TX.
E-mail address: zgonis@uthscsa.edu

Clin Podiatr Med Surg 28 (2011) 203–209
doi:10.1016/j.cpm.2010.10.003   **podiatric.theclinics.com**
0891-8422/11/$ – see front matter © 2011 Elsevier Inc. All rights reserved.

reconstruct all joint surfaces, and permit function by primary stable osteosynthesis. It is imperative that the foot and ankle specialist recognizes the kinematic impact the calcaneus accounts for in the lower extremity and thus the importance of restoration. Concomitant injuries elsewhere in the body have also be recognized, such as injuries to the lumbar spine, ankles, femurs, and upper extremities.[4,5] It is paramount that a comprehensive evaluation be performed to appreciate any proximal condition.

TECHNICAL CONSIDERATIONS

The anatomy of the calcaneus is complex because of its 4 facets articulating with the talus and cuboid, 3 for the talus, the fourth for the cuboid. The surgeon must respect the talocalcaneal and calcaneocuboid articulations and their related motion, in addition to the ligamentous attachments within this region. The arterial supply to the calcaneus and adjacent soft tissue structures is through the anterior tibial, posterior tibial, and peroneal arteries. The vital neurovascular structures are located medially and laterally, at risk during surgery either directly or iatrogenically.

The topographic contour comprises 6 surfaces and a thin corticocancellous shell enclosing cancellous bone, where the static and dynamic stress patterns can be seen throughout. The neutral triangle is of particular interest, defined as an area of scant trabecular bone that resides between the compression and traction trabeculae. It is considered the weakest portion of the calcaneus.[6] Radiographic examination and other imaging modalities are essential for the diagnosis and treatment of these fractures. Sanders' classification is a popular scheme for surgical planning, detailing the number and location of articular fracture fragments involving the posterior facet of the subtalar joint.[7]

Diabetes mellitus is of particular interest when contemplating the risk assessment for surgical intervention. A thorough history and physical examination, vascular assessment, review of radiographs and/or imaging studies, and critique of laboratory testing serve as the foundation in any surgical preparation but more so in the person with diabetes. Diabetes mellitus has been found to affect bone status with resultant increase in fractures.[8,9] Delayed bone and soft tissue healing are well known impairments associated with diabetes.[10] Tight glycemic control is essential in these patients.

Open reduction with internal fixation (ORIF) has notoriously been performed through an extensile lateral approach for fracture visualization and reduction of both the subtalar and calcaneocuboid joints. Recommendations for internal fixation have varied, some examples of which include, but are not limited to, small and large interfragmentary screws, locking plate technology, Kirschner wires, Steinmann pins, and staples.[11–13] When selecting the relevant instrumentation, the appropriate size and contour are essential to endorse meticulous fit and stabilization. Percutaneous reduction with internal fixation has been shown to restore calcaneal and subtalar joint anatomy, which may reduce wound complications, posttraumatic arthrosis, infectious processes, and overall morbidity seen with extensive dissection and manipulation when traditional ORIF is performed.[13]

External fixation for bony realignment has been in practice since the early twentieth century, primarily used for trauma but also used for various applications, such as deformity correction and arthrodesis.[14] The associated advantages include relative ease of application for surgeons well trained in the technique, adjustability of the construct, and increased access for wound care and monitoring. External fixation configuration requires a combination of pins, wires, rings, rods, clamps, and hinges to ultimately achieve a sturdy device to allow neutralization, compression, and/or distraction forces. When placing an external fixator, preoperative planning is essential so that compromise to surrounding anatomic structures, including muscles, tendons, and neurovascular structures, must be avoided or minimized at all costs.

The treatment methods of calcaneal fractures continue to be a frequently discussed topic. It is beyond the scope of this article to further elaborate on the numerous internal and external fixation patterns. The following is a case report detailing our approach for combined internal and external fixation for successful treatment of a comminuted calcaneal fracture in a patient with diabetes.

CASE REPORT

A 54-year-old woman presented to our outpatient clinic with chief complaint of progressively increasing swelling and severe pain in the left heel. She reported sustaining a twisting injury while walking on an even surface 2 weeks previously and had pain with ambulation ever since, but had not sought prior medical treatment. Her past medical history was significant for poorly controlled diabetes mellitus type 2, proliferative retinopathy, coronary artery disease, hypertension, hyperlipidemia, peripheral neuropathy, and asthma. Past surgical history included bilateral laser eye surgery under general anesthesia without complications. She admitted to an active lifestyle with current occupation in food services requiring standing for long periods. She admitted to a 35-pack-year history of smoking, but no alcohol or illicit drug use. A review of systems was significant only for the chief complaint.

General examination revealed a pleasant, obese woman in no apparent distress and with stable vital signs. Her cardiopulmonary examination revealed no abnormalities. The focused left lower extremity examination demonstrated palpable dorsalis pedis and posterior tibial pulses, loss of sensation per Semmes-Weinstein 5.07 monofilament, markedly diminished vibratory sensation, and nonpitting edema to the rear foot. There was noticeable collapse of the hindfoot compared with the contralateral side. The clinical findings were suggestive of subacute Charcot neuroarthropathy. There were no open wounds or signs of acute infection. Radiographs of the foot and ankle showed a comminuted, depressed, intra-articular calcaneal fracture. Computed tomography scan confirmed heavy comminution involving extension into the anterior, middle, and posterior subtalar joint with impaction and anterior rotation of the posterior facet. Because of the patient's history of diabetes, coronary artery disease and smoking, noninvasive vascular testing was ordered and showed no evidence of arterial occlusive disease. Laboratory testing was unremarkable except for increase in both serum glucose (181 mg/dL) and glycosylated hemoglobin (11.1%). Chest radiograph, electrocardiogram, and cardiac stress test were within normal limits.

After thorough discussion with the patient regarding all possible treatment options and perioperative considerations, the patient elected to have surgical correction. She was medically optimized and cleared for surgery by her primary care physician and cardiologist. She was given a preoperative dose of intravenous cefazolin for infection prophylaxis. Under general endotracheal anesthesia and ipsilateral pneumatic thigh tourniquet, a 3-cm curvilinear incision was made at the lateral aspect of the subtalar joint. Atraumatic technique was maintained in dissection to avoid excessive soft tissue injury and protect vital structures. Extensive comminution to the articular surface of the calcaneus was visualized. Allogenic bone graft was interpolated at the subtalar joint following articular resection via curettage. Two 6.5-mm cannulated partially threaded screws were placed across the subtalar joint for arthrodesis under fluoroscopic guidance with adequate compression noted. The incision was closed in layered fashion, followed by application of a modified circular off-loading external fixation system. Postoperatively, the patient was hospitalized for 4 days for continued medical stability, pain control, infection prophylaxis, progressive physical therapy to maintain non–weight-bearing status of the operative limb, and deep vein thrombosis prophylaxis. She was discharged to her home on oral pain and antibiotic medications with strict instructions for maintenance of non–weight bearing to the left foot.

The patient was closely followed at our outpatient clinic every 2 weeks for incision and external fixation care, as well as serial radiographs. Radiographs demonstrated consolidation at the fusion site noted at postoperative week 6 She had an unremarkable postoperative course. She was taken back to the operating room at postoperative week 7 for removal of the external fixator and application of a non–weight-bearing short leg fiberglass cast. She remained non–weight bearing for 8 weeks, and subsequently began progressive weight bearing in a walking boot for 6 additional weeks. At week 12 after removal of the external fixator, the patient was transitioned into custom extra depth shoes with soft inlays and double-upright brace, and underwent incremental increases in activity level for the next 6 months. At 13 months after the initial surgery, the patient was fully ambulatory and without evidence of soft tissue or osseous breakdown (**Fig. 1**).

DISCUSSION

Aside from trauma, patients with diabetes can be prone to calcaneal fractures as a result of various systemic processes such as peripheral vascular disease, renal impairment, soft tissue infections, and neuropathic joint fracture/dislocation. Spontaneous calcaneal fractures in patients with diabetes has also been reported.[15,16] In those patients who are neuropathic, a level of pain is typically experienced following further progression of deformity.

The literature is replete with numerous methods of fixation for calcaneal fracture reconstruction.[17–21] Hüfner and colleagues[22] performed a retrospective study on 434 patients and found primary subtalar joint arthrodesis for comminuted calcaneal fractures resulted in good to very good outcomes based on American Orthopaedic Foot and Ankle Score (AOFAS). Their goal was to prevent or minimize the extent of posttraumatic arthrosis commonly seen in this injury. Li and Liu[23] found that after operating on 32 feet with both external fixation and limited internal fixation, Böhler and Gissane angles improved significantly; they concluded that this combined treatment offers good recovery with limited complications in complex fractures.

Primary subtalar joint arthrodesis has been advocated for calcaneal fracture patterns involving extensive comminution at the posterior facet of the subtalar joint. Primary subtalar joint arthrodesis can provide more optimal stability than isolated ORIF in patients with multiple comorbidities including diabetes, peripheral neuropathy, and obesity.[19] This technique offers a limited incision that avoids the high morbidity that is usually associated with a traditional extensile lateral approach.[17,19] In addition, arthrodesis provides stable reduction of the deformity and prevention of further collapse. Circular external fixation complements the mechanical stability of internal fixation, thereby preventing motion that can compromise the surrounding soft tissue and delay or inhibit osseous healing. External fixation can be a viable alternative to traditional casting or splinting techniques in patients with conditions that predispose them to skin breakdown such as diabetes, peripheral vascular disease, peripheral neuropathy, and smoking history. Other advantages of external fixation include easy access to incisions for frequent evaluation and care, as well as promotion of non–weight-bearing status. This protocol of fixation is ideal for patients who may have contraindications to traditional ORIF techniques or when limited approaches are used.

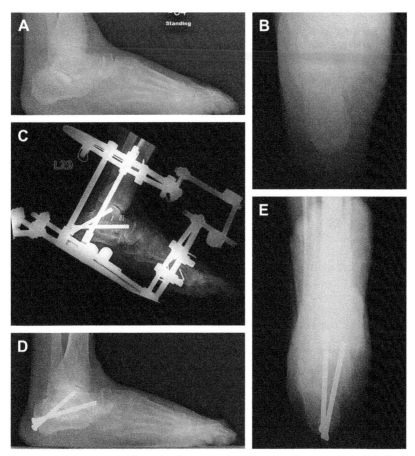

Fig. 1. Preoperative lateral (*A*) and calcaneal axial (*B*) views showing the diabetic intra-articular calcaneal fracture with joint depression and displacement. Immediate postoperative lateral view (*C*) showing the primary subtalar joint arthrodesis with internal fixation supplemented with a modified circular external fixation device, which was kept for 7 weeks. Final postoperative lateral (*D*) and calcaneal axial (*E*) views at 13 months follow-up.

The postoperative timeline after calcaneal fracture repair may include various complications, the severity of which depends on the extent of injury, preexisting conditions, soft tissue handling, and compliance level. The patient is normally kept immobilized and non–weight bearing for a period of 8 to 12 weeks. Limited ambulation with appropriate bracing is then used. If premature removal of hardware is warranted, continued meticulous care is essential for added protection and prevention of skin compromise, malunions, and/or nonunions. Complications of fracture treatment in patients with diabetes often have multifactorial causes, therefore conscientious perioperative management is critical to overall success.

SUMMARY

Controversy continues to exist concerning the appropriate treatment of displaced comminuted intra-articular fractures of the calcaneus. We promote the use of combined internal and external fixation for certain comminuted diabetic calcaneal fractures because the procedure offers the benefits of deformity correction and maximum stability while promoting non–weight-bearing activity throughout the healing period. Appropriate patient and procedure selection, as well as punctual treatment, remain hallmarks for favorable outcomes.

REFERENCES

1. Mitchell MJ, McKinley JC, Robinson CM. The epidemiology of calcaneal fractures. Foot (Edinb) 2009;19:197–200.
2. Rockwood CA Jr, Greene DP. Rockwood and Green's fractures in adults. 4th edition. Philadelphia: Lippincott-Raven; 1996. p. 2405–62.
3. Crosby LA, Kamins P. The history of the calcaneal fracture. Orthop Rev 1991;20: 501–9.
4. Essex-Lopresti P. The mechanism, reduction technique, and results in fractures of the os calcis, 1951–52. Clin Orthop Relat Res 1993;290:3–16.
5. O'Connell F, Mital MA, Rowe CR. Evaluation of modern management of fractures of the os calcis. Clin Orthop Relat Res 1972;83:214–23.
6. Harty M. Anatomic considerations in injuries of the calcaneus. Orthop Clin North Am 1973;4:179–83.
7. Sanders R, Fortin P, DiPasquale T, et al. Operative treatment in 120 displaced intraarticular calcaneal fractures. Results using a prognostic computed tomography scan classification. Clin Orthop Relat Res 1993;290:87–95.
8. Lecka-Czernik B. Bone loss in diabetes: use of antidiabetic thiazolidinediones and secondary osteoporosis. Curr Osteoporos Rep 2010;8:178–84.
9. Barbaro D, Orsini P, Lapi P, et al. Foot bone mass and analysis of calcium metabolism in diabetic patients affected by severe neuropathy. Minerva Endocrinol 2008;33:283–8.
10. Mehta SK, Breitbart EA, Berberian WS, et al. Bone and wound healing in the diabetic patient. Foot Ankle Clin 2010;15:411–37.
11. Demcoe AR, Verhulsdonk M, Buckley RE. Complications when using threaded K-wire fixation for displaced intra-articular calcaneal fractures. Injury 2009;40: 1297–301.
12. Zeman P, Zeman J, Matejka J, et al. [Long-term results of calcaneal fracture treatment by open reduction and internal fixation using a calcaneal locking compression plate from an extended lateral approach]. Acta Chir Orthop Traumatol Cech 2008;75:457–64 [in Czech].
13. Schepers T, Vogels LM, Schipper IB, et al. Percutaneous reduction and fixation of intraarticular calcaneal fractures. Oper Orthop Traumatol 2008;20:168–75.
14. Naden JR. External skeletal fixation in treatment of fractures of the tibia. J Bone Joint Surg Am 1949;31:586–98.
15. Kathol MH, El-Khoury GY, Moore TE, et al. Calcaneal insufficiency avulsion fractures in patients with diabetes mellitus. Radiology 1991;180:725–9.
16. Chagares W, Stepanczuk P, Pandit JK, et al. Bilateral, spontaneous calcaneal fractures in a diabetic. J Foot Surg 1981;20:38–40.
17. Harvey EJ, Grujic L, Early JS, et al. Morbidity associated with ORIF of intraarticular calcaneus fractures using a lateral approach. Foot Ankle Int 2001;22: 868–73.
18. Zgonis T, Roukis TS, Polyzois VD. The use of Ilizarov technique and other types of external fixation for the treatment of intra-articular calcaneal fractures. Clin Podiatr Med Surg 2006;23:343–53.

19. Stapleton JJ, Kolodenker G, Zgonis T. Internal and external fixation approaches to the surgical management of calcaneal fractures. Clin Podiatr Med Surg 2010;27:381–92.
20. McGarvey WC, Burris MW, Clanton TO, et al. Calcaneal fractures: indirect reduction and external fixation. Foot Ankle Int 2006;27:494–9.
21. Rammelt S, Gavlik JM, Barthel S, et al. The value of subtalar arthroscopy in the management of intra-articular calcaneus fractures. Foot Ankle Int 2002;23: 906–16.
22. Hüfner T, Geerling J, Gerich T, et al. Open reduction and internal fixation by primary subtalar arthrodesis for intraarticular calcaneal fractures. Oper Orthop Traumatol 2007;19:155–69.
23. Li MH, Liu Y. [Treatment of complex calcaneal fractures with external fixator and limited internal fixation]. Zhongguo Gu Shang 2010;23:217–9 [in Chinese].

External Fixation for Surgical Off-Loading of Diabetic Soft Tissue Reconstruction

Crystal L. Ramanujam, DPM[a], Zacharia Facaros, DPM[b],
Thomas Zgonis, DPM[c,d],*

KEYWORDS

- Diabetic foot • Local flaps • Soft tissue coverage
- External fixation • Surgical off-loading

Reconstructive procedures for the foot and ankle have progressively evolved over the years since the first written description of techniques used during surgery in the ancient roman war.[1] With the advent of concepts including antisepsis and analgesia combined with detailed anatomic studies of the foot and ankle, functional reconstruction rather than amputation has become the goal of treatment of surgeons for the management of complicated wounds. Wounds are common in the diabetic foot yet challenging to heal and maintain long-term closure. The skin of the foot and ankle has unique characteristics based on the specific regions; likewise, certain locations require special considerations for closure. The sole of the foot is highly specialized with minimal subcutaneous tissue and multiple fibrous septations between the dermis and plantar fascia to help absorb shock and withstand weight-bearing forces. In contrast, the skin of the dorsal foot is thin and pliable, providing an increased range of extensibility while demanding further delicate tissue handling.

The concept of the "reconstructive ladder" has provided surgeons with options for wound closure to help match the complexity of the wound with the appropriate level of treatment.[2,3] Primary closure is often precluded in diabetic foot wounds that lack

[a] Division of Podiatric Medicine and Surgery, Department of Orthopaedic Surgery, University of Texas Health Science Center at San Antonio, San Antonio, TX, USA
[b] Reconstructive Foot and Ankle Surgery, Division of Podiatric Medicine and Surgery, Department of Orthopaedic Surgery, University of Texas Health Science Center at San Antonio, San Antonio, TX, USA
[c] Division of Podiatric Medicine and Surgery, Department of Orthopaedic Surgery, University of Texas Health Science Center at San Antonio, San Antonio, TX, USA
[d] Research and Reconstructive Foot and Ankle Fellowships, University of Texas Health Science Center at San Antonio, San Antonio, TX, USA
* Corresponding author. Division of Podiatric Medicine and Surgery, Department of Orthopaedic Surgery, University of Texas Health Science Center at San Antonio, San Antonio, TX.
E-mail address: zgonis@uthscsa.edu

Clin Podiatr Med Surg 28 (2011) 211–216
doi:10.1016/j.cpm.2010.10.004
0891-8422/11/$ – see front matter © 2011 Elsevier Inc. All rights reserved.

podiatric.theclinics.com

adequate viable margins and mobility. Healing by secondary intention is slow, which can leave wounds prone to infection and may lead to extensive scarring. Split-thickness or full-thickness skin grafts are inadequate for closure at weight-bearing surfaces because of their inability to withstand high pressures inflicted on the tissues during ambulation.[4] In the correct setting, local advancement flaps are ideal for diabetic foot wounds because they provide surgeons the ability to replace like with like tissue, thereby preserving both the morphology and function. Off-loading of these delicate soft tissue reconstructions with external fixation ensures a stable protective construct during the initial healing period.

TECHNICAL CONSIDERATIONS

The blood supply for advancement flaps comes from the dermal-subdermal plexus, therefore dissection should avoid extensive undermining. Movement of advancement flaps is usually in a single direction. These flaps are ideal for small- to moderate-sized defects and are used for closure of wounds both on the dorsal and plantar aspects of the foot.[5] Careful preoperative planning should be undertaken to evaluate the elasticity of the surrounding tissue for closure of wounds without tension once the flap is advanced. A firm knowledge of the vascular anatomy of the foot is required for proper selection of the specific anatomic flap, its location, and the incisional approach.[6] Advancement flaps encompass a broad category, which includes single or double advancement flaps, rotational flaps, M-plasty, T-plasty, crescentic advancement flaps, V-Y or double V-Y advancement flaps, and oblique sigmoid island flaps.[7] These flaps can also be used in conjunction with other reconstructive soft tissue and osseous procedures.[8,9]

As with treatment of any diabetic foot or ankle wound, the medical status of the patient should be optimized preoperatively. Comorbidities of diabetes, particularly peripheral vascular disease and peripheral neuropathy, should be addressed because these have a significant effect on wound healing.[10] Vascular assessment of the lower extremities should include ankle-brachial index, toe-brachial index, Doppler waveforms, and pulse volume recordings to determine whether a vascular surgical consultation is warranted to improve perfusion. Formal surgical debridement of infected wounds should be performed along with appropriate antibiotic therapy assigned based on intraoperative cultures, followed by performance of staged reconstruction when indicated. Only foot and ankle wounds free of infection and with adequate perfusion may be considered for flap closure.

Intraoperatively, atraumatic technique is required so as not to compromise viability of the flap and surrounding tissues.[6] Incision design depends on the wound itself, anatomic location, and regional blood supply. Meticulous hemostasis before insetting of the flap to the donor site reduces the risk of hematoma formation. Most commonly, suture of lower strength, such as 3-0 or 4-0 nylon or less, is ideal for reapproximation of the flap. Dog-ears created by redundant tissue adjacent to the flap can be corrected using Burrow triangles. Surgeons may leave sutures intact for prolonged periods in diabetic patients, especially with plantar flaps to prevent dehiscence.

In any case, appropriate off-loading methods for survivability of the flap must be considered. Simple casting or splinting may provide immobilization of the foot and ankle; however, these methods often make it difficult to regularly monitor flap viability. In addition, the casting material can cause pressure and irritation directly to the flap, and caution should be implemented accordingly. In selected patients, external fixation devices can provide excellent immobilization of the joints while also allowing access to the flap for periodic care.[11] Furthermore, external fixation may be advantageous when considering the use of an advancement flap with or without concomitant osseous reconstruction.[12]

Because it is beyond the scope of this article to discuss the detailed technical aspects for all types of local advancement flaps, the authors provide a case report to share their experience in a multidisciplinary setting.

CASE REPORT

A 58-year-old woman presented to the authors' outpatient clinic with nonhealing ulceration at the central lateral plantar aspect of the right foot for more than a year. The ulceration was secondary to a chronic lateral column Charcot deformity with plantar subluxation. The patient had a history of poorly controlled diabetes, hypertension, anemia, chronic kidney disease, and hyperlipidemia. Noninvasive vascular testing showed no indication for revascularization before staged reconstruction. The patient was treated with medicines and cleared for surgical reconstruction. An initial circular surgical excision of the ulcer was performed, making sure to note for any osseous pathologic condition. No underlying exposure of bone or joint was noted, and the soft tissue cultures obtained were negative for bacterial growth. The patient was maintained on broad-spectrum intravenous antibiotic therapy consisting of piperacillin/tazobactam and vancomycin. Based on the location of the wound, osseous deformity, and extensibility of the surrounding tissues, revisional surgery consisting of plantar ostectomies of the calcaneus and cuboid, bursa excision, and local advancement flap closure was planned for 2 days later. Under general anesthesia and with the thigh tourniquet inflated to 325 mm Hg, the bursa located just inferior to the wound was excised to eliminate chronic pressure to the site and a partial plantar ostectomy of the calcaneocuboid joint was performed. A curvilinear full-thickness skin incision was created extending from the base of the triangular defect to provide adequate movement of the flap about the pivot point. Atraumatic technique with minimal retraction was used during dissection, and the tourniquet was released on completion of flap elevation. Once local hemostasis was achieved with electrocautery and topical thrombin, the flap was inset with 3-0 nylon simple interrupted sutures. To provide maximum stability and immobilization of the foot and ankle, a modified circular off-loading external fixation system was applied. The external fixator was removed approximately 6 weeks later, revealing complete healing of the flap with a durable soft tissue reconstruction. The foot was eventually placed in extradepth diabetic shoes and accommodative inserts at approximately 4 months after the initial surgery (**Fig. 1**).

DISCUSSION

Local advancement flaps are advantageous in providing durable closure without sacrificing the structure and function of the soft tissues. These flaps are especially useful for diabetic wounds in weight-bearing locations of the foot. Careful attention to the vascular supply of the lower extremity coupled with meticulous atraumatic technique is paramount for the success of these flaps.

In 1986, Shaw and Hidalgo[6] outlined the anatomic basis of plantar flaps and described the outcomes of 10 patients, although not all wounds included were of a diabetic cause. The investigators emphasized careful technique in flap elevation to maintain vascular supply originating from the subcutaneous plexus and to restore sensation in weight-bearing surfaces of the foot. In diabetic patients, the presence of peripheral neuropathy obviates the need to preserve sensation; however, the same technical proficiency is required for flap viability. Colen and colleagues[13]

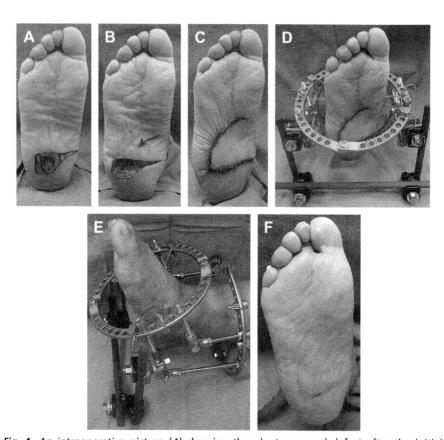

Fig. 1. An intraoperative picture (*A*) showing the plantar wound defect after the initial surgical excision of the full-thickness ulceration. The patient subsequently underwent further reconstruction with a plantar partial ostectomy and local rotational flap closure (*B, C*). Please note that the defect was surgically revised in a triangular manner, which allowed the flap to rotate toward its base at the proximal lateral aspect of the foot (*B*). A modified circular external fixator was used for stabilization and surgical off-loading of the lower extremity (*D, E*). The final clinical picture at approximately 4 months' follow-up (*F*).

reported on 38 plantar forefoot wounds, including 71% diabetic neuropathic wounds, treated via V-to-Y advancement flaps. Their findings promoted the use of corrective forefoot osseous procedures in conjunction with local flaps to prevent reulceration. Bharathi and colleagues[14] described the use of V-Y advancement flaps for the reconstruction of distal toe defects in 10 patients, showing that adequate contour and padding at toe amputation sites can be provided with this method. Roukis and colleagues[15] recommended the use of local advancement flaps even amongst high-risk patients.

Although several types of local advancement flaps exist, the success of their use in the diabetic population is highly dependent on careful patient selection with medical optimization of comorbidities.[16,17] As exemplified by the authors' patients, a multidisciplinary approach is recommended for successful limb salvage.[18] These flaps can be used for a variety of wounds, ranging from simple neuropathic ulcerations to traumatic wounds to defects left after resection of the infected bone. Staged reconstruction may be used in the event of soft tissue and/or bone infection. Special considerations to address underlying osseous abnormalities, such as deformities created by Charcot neuroarthropathy, need to be incorporated into the reconstructive surgical plan.

There must be close postoperative monitoring to maintain flap viability and prevent complications. Hematoma, venous congestion, tight postoperative dressings, and uncontrolled edema can compromise the flap leading to ischemia and subsequent dehiscence.[19] These flaps may require prolonged immobilization in the diabetic patient with adequate off-loading devices. Traditional cast or splint techniques can be effective in immobilizing the lower extremity, however, these can compromise flap viability if incorrectly applied because of tension and compression directly against the surgical site. External fixation offers a major advantage by providing suspension of the extremity with a stable construct that protects the flap from shear and compressive forces.[20] This technique is especially helpful for complex cases such as Charcot reconstruction requiring simultaneous stabilization of osseous procedures and off-loading of local or pedicle flaps.[21] Circular external fixation devices also allow easy access to the flap sites for frequent postoperative care and may help to discourage weight-bearing status.[12] The disadvantages of external fixation, such as high cost and difficult maintenance with increased risk of complications, need to be carefully considered for proper patient selection.[11] Long-term observation and maintenance in an effort to prevent flap failure and reulceration is of great importance for local advancement flaps in diabetic patients. For these patients, custom-molded extra-depth shoes with multidensity inlays help to accommodate the resultant foot structure and decrease shear forces encountered during ambulation. Additional durable bracing constructs may be required for further correction and stabilization.

SUMMARY

A variety of local advancement flap designs that may be ideal for simple to complex wounds exist. With appropriate patient selection and preoperative considerations, these flaps may help to decrease the cost and duration of hospital stay in diabetic patients. Further prospective and long-term studies should be undertaken to determine more information regarding the efficacy of this treatment. Although these techniques may not be applicable to all patients, reconstructive surgeons may consider the use of local advancement flaps with external fixation for closure of certain diabetic wounds because this option allows for replacement of tissue in a manner that most closely preserves optimal structure and function of the foot and ankle.

REFERENCES

1. Broughton G 2nd, Janis JE, Attinger CE. A brief history of wound care. Plast Reconstr Surg 2006;117:6S–11S.
2. Levin LS. The reconstructive ladder: an ortho-plastic approach. Orthop Clin North Am 1993;24:393–409.
3. Boyce DE, Shokrollahi K. ABC of wound healing. Reconstructive surgery. BMJ 2006;332:710–2.
4. Malizos KN, Gougoulias NE, Dailiana ZH, et al. Ankle and foot osteomyelitis: treatment protocol and clinical results. Injury 2010;41:285–93.
5. McCraw JB. Selection of alternative local flaps in the leg and foot. Clin Plast Surg 1979;6:227–46.
6. Shaw WW, Hidalgo DA. Anatomic basis of plantar flap design: clinical applications. Plast Reconstr Surg 1986;78:637–49.

7. Blume PA, Key JJ. Local random flaps for soft tissue coverage of the diabetic foot. In: Zgonis T, editor. Surgical reconstruction of the diabetic foot and ankle. Philadelphia: Lippincott Williams & Wilkins; 2009. p. 140–64.

8. Zgonis T, Stapleton JJ, Roukis TS. Advanced plastic surgery techniques for soft-tissue coverage of the diabetic foot. Clin Podiatr Med Surg 2007;24:547–68.

9. Capobianco CM, Ramanujam CL, Zgonis T. A simple adjunct to a plantar local random flap for submetatarsal ulcers. Clin Podiatr Med Surg 2010;27:167–72.

10. Aust MC, Spies M, Guggenheim M, et al. Lower limb revascularisation preceding surgical wound coverage—an interdisciplinary algorithm for chronic wound closure. J Plast Reconstr Aesthet Surg 2008;61:925–33.

11. Clemens MW, Parikh P, Hall MM, et al. External fixators as an adjunct to wound healing. Foot Ankle Clin 2008;13:145–56.

12. Oznur A, Zgonis T. Closure of major diabetic foot wounds and defects with external fixation. Clin Podiatr Med Surg 2007;24:519–28.

13. Colen LB, Replogle SL, Mathes SJ. The V-Y plantar flap for reconstruction of the forefoot. Plast Reconstr Surg 1988;81:220–8.

14. Bharathi RR, Jerome JT, Kalson NS, et al. V-Y advancement flap coverage of toe-tip injuries. J Foot Ankle Surg 2009;48:368–71.

15. Roukis TS, Schweinberger MH, Schade VL. V-Y fasciocutaneous advancement flap coverage of soft tissue defects of the foot in the patient at high risk. J Foot Ankle Surg 2010;49:71–4.

16. Krishnan ST, Quattrini C, Jeziorska M, et al. Neurovascular factors in wound healing in the foot skin of type 2 diabetic subjects. Diabetes Care 2007;30:3058–62.

17. Liu ZJ, Velazquez OC. Hyperoxia, endothelial progenitor cell mobilization, and diabetic wound healing. Antioxid Redox Signal 2008;10:1869–82.

18. Baumeister S, Dragu A, Jester A, et al. [The role of plastic and reconstructive surgery within an interdisciplinary treatment concept for diabetic ulcers of the foot]. Dtsch Med Wochenschr 2004;129:676–80 [in German].

19. Browne EZ. Complications of skin grafts and pedicle flaps. Hand Clin 1986;2: 353–9.

20. Lowenberg DW, Sadeghi C, Brooks D, et al. Use of circular external fixation to maintain foot position during free tissue transfer to the foot and ankle. Microsurgery 2008;28:623–7.

21. Zgonis T, Roukis TS, Stapleton JJ, et al. Combined lateral column arthrodesis, medial plantar artery flap, and circular external fixation for Charcot midfoot collapse with chronic plantar ulceration. Adv Skin Wound Care 2008;21:521–5.

Index

Note: Page numbers of article titles are in **boldface** type.

Clin Podiatr Med Surg 28 (2011) 217–227
doi:10.1016/S0891-8422(10)00116-3
0891-8422/11/$ – see front matter © 2011 Elsevier Inc. All rights reserved.

podiatric.theclinics.com

Moving?

Make sure your subscription moves with you!

To notify us of your new address, find your **Clinics Account Number** (located on your mailing label above your name), and contact customer service at:

Email: journalscustomerservice-usa@elsevier.com

800-654-2452 (subscribers in the U.S. & Canada)
314-447-8871 (subscribers outside of the U.S. & Canada)

Fax number: 314-447-8029

Elsevier Health Sciences Division
Subscription Customer Service
3251 Riverport Lane
Maryland Heights, MO 63043

*To ensure uninterrupted delivery of your subscription, please notify us at least 4 weeks in advance of move.

Printed and bound by CPI Group (UK) Ltd, Croydon, CR0 4YY

03/10/2024

01040456-0005